Treatment of Cerebral Palsy and Motor Delay

Fourth edition

Sophie Levitt

BSc (Physiotherapy) Wits, FCSP
Consultant paediatric physiotherapist
Tutor on developmental therapy

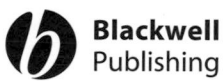
Blackwell
Publishing

© 1977, 1982, 1995, 2004 Sophie Levitt

Published by Blackwell Publishing Ltd
Editorial offices:
Blackwell Publishing Ltd, 9600 Garsington Road, Oxford OX4 2DQ, UK
   Tel: +44 (0)1865 776868
Blackwell Publishing Inc., 350 Main Street, Malden, MA 02148-5020, USA
   Tel: +1 781 388 8250
Blackwell Publishing Asia Pty Ltd, 550 Swanston Street, Carlton, Victoria 3053, Australia
   Tel: +61 (0)3 8359 1011

First published 1977
Second edition published by Blackwell Scientific Publications 1982
Third edition published by Blackwell Science 1995
Fourth edition published by Blackwell Publishing 2004

Library of Congress Cataloging-in-Publication Data
Levitt, Sophie
  Treatment of cerebral palsy and motor delay / Sophie Levitt.—5th ed.
    p. cm.
  Includes bibliographical references and index.
  ISBN 1-4051-0163-6 (sc : alk. paper)
   1. Cerebral palsied children—Rehabilitation. 2. Physical therapy for children.
  3. Movement disorder in children. 4. Cerebral palsied. I. Title.
RJ496.C4L43 2003
618.92′83603—dc22

                                                       2003060516

ISBN 1-4051-0163-6

A catalogue record for this title is available from the British Library

Set in 10/12.5 pt Sabon by
SNP Best-set Typesetter Ltd., Hong Kong
Printed and bound in the UK using acid-free paper
by Ashford Colour Press, Gosport

For further information on Blackwell Publishing, visit our website:
www.blackwellpublishing.com

Contents

Foreword to Fourth Edition

It is a great pleasure to welcome the fourth edition of this book, which gives a detailed account of the important issues within the treatment of the cerebral palsies. It is comprehensive from various perspectives. Having described each approach, there is a clear analysis of the conceptual framework for the therapies leading logically to an eclectic personal approach, i.e. what a therapist can do in terms of assessment and treatment. Such a masterly synthesis could only be carried out by someone of great theoretical and practical experience of the subject and Sophie Levitt is certainly that.

The section on research methodology is most welcome, indicating the inevitable gulf between good scientific evidence and the need to help families and children. It has always been easy to criticize therapies that are based upon studies with low statistical power, on qualitative approaches, and even on 'experience'. However, with a group of conditions that show almost infinite variations and that are successively modified by the child's development, these problems are integral to both our difficulties and the fascination of this field of medicine.

Although a strong case can be made for abandoning the use of the term cerebral palsy now that modern investigations, particularly MRI, are defining more precise pathogenic sequences, the practical issue is that all children who show motor delay and deviance need help, whether or not they strictly fit a cerebral palsy diagnosis. Perhaps even more importantly, the parents with a motor delayed child need the support of therapists who have shared such predicaments with parents, and who can help by giving both their professional insights and that derived from parents over the years.

A unique feature of the book is the historical perspective of the development of our understanding of the cerebral palsies, including the contributions of so many people over the last 100 years to what is undoubtedly one of the most difficult areas of medicine. This book is an amazing compendium of information, which I think is essential reading for the developmental therapist and doctor. Sophie is to be congratulated on pulling it together in such a readable volume.

Brian Neville
Professor of Paediatric Neurology
Institute of Child Health/Great Ormond
Street Hospital for Children NHS Trust

Extract from Foreword to Second Edition

Dr Mary D. Sheridan

The happy accident of being a fellow lecturer on a course in developmental paediatrics some years ago brought about my first introduction to Sophie Levitt's work. My attention was immediately engaged by the gentle but firm authority with which she expounded her message to us, an experienced professional audience, and by her well-chosen slides. Later I was impressed by her ease in rapidly establishing good relationships with half a dozen young handicapped children and their mothers who had been called for demonstration, and were previously unknown to her; but above all the lovely competence of her 'laying on of hands' filled me with admiration. Since then I have welcomed any opportunity open to me to see and listen to her in action. No greater compliment than this can be paid by one teacher to another.

Experience has taught Sophie the importance of a host of other influences which must be taken into serious consideration in treatment of a child and the counselling of parents. She stresses the importance of a comprehensive assessment which is not mere 'reflex hunting' but takes into account a child's present levels of visual, auditory and language development, his intelligence and personality, and, very importantly, the prognosis of his disability. She points out the parents' needs for consistent, sympathetic, knowledgeable guidance and the necessity for adequate local services for follow-up supervision and education.

The book cannot fail to inform and inspire many other workers in the field of developmental paediatrics as it has informed, inspired and indeed comforted me.

Preface

'What makes a child move?' is a crucial question for the treatment and management of children with cerebral palsy and children with developmental motor delay. I have sought the answers to this question from a variety of treatment systems and from different professionals with whom I worked in teams and in multi-disciplinary education. The first edition of this book (1977) proposed an eclectic approach drawing on topics in neurology, orthopaedics and normal and abnormal child development. In addition, there was always the recognition that children 'do not move by neurophysiology alone' but that learning processes enable a child to progress through stages of motor development. Therefore, ideas from psychology and special education were also adapted for physiotherapy. The second edition continued to elaborate learning principles to develop children's motor function. The third edition contained a specific chapter on learning motor function and also one on a Collaborative Learning Approach. I had developed this approach over some years for working with parents, carers and others involved with a child with cerebral palsy. This 'client-centred' approach depends on their participation in a learning process. Unlike some learning models, this model also includes the therapist's own participation in learning as well as the emotional issues affecting learning of parent and therapist in collaborative work. The quality of positive relationships between a parent and therapist is emphasized with consideration of the views and needs of both of them.

Respect for a family's cultural and social values is also facilitated. The Collaborative Learning Approach depends on daily tasks chosen by people with disabilities and their parents, carers and teachers in different communities. This promotes *inclusion* in mainstream schools and in the specific cultural communities in which a child or older person find themselves. The collaborative approach allows parents and others involved to learn at their own pace, so adjusting their expectations and attitudes while maintaining hope.

This fourth edition crystallizes ideas from earlier editions for further development of the Collaborative Learning Approach in the following framework:

(1) The task(s) (e.g. a daily activity, self-care, play, or social interaction) are chosen by the person with cerebral palsy, together with his parents or other people involved in their familiar environments of home and community.
(2) The motor functions for the chosen task are selected.
(3) The components (abilities, skills, prerequisites) of the motor function are analysed, e.g. specific postural mechanisms, voluntary movement, perception and understanding (cognitive and emotional).
(4) The motor impairments which constrain motor function are assessed, e.g., limited joint range, weakness, abnormal postural alignment, limited repertoire of movements, abnormal movement patterns (synergies) or abnormal reflex reactions as well as general health.
(5) The non-motor impairments which constrain motor function and task are

considered, e.g. problems of vision, perception, understanding and communication.

(6) The residual abilities in all areas of function are identified, so they can be augmented to increase achievement through different strategies.

The individual person and those assisting him/her in home, school or community, contribute most to items 1 and 2, while the physiotherapist and her multidisciplinary colleagues contribute most to items 3 to 6. The clinician will find there are overlaps between items, which are addressed in the practical chapters. Therapy goals can be clarified in this framework so that methods can be selected to activate components and minimize impairments at the same time. Methods for active postural control, in the best possible alignments, and movements themselves all minimize impairments. When this is not possible additional specific treatment procedures and specialized medical procedures are also outlined.

The framework above also offers a current perspective on neuro-facilitation methods which is within the context of motor function. Despite current theories calling into question neurophysiological bases underlying neuro-facilitation, the methods themselves, which need to be appropriately selected, are used within new approaches. As an eclectic worker I have continued to draw on contributions from different new approaches in motor control and motor learning. This differs from some who use an eclectic approach which only draws on methods from different systems of neuro-facilitation without use of learning principles.

The Older Person. The fourth edition suggests use of the framework of my Collaborative Learning Model in the new chapter on 'The Older Person with Cerebral Palsy'. Similarly, as with child and parents, it offers mutual respect between individuals and therapists and develops self-esteem and confidence in adolescents and adults. Meaning is given for their daily lives so

that the procedures suggested can improve their participation in a better quality of life. Therapy methods and recreational therapeutic activities are included to add to their quality of life.

Evidence-Based Practice. The fourth edition has many revisions in the light of new knowledge, research studies and clinical evidence. Unfortunately, in this complex field and with this heterogeneous population, reliable scientific evidence to support interventions that we make can be difficult to obtain. Therefore, we still rely on long experience and expert opinion. Fortunately, research studies have increased and are becoming more rigorous and we look forward to further clinical progress as a result. This edition contains sections on current 'Assessment Measures' and 'Appraisal of Research Studies', indicating the current problems in accepting evidence for clinical work.

It is worth pointing out that there is a tendency to overrate numerical data which is the norm in the physical sciences. However, while science may often involve numbers, this is not always necessary but good research must always involve careful systematic observation and detailed analysis, i.e. a lot of hard thinking.

Again, even when the research is thorough it is often reported in obscurely written papers where little attempt seems to be made to communicate the findings to clinicians who are seeking to use results to improve their practice. On behalf of therapists, I would plead with researchers to keep their findings clear and reasonably simple, and to realize that most practising therapists have little training in or aptitude for statistical analysis. Please spell out what your statistical tests are testing and also what assumptions are made. It is well known that medical research can be harmed by poorly applied statistics.

Previous editions and recent advances. Since publication of earlier editions of this book it is rewarding to find an increase in an eclectic viewpoint and in more functional physiotherapy, which were so controversial in the past. Recent advances in motor learning and motor control support and extend specific ideas presented previously as well as in the fourth edition. For example, recent studies now support my long-held view that spasticity and reflex reactions or 'reflex-hunting' were over-emphasized. Spasticity has more relevance to deformities than to direct causation of most of the motor dysfunction. More recognition and studies are now available on the importance of postural control – a subject given particular emphasis in all editions that use the terminology of 'the postural mechanisms'. The terminology throughout the book is updated, although in some cases terminology has changed but not the meanings originally presented. There are also new research studies on the value of strengthening people with cerebral palsy. In the past, my inclusion of strengthening methods was considered controversial. This book continues to suggest strengthening methods using manual resistance, selected from proprioceptive neuromuscular facilitation. The methods are selected for use in the context of developmental motor functions. The treatment of deformities also continues to employ strengthening of agonists and antagonists.

There remain many methods suggested from long clinical experience which still await research studies as to their value for specific problems, at different ages or developmental stages. This is not a book of 'recipes' but of suggestions for therapy and daily care based on assessment of an *individual* person with cerebral palsy and/or motor delay. They are presented with any evidence that exists at this time.

Not all methods are given, as some are difficult to describe and need demonstration. However, wherever possible, the principle has been given as to why, when and when not to use methods, which also allows a therapist to invent her own besides those suggested in this book. Not all possibilities for each person with cerebral palsy can be covered, so the therapist will also need to solve problems in each case and draw on his or her clinical experience. This book should be used with practical courses, further study and supervision by senior colleagues.

Dynamical Systems Theory. Since the third edition this topic has become more important. The theory originated in the field of motor control, where it was hoped that making analogies with the physics of complex systems (a notoriously difficult subject I am told) would lead to advances. The main conclusion seems to be that 'we should be aware that many factors are involved in the development of motor control'. This is an excellent notion. In fact, many thoughtful clinicians, particularly those working in interdisciplinary teams, have long been aware of this. For example, they have recognized factors such as vision, sensory-perception, biomechanics and postural mechanisms, deformities and growth. In addition, motivation and attention to the human and physical environment in a child's home, or outside it, were particularly addressed by community therapists in Britain and elsewhere.

Unfortunately, Dynamical Systems Theory does not yet offer much guidance as to which of the varied factors are most important and how they interact in any particular circumstance. In addition, many of the studies on this topic relate to able-bodied subjects, to normal cognition and to adults with or without brain damage. Moreover, the writing on Dynamical Systems Theory can be obscure and lead to different clinical interpretations. Practical methods based on this theory have understandably not yet developed.

THE PLAN OF THE BOOK

The first chapter gives the clinical picture in direct relationship with principles of management. The second chapter reviews the different treatment approaches with some current additions. The historical background shows how we arrived at some of our current good practice and perhaps avoids unnecessary energy to 're-invent the wheel'. The third chapter suggests how a synthesis of different approaches can be obtained. This eclectic approach has grown out of my studies, and especially from the privilege of discussions and observations or courses with Dr Phelps, Dr and Mrs Bobath, Dr Fay, Dr Vojta, Miss Knott, Mrs Collis and Dr Hari. Chapters 4 and 5 integrate the learning principles into an eclectic viewpoint. Chapter 6, on the older person, suggests modifying or selecting methods described for a child's motor function, as well as other issues of specific relevance to this age group.

Chapters 7 to 10 offer practical assessments and methods of treatment and management. As this book emphasizes that equipment needs to be associated with motor training and not substituted for it, equipment is described in Chapter 8 (Treatment Procedures and Management) and in Chapter 9 (Motor Function and the Child's Daily Life). An Appendix (Appendix 2) on equipment is given for reference and useful addresses include organizations which have information on current suppliers.

Swimming, horse-riding, skiing, abseiling, angling, wheelchair-dancing and other therapeutic and recreational leisure activities are highly recommended and the list of useful addresses includes those specializing in these areas.

It is hoped that this book will respond to some extent to the remarks of my post-graduate students and colleagues who suggested I write it – remarks such as:

'I agree with your eclectic approach, but how do I go about doing it?'

'How is it possible to combine such different viewpoints in our field?'

'I have followed one system but would like to extend my repertoire of methods and I am open to hearing other views.'

But especially to the remark:

'Help me to help these people and their families.'

Sophie Levitt
London

Acknowledgements

This fourth edition updates this book with acknowledgements to my reviewers and colleagues who have given me constructive criticism and much encouragement. I would particularly like to thank Alison Wisbeach, paediatric occupational therapist, for all the drawings and useful discussions. Dr Richard Lovell (physicist) has been a great help and support in facing and critically appraising the enormous number of research studies now available for physiotherapists. I am grateful for useful clinical comments from Gillian Hill, Eva Bower, Di Coggings, Terry Pountney, Helen Stevens, Maria Ash, Paulette van Vliet, Vivienne Funke, Michele Lee, Lesley Carroll-Few, April Winstock, Katrin Stroh, Elinor Goldschmied and from many of my post-graduate students in both the United Kingdom and overseas.

I feel privileged to have been awarded a Folke Bernadotte Fellowship supported by the Paediatric group of the Swedish Physiotherapy Association and their chairperson Elisabeth Price in 1990. Their encouragement of my eclectic approach and work with parents has been an inspiration. My thanks are also due to Dr Patricia Sonksen, Dr Joan Reynell, Dr Pam Zinkin, the late Mary Kitzinger and others with whom I worked on severely visually impaired children at the Wolfson Centre, Institute of Child Health. I am grateful to Mrs J.E. Perks and physiotherapy staff of the Treloar School for their hospitality and helpful discussions on cerebral palsy in adolescence and to Dr Lucinda Carr and physiotherapy staff for observation at the clinic on Botulinum Toxin at the Wolfson Centre.

This book was originally commenced when I was Director of Studies at The Cheyne Centre for Children with Cerebral Palsy, London, where I was given encouraging support from Dr John Foley and the staff. The foundation of this book was the correlation of the neurology of Dr Foley and Dr J. Purdon Martin with the child development studies of the late Dr Mary Sheridan. My eclectic approach was generously encouraged by Dr Foley and subsequently by Professor Kenneth Holt, with whom I worked at the Wolfson Centre, Institute of Child Health, by Professor Robert Collis and Professor G. Tardieu.

I am grateful to the Leverhulme Trust Fund, who kindly awarded me a Research Fellowship for part of my studies on the synthesis of treatment systems in cerebral palsy, which formed the basis of this book in all its editions.

I remain particularly appreciative of the privilege of many observations, discussions or courses in the past with Dr Phelps, Dr Fay, Dr Vojta, Maggie Knott, Eirene Collis, Dr and Mrs Bobath, Ester Cotton and Dr Hari. They have inspired and influenced me and without them this book would not have been written.

Thanks for photographs are given to Ted Remington, previously Assistant Head of the Richard Cloudsley School, London, who patiently photographed them with help from Christine White, former Head Ms Suckling and staff at the time. Photographs for Figs 8.62, 8.76, 8.130, 8.132, 8.133 and 11.1 kindly given by Cheyne Centre, Figs 8.92, 8.93, 8.114 and 8.120–8.124 by Alison Wisbeach, Figs 5.2, 5.6, 8.168 and 8.171 by the Wolfson Centre, Figs 5.1, 5.3 and 5.7 by the Indian Spastics Society, and Figs 8.125 and 8.126 by The Foxdenton School, England. Many new photographs were taken by David Halpern, with enormous organization by Helen Stevens, Superintendent Paediatric Physiotherapist, Winchester and Eastleigh Healthcare NHS Trust and wonderful cooperation of parents and young people. Thanks for Figs 8.68, 8.111, 8.154, 8.174, 8.210–8.212 and 9.3.

A special thanks to my son David Halpern who as a boy showed much patience and understanding, with skill in supplying numerous cups of coffee, and now a great help with advice on editing and discussing my manuscripts.

I am deeply grateful to all the children, adolescents and their parents who cooperated so amazingly with all the long sessions of photography used throughout the book. My special appreciation goes to all the children and older people with cerebral palsy, their parents and families, with whom I have been privileged to work and from whom I have learnt so much.

My publishers have been particularly kind, helpful and sensitive and I thank Caroline Connelly and Lisa Whittington and the staff of Blackwells for all their help and support.

Professor Brian Neville has honoured and encouraged me by writing the Foreword and generously sharing his ideas.

The Clinical Picture for Therapy and Management

1

Cerebral palsy is the commonly used name for a group of conditions characterized by motor dysfunction due to non-progressive brain damage early in life. There are usually associated disabilities as well as emotional and social family difficulties. The range of severity may be from total dependency and immobility to abilities of talking, independent self-care and walking, running and other skills, although with some clumsy actions.

THE MOTOR DYSFUNCTION

The brain damage results in disorganized and delayed development of the neurological mechanisms of postural control or balance and movement. The muscles activated for these motor aspects are therefore inefficient and incoordinated. Individuals have hypertonic or hypotonic muscles with weakness. Besides neuromuscular components the motor dysfunction has musculo-skeletal components. Therapy aims to improve postural control and movement as well as provide for specific abnormal muscles and joints.

The motor components change both with growth and a child's development. Change also depends on how an individual uses his body. However, the brain damage is not progressive, though the motor behaviour changes. What matters most to a child and his family is the overall functional delay and abnormal performance. Therapists need to address these daily functional difficulties together with a child and his parents or directly with an older person with cerebral palsy. Therapists will assess and assume which of the abnormal motor compo-

nents are responsible for any functional absence and abnormal performance.

There are different views as to which abnormal motor components are responsible for the total motor dysfunction and what correlation exists between various components. The underlying motor dyscontrol is controversial. This is not surprising as not all the normal and abnormal neurological mechanisms are fully understood. Additional biomechanical problems result from these abnormal mechanisms which also provide controversies. Research continues on the basic dyscontrol and biomechanics.

The new edition of this book continues my synthesis of valuable contributions from different therapy systems, some of which have hitherto been regarded as mutually exclusive. As many of my colleagues are now not wedded to any one system of therapy, many of their views are presented as well as those from my own studies and experience.

As a child does not 'move by neurophysiology alone', various ideas on learning motor control have been integrated into the general therapy framework so that 'what to do' is combined with 'how to do it'. The associated impairments and disabilities influence the motor function and the learning of motor control. Motor learning and learning daily functions need to be considered in the context of a child's whole development, which takes place in his home, school and community.

ASSOCIATED IMPAIRMENTS AND DISABILITIES

Brain damage in cerebral palsy may also be responsible for special sense defects of vision and hearing, abnormalities of speech and language and aberrations of perception. Perceptual defects or *agnosias* are difficulties in recognizing objects or symbols, even though sensation as such is not impaired, and the patient can prove by other means to know or have known what the object or symbol is. There may also be *dyspraxias*, some of which are also called visuo-motor defects. This means that the child is unable to perform certain movements even though there is no paralysis, because the patterns or *engrams* have been lost or have not developed. Dyspraxia can involve movements of the limbs, face, eyes, tongue or be specifically restricted to such acts as writing, drawing, and construction or even dressing. In other words there seems to be a problem in 'motor planning' in those children who are dyspraxic. Some children may also have various behavioural problems such as distractibility and hyperkinesis which are based on the brain damage. All these defects result in various learning problems and difficulties in communication. In addition there may also be various epilepsies or intellectual impairment (Foley 1977b; Hall 1984; Neville 2000).

Not every child has some or all of these associated impairments. Even if the impairment were only motor, the resulting paucity of movement would prevent the child from fully exploring the environment. He is therefore limited in the acquisition of sensations and perceptions of everyday things. A child may then *appear* to have defects of perception, but these may not be due to the brain damage but caused by lack of experience. The same lack of everyday experiences retards the development of language and affects the child's speech. His general understanding may suffer so that he appears to be intellectually retarded. This can go so far that normal intelligence has been camouflaged by severe physical disability. Furthermore the lack of movement can affect the general behaviour of the child. Thus some abnormal behaviour may be due to the lack of satisfying emotional and social experiences for which movement is necessary. It is therefore important for any therapist to recognize that motor function cannot be isolated from other functions and that she is treating a child who is not solely physically but multiply disabled.

Motor problems create difficulties for a child in social activities and in being able to access educational activities. A therapist needs to address the motor problems in these situations. In order to manage the multiple disabilities and lack of related learning experiences which interfere with a child's development, a physiotherapist or occupational therapist needs to be part of a team. The teamwork varies in different places such as community centres, child development centres, units in hospitals or within educational settings. Teamwork is discussed in Chapters 4, 5, 9 and 11.

AETIOLOGY

Premature infants are at greater risk of brain dysfunction. There are many causes of the brain damage, including abnormal development of the brain, anoxia, intracranial bleeding, excessive neonatal asphyxia (hypoxic ischaemic neonatal encephalopathy), trauma, hypoglycaemia and virus and other infections. These have been extensively discussed in the medical literature (Stanley & Alberman 1984; Gordon & McKinlay 1986; Rosenbloom 1995; Hagberg *et al.* 1996). The therapist is, however, rarely guided by the aetiology in her treatment planning. In some cases the cause is not certain and in many cases knowing the cause does not necessarily indicate a specific diagnosis or specific treatment. Nevertheless, the therapist should acquaint herself with the history of the case. Many of these children have been affected from infancy and have been difficult to feed and handle. Many hospitalizations and separations of babies from parents may happen in the early period. This may easily have influenced the parent–child relationships. Furthermore the history may sometimes give an indication of the prognosis, e.g. with marked microcephaly with severe multiple impairments the prognosis would be poor.

CLINICAL PICTURE AND DEVELOPMENT

It is important to recognize that the causes of cerebral palsy take place in the prenatal, perinatal, and postnatal periods. In all cases, it is an immature nervous system which suffers the insult and the nervous system afterwards continues to develop in the presence of the damage. The therapist must therefore not think of herself as treating an upper motor neurone lesion in a 'little adult' nor can she regard the problem solely as one of retardation in development. What the therapist faces is a complex situation of pathological symptoms within the context of a developing child (Twitchell 1961, 1965; McGraw 1989; Griffiths 1967; Sheridan 1973, 1975; Egan 1990; Holt 1975; Van Blankenstein *et al*. 1975; Illingworth 1975, 1983; Drillien & Drummond 1977, 1983). There are three main aspects to the clinical picture:

(1) Retardation in the development of new skills expected at the child's chronological age.
(2) Persistence of infantile behaviour in all functions, including infantile reflex reactions.
(3) Performance of various functions in patterns never seen in normal babies and children. This is because of the pathological symptoms or impairments due to upper motor neurone lesions such as hypertonus, hypotonus, involuntary movements and biomechanical difficulties confronting children with cerebral palsy.

In order to recognize abnormal motor and general behaviour, the therapist should know what a normal child does and how he does it at the various stages of his development. Information on each individual child's developmental levels should be sought from the consultants and other members of the cerebral palsy team. Reference will have to be made to the extensive literature on the field of child development.

Although normal child development is the basis on which the abnormal development is appreciated, it does not follow that assessment and treatment should rely upon a strict adherence to normal developmental schedules. Even 'normal' children show many variations from the 'normal' developmental sequences and patterns of development which have been derived from the *average* child. The cerebral palsied child will show additional variations due to neurological and mechanical difficulties. If one considers, say, the normal developmental scales of gross motor development, the cerebral palsied child has frequently achieved abilities (components) and motor functions at one level of development, omitted abilities at another level and only partially achieved motor abilities and functions at still other levels. There is thus a scatter of abilities and whole motor functions. The analysis of motor function into components is discussed in Chapters 3, 7 and 8.

If the gross motor development is generally considered to be around a given age, the development of hand function, speech and language, social and emotional and intellectual levels may all be at different ages. None of these ages may necessarily coincide with the child's chronological age.

Therefore the developmental schedules in normal child development should only be used as *guidelines* in treatment and adaptation should be made for each child's disabilities and individuality (Chapter 8).

More attention is usually given to motor development rather than other avenues of development, as it is the motor dysfunction which characterizes cerebral palsy. Here again, the therapist should remember that abnormal motor behaviour may interfere with other functions. Each area of development – such as gross motor, manipulation, speech and language, perception, social and emotional and mental – interacts as well as each having its own pattern or avenue of development. Therefore a total habilitation programme is necessary and should be planned to deal with the total development of the child.

Whilst aiming at the maximum function possible, the therapists concerned must take account of the *damaged* nervous system and adjust their expectations of achievements by the child which involve:

(1) Late acquisition of motor skills and slow rate of progress from one stage to the next.
(2) A smaller variety of skills than in the normal child.
(3) Variations in normal sequences of skills.
(4) Abnormal and unusual patterns of some of the skills.

Furthermore, the potential for function is dependent not only on the disabilities present but also on the emotional and social adjustment of the child, his personality and 'drive' as well as his capacity to learn.

CHANGE IN CLINICAL PICTURE

As the lesion is in a developing nervous system the clinical picture is clearly not a static set of signs and symptoms for treatment. But whilst the lesion itself is non-progressive its manifestations change as the nervous system matures. As more is demanded of the nervous system the degree of the handicap appears to be greater. For example, a 3-year-old is expected to do more than a baby, and therefore his difficulties are greater for the same lesion.

In addition, the pathological symptoms may develop with the years. Spasticity may increase, involuntary movements may only appear at the age of 2 or 3 years, and ataxia may only be diagnosed when the child walks or when grasp is expected to become more accurate.

Diagnoses may change as the baby develops to childhood, and especially as the child becomes more active. For example, a monoplegia reveals itself as a hemiplegia. Later a triplegia reveals itself as a tetraplegia. Cerebral palsies have an evolving diagnosis. Later, especially in adolescence, growth and increase in weight contribute to apparent deterioration as the child matures.

Treatment and management in infancy. The earlier treatment is started the more opportunity is given for whatever potential there may be for developing any normal abilities and for decreasing the abnormal movement patterns and postural difficulties (Kong 1987; de Groot 1993). A baby or young child may make his own efforts to move using compensatory or adaptive patterns which can be 'good enough' but block the development of more efficient patterns or result in 'learned disuse' of a body part. Any immobility threatens musculoskeletal growth. Early physiotherapy minimizes such problems.

The value of early developmental intervention is to provide an increase in a baby's everyday experiences and interaction with his mother. The sooner a baby can be helped to move, the sooner he can explore, the sooner he can communicate the information he gains through such exploration. The therapist is in fact contributing to his learning and understanding as well as enabling him to bond with his mother.

Although the clinical picture is known to change with the years it is not yet possible to predict the natural history of the condition in each particular child. Infants and babies with marked early neurological signs may later prove to be only mildly affected, or even normal (Ellenberg & Nelson 1981; Nelson & Ellenberg 1982). On the other hand, apparently mildly affected ones may become progressively worse with the years. It is therefore difficult to prove the value of a number of different early treatment approaches (Morris 1996; Campbell

1999). Nevertheless, until we know which babies are going to 'come right' on their own, it is better to let them have the benefit of treatment so that any potentials for improvement are not lost. Despite the controversy as to the value of early treatment, there is clearly no doubt about its importance to the parents, who receive a great deal of practical advice and support from the therapists. Among others, Goodman *et al.* (1991) found that if their research could not firmly state that neonatal physiotherapy was responsible for babies' motor developmental progress, all mothers confirmed their great appreciation for the support and practical ideas from their physiotherapists. Olow (1986) emphasizes that early intervention reduces the frustration of early rearing of children with disabilities. Whilst medical practitioners are watching the development of the child in order to make a reliable diagnosis, the parents have to live with that child throughout each day of those months and years. Parents need support and practical ideas for feeding, child care and motor activities for their child throughout the evolving diagnoses.

Treatment and management in childhood, adolescence and adulthood. During these changes in the clinical picture, treatment and management programmes need to relate to an individual's wider environments of the playgroup, nursery, pre-school, schools, adult day care centres and work places. The persons with cerebral palsy at different ages also change through interaction with the variety of personnel in environments in which they find themselves. Physiotherapy and occupational therapy as well as other therapies are therefore being planned across a lifespan of each person with cerebral palsy.

CLASSIFICATION

Numerous classifications and subclassifications have been proposed by different authorities, but none of these diagnostic labels suffice to formulate adequate treatment plans. The therapist must also have a detailed assessment based primarily on motor functions, in order to work out a treatment programme.

Classifications of Topography and Types of Cerebral Palsy

The topographical classifications frequently used are as follows:

Tetraplegia (quadriplegia) Involvement of all limbs. Arms are equally or more affected than the legs. Many are asymmetrical (one side more affected) and called double hemiplegia.
Diplegia Involvement of limbs, with arms much less affected than legs.
Hemiplegia Limbs on one side affected.

These topographical classifications are imprecise as they may change with a child's development. One useful upper limb may convey a triplegia which becomes a tetraplegia. Upper limbs may appear unaffected suggesting a paraplegia but being really a diplegia with only fine-hand use being affected when this is later expected. Hemiplegia may have minor involvement on the unaffected side. A monoplegia usually becomes a hemiplegia with increased activity.

Classification of Types of Cerebral Palsy

There are spastic types, athetoid (dyskinetic) types and a rare ataxic type. There is a hypotonic type which either becomes a spastic, athetoid or ataxic type. Tetraplegias usually have either spasticity, dystonia, dyskinesia (athetosis), hypotonia or ataxia. Hemiplegia usually is a spastic type often starting out hypotonic. Hemi-athetoids with or without dystonia are occasionally seen. Once again, classifications are not always clear-cut and the therapist may have to treat impairments of one type in another type. The predominant impairments will contribute to the diagnostic type referred for therapy.

SPASTIC CEREBRAL PALSY

Main motor characteristics are:

Hypertonus of the *clasp-knife* variety. If the spastic muscles are stretched at a particular speed they respond in an exaggerated fashion. They contract, blocking the movement. This hyperactive stretch reflex may occur at the beginning, middle or near the end of the range of movement. There are increased tendon jerks, occasional clonus and other signs of upper motor neurone lesions.

Abnormal postures (see Figs 1.1–1.3). These are usually associated with the antigravity muscles

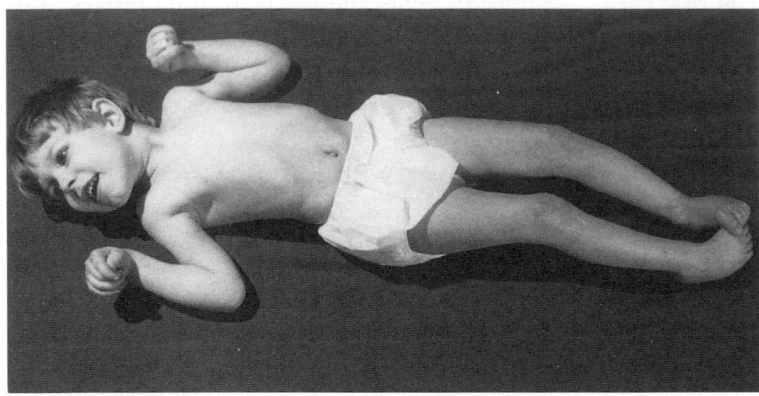

Fig. 1.1 Child with spastic quadriplegia. Head preference to right, shoulders protracted, semi-abduction, elbows flexed-pronated, wrists and fingers flexed, thumb adducted. Hips and knees flexed, tendency to internal rotation-adduction with feet in equino-varus, toes flexed.

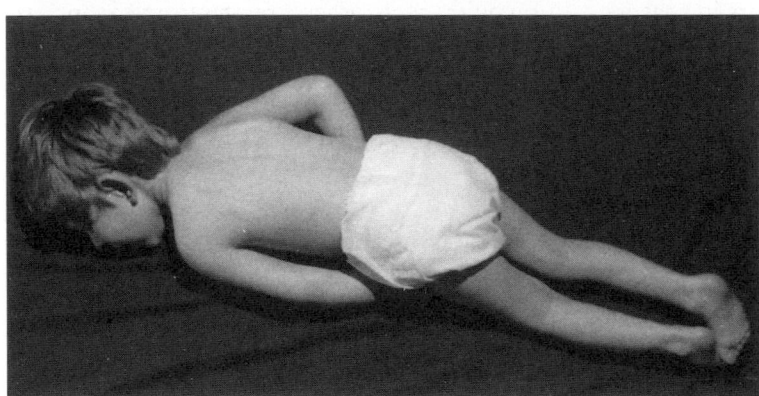

Fig. 1.2 Same child with quadriplegia with postural changes in prone. Asymmetry of arms caught under body. Hips and knees flexed, feet in equino-varus. Head preference is now to left.

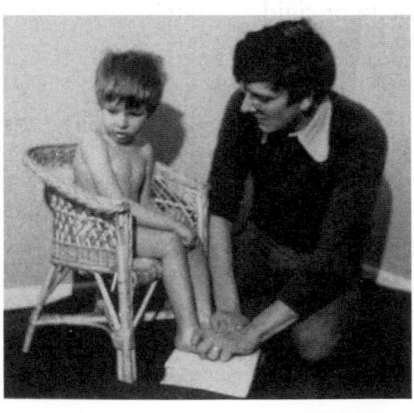

Fig. 1.3 Same child being taught to sit by his father. Head preference to right, shoulders protracted, elbows flexed-pronated, hands flexed, knees and feet held symmetrical with hips. Symmetrical trunk.

which are extensors in the leg and the flexors in the arm. The therapist will find *many* variations on this especially when the child reaches different levels of development (Bobath & Bobath 1972). Common abnormal postures in supine, prone, sitting, standing, walking and in hand function are described in Chapters 8 and 10.

The abnormal postures are held by tight shorter spastic muscle groups whose antagonists are weak, or apparently weak in that they cannot overcome the tight pull of the spastic muscles and so correct the abnormal postures. There are various other causes of abnormal postures which are discussed in relation to abnormal postural mechanisms of control in Chapters 3, 7 and 9. Spasticity is therefore not over-emphasized as a cause. Abnormal postures appear as unfixed deformities which may become fixed deformities or contractures.

Changes in spasticity and postures may occur with excitement, fear or anxiety and pain which increase muscle tension. Shifts in spasticity occur in the same affected parts of the body or from one part of the body to another in, say, stimulation of abnormal reactions such as 'associated reactions' or remnants of tonic reflex activity. Changes in spasticity are seen with changes of position in some children. Position of the head and neck may affect the distribution of spasticity. The latter are due to abnormal reflexes which may sometimes be found in these children. Sudden or fast movements, rather than slow movements, increase spasticity.

Hypertonus may be either spasticity or rigidity (dystonia). The overlap between the two is almost impossible to differentiate when severe. Rigidity is recognized by a *plastic* or continuous resistance to passive stretch throughout the full range of motion. This *lead-pipe* rigidity differs from spasticity as spasticity offers resistance at a point or small part of the passive range of motion. For treatment planning the type of hypertonus is rarely important and techniques for motor development and prevention of deformity are the same.

Voluntary movement. Spasticity does not necessarily mean paralysis. Voluntary motion is present and may be laboured. There may be weakness in the initiation of motion or during movement at different parts of its range. If spasticity is decreased or removed by treatment or drugs, the spastic muscles may be found to be strong, or may be weak. Spastic muscles may have specific structural changes due to adaptability to abnormal use or disuse (Tabary *et al.* 1981). Initially spastic muscles are however *structurally* normal though not normally extensible (Tardieu *et al.* 1982). Once spasticity is decreased the antagonists may also be stronger once they no longer have to overcome the resistance of tight spastic muscles. However, in time these antagonists may have become weak with disuse.

The groups of muscles or *chains* of muscles used in the movement patterns are different from those used in normal children of the same age. Either the muscles which work in association with each other are stereotyped and are occasionally seen in the normal child, usually at an infantile level of movement, or the association of muscles is abnormal. For example, hip extension-adduction-internal rotation is used in creeping movements or in the push-off in walking but many other combinations must be used during the full execution of creeping and walking. This may be impossible and a child only uses the same pattern at all times in the motor skill. One example of a normal arm pattern is shoulder flexion-adduction with some external rotation for feeding or combing one's hair. In the case of the child with spasticity, the arm pattern is usually flexion-adduction with *internal* rotation and *pronation* of the elbow.

Co-contraction of the agonist with the antagonist instead of the normal reciprocal relaxation persists in the spastic type. Normal co-contraction is also evident in any person attempting a new and difficult skill. Before the postural control develops in normal infants there is co-contraction of a positive supporting response in weight-bearing and co-contraction features in early stages of walking. These patterns persist in cerebral palsy (Leonard *et al.* 1991; Foley 1998; Lin 2000) so that training of postural control is essential. Voluntary movements are directly affected as poor postural control interferes with their efficiency creating weakness of both postural muscles and voluntary synergies (movement patterns).

Lack of isolated or discrete movements and fine motor coordination are also delayed in younger able-bodied children as well as in older children with this type of cerebral palsy.

Treatment is therefore needed for abnormalities of voluntary movement such as weakness, abnormal movement patterns (synergies), lack of isolated (discrete, selective) movements and abnormal co-contractions. Deformities develop due to abnormal postures and abnormal repetition of a few stereotyped movements which are only available to a child with this condition.

Associated impairments

(1) Intelligence varies and is usually more impaired in tetraplegia.
(2) Sensory loss occasionally occurs in hemiplegia with visual field loss and lack of sensation in the hand (Tizard *et al.* 1954). Sensory dysfunction such as sensory discrimination and sensory integration rather than sensory loss is present in individuals (Lesny 1993; Yekutiel *et al.* 1994). Children may be hyposensitive or hypersensitive to sensory input so that sensory-motor therapy needs to be carefully assessed.
(3) Perceptual problems especially of body and spatial relationships are more common in the spastic type. They relate to sensory dysfunction and cognitive problems as well as to poor sensory-motor experiences.
(4) Poor respiration with later rib cage abnormalities may exist. Feeding problems exist.
(5) Growth of hemiplegic limbs or severely affected lower limbs in bilateral cases can be less than the other limbs.

(6) Epilepsies are more common in tetraplegia and hemiplegia but minimal in diplegia (Neville 2000).
(7) A congenital suprabulbar palsy is found in some tetraplegias with mild spasticity (Neville 2000) or severe involvement.

ATHETOID (DYSKINETIC) CEREBRAL PALSY

Main motor characteristics are:

Involuntary movements – athetosis. These are bizarre, purposeless movements which may be uncontrollable. The involuntary movements may be slow or fast; they may be writhing, jerky, tremor, swiping or rotary patterns or they may be unpatterned. They are present at rest in some children. The involuntary motion is increased by excitement, any form of insecurity, and the effort to make a voluntary movement or even to tackle a mental problem. Factors which decrease athetosis are fatigue, drowsiness, fever, prone lying or the child's attention being deeply held. Athetosis may be present in all parts of the body including the face and tongue. Athetosis may only appear in hands or feet or in proximal joints or in both distal proximal joints. Generally the child finds great difficulty in being still.

Postural control. The involuntary movements or dystonic spasms may throw a child off balance. However, the well-known instability in athetoids is often directly connected with the postural mechanisms discussed in Chapter 3 (Foley 1983). Foley (1998) relates involuntary motion with abormal tilt reactions.

Voluntary movements. These are possible but there may be an initial delay before the movement is begun. The involuntary movement may partially or totally disrupt the willed movement making it uncoordinated. There is a lack of finer movements and weakness.

Hypertonia or hypotonia. Either may exist or there may be fluctuations of tone. The hypertonus or dystonia is a 'lead-pipe' or 'cog-wheel' rigidity. There is a continuous resistance to passive stretch throughout full range of motion. Dystonia can be particularly disabling especially if combined with spasticity. Arousal of emotions increases tone. Sudden flexion or extensor spasms could occur. Sleep decreases spasms or dystonic postures.

The athetoid dance. Some athetoids are unable to maintain weight on their feet and continually withdraw their feet upwards, or upwards and outwards, in an athetoid dance. They may take weight on one foot whilst pawing or scraping the ground in a withdrawal motion with the other leg. This has been attributed to a conflict between grasp and withdrawal reflexes. This conflict of reflexes may also be seen in the hands (Twitchell 1961, 1963).

Paralysis of gaze movements may occur so that athetoids may find it difficult to look upwards and sometimes also to close their eyes voluntarily. Poor head control also disrupts use of eyes.

The dyskinetic types change with time. They may be floppy in babyhood and only exhibit the involuntary movements when they reach 2 or 3 years of age. Adult athetoids do not appear hypotonic but have muscle tension. Muscle tension also seems to be increased in an effort to control involuntary movements.

Subclassifications of athetoids vary from clinic to clinic. It is therefore particularly inaccurate to discuss the 'treatment of athetoids'. As mentioned above any classification changes with time. The therapist should treat the symptoms found rather than the subclassification.

Associated impairments

(1) Intelligence is frequently good and may be very high. Intellectual impairment is occasionally present.

(2) Hearing loss of a specific high frequency type is associated with athetoids caused by kernicterus, though it is now a rare cause.
(3) 'Drive' and outgoing personalities are often observed among athetoids. Emotional lability is more frequent than in other cerebral palsies.
(4) Articulatory speech difficulties and breathing problems may be present, and the child's oro-motor problems create feeding difficulties.

ATAXIC CEREBRAL PALSY

Main motor characteristics are:

Disturbances of balance. There is poor fixation of the head, trunk, shoulder and pelvic girdles. Some ataxics overcompensate for this instability by having excessive balance-saving reactions in the arms. Instability is also found in children with any type of cerebral palsy. Unsteady gaits arise from the brain lesion affecting motor control (Neville 2000; Foley 1998).

Voluntary movements are present but clumsy or uncoordinated. The child overreaches or underreaches for an object and is said to have 'dysmetria'. This inaccurate limb movement in relation to its objective may also be accompanied by intention tremor. Poor fine hand movements occur.

Hypotonia is usual. There is excessive flexibility of joints and poor muscle power.

Nystagmus may exist.

Associated impairments

(1) Intellectual impairment appears, especially in the presence of visual and perceptual problems.
(2) 'Clumsy' intelligent children are sometimes diagnosed as having ataxic cerebral palsy.

(3) A 'pure' ataxic is rarely diagnosed except for a group of genetic origin called 'dys-equilibrium' syndrome (Neville 2000).

COMMON FEATURES IN ALL TYPES OF CEREBRAL PALSY

The classification into types of cerebral palsy tends to obscure the fact that there are important motor features which are common to all types. For instance, all cerebral palsied children are retarded in motor development. However the symptoms of the different types of cerebral palsy, such as hypertonus and the various involuntary movements, only play a part in this disturbance of development. Retarded or abnormal development of the postural-balance mechanisms disturbs the motor development. Postural mechanisms are an intrinsic part of motor skills. When they are absent or abnormal, this leads to absent or abnormal motor skills.

Chapter 3 discusses these aspects in detail as they are fundamental to the framework for therapy.

In cerebral palsied children floppiness of the head and trunk are also seen together with hypertonic limbs. This lack of development of head and trunk control is usually attributed to retardation of motor development. But this is in effect due to retarded development of the mechanisms of postural stabilization of the head and trunk.

Another common feature is the appearance of certain abnormal reflexes which have no predilection for a specific type of cerebral palsy.

Abnormal Reflexes (see Table 7.2)

Besides the desirable postural reactions, there are also reflexes which are undesirable. Many such pathological reflexes have been described in cerebral palsied children of all types. Diagnostic reflexes such as the tendon jerks, however, are of little relevance to treatment planning. Those reflexes which concern the therapist are some of the infantile or primitive reflexes. These are reflexes which are present in the normal newborn and which become integrated or disappear as the baby matures. In cerebral palsied children infantile reflexes are still present long after the ages when they should have become integrated within the nervous system. Whilst there are many infantile reflexes, those of most interest to the therapist are the Moro reflex, the palmar and plantar grasp reflexes, automatic stepping, excessive neck righting reflex, positive supporting, extensor thrust and feeding reflexes (Capute *et al.* 1978, 1984).

There are also the tonic reflexes, which are the tonic labyrinthine reflexes (TLR), the asymmetrical tonic neck reflex (ATNR) and the symmetrical tonic neck reflexes (STNR). Some neurologists group these tonic reflexes amongst the infantile reflexes whereas others argue that they are not present in the normal infant and are always pathological. These tonic reflexes are sometimes called *postural reflexes* but they are *abnormal* postural reflexes and should not be confused with the normal postural mechanisms as described by Rushworth (1961), Martin (1967), Foley (1977a), Roberts (1978) and others.

The principle of treatment which therapists should follow in relation to the complicated collection of reflexes is *not* to go 'reflex hunting'. Reflexes only concern the therapist when they interfere with motor function and speech. This does *not* always occur. The approach is to examine the function of the child first and, only when abnormality has been detected, to then consider whether *one* of the reasons for this abnormality seems to be a pathological or primitive reflex.

Tonic reflexes are only seen in the most severely impaired children (Foley 1977a), especially if obligatory. Table 7.2 and Fig. 7.4 of primitive and tonic reflex reactions are given so that a therapist recognizes any total or remnants of these reflex reactions or infantile (primitive) responses in individual children. These reactions may be stimulated by either peripheral or cortical activations. Some children with severe multiple disabilities activate some of these reflex responses in their efforts to balance, move or communicate non-verbally. A therapist needs to include knowledge of how her peripheral stimulation and handling might cause undesirable reflex responses. However it is the therapist's work in building postural and movement control that does at the same time modify or overcome any undesirable reflex reactions.

Recent research calls into question the importance of primitive (infantile) reflexes. They are no longer considered a substrate for motor control and are not reliable predictors of future motor development. New ideas on theoretical bases of motor training disagree with using the 'hierarchical lists' of primitive and tonic reflexes followed by more mature reactions (Cioni *et al.* 1989, 1992; Horak 1992; Prechtl *et al.* 1997, 2001). This increasing research on reflexes lends support to my view against reflex hunting expressed in this book since the First Edition in 1977.

MOTOR DELAY

Cerebral palsy consists of both motor delay and motor disorder. There are many other conditions which present similar problems of motor delay or of delay and disorder. All these conditions are also called the *developmental disabilities* (Pearson & Williams 1972).

They may be due to:

Intellectual impairment which is caused by various metabolic disorders, chromosome anomalies, leucodystrophies, microcephaly and other abnormalities of the skull and brain, endocrine disorders and the causes of brain damage given for the cerebral palsies. Down's syndrome also creates motor delay.

Deprivation of normal stimulation associated with social, economic and emotional problems, including maternal depression.

Malnutrition alone, but usually together with deprived environments. Once malnutrition is treated, lack of normal stimulation may still retard the child's development.

The presence of non-motor impairments which may lead to motor delay, e.g. severe visual impairments, severe perceptual defects, apraxias, as well as intellectual disabilities mentioned above. Children with delay in any developmental area may have an associated delay in motor development (see the section on motor development and the visually impaired child in Chapter 8).

Presence of motor impairments other than the cerebral palsies. For example spina bifida, the myopathies, myelopathies and various progressive neurological diseases and congenital deformities may obviously delay development, e.g. hand function has been delayed in children with spina bifida (Holt 1975) as well as gross motor development.

Principles of treatment and organization of treatment will be similar to that discussed in Chapters 3, 4, 5 and 8. *Specific problems* in the conditions above are considered in other publications (Levitt 1984; Eckersley 1993; Shepherd 1995; Burns & MacDonald 1996; Tecklin 1999; Campbell *et al.* 2000).

PRINCIPLES OF LEARNING AND THERAPY

Speech therapy and occupational therapy obviously overlap with education in drawing on principles of learning. Physiotherapy has 'grown up' predominantly within the fields of orthopaedics and neurophysiology. In recent years physiotherapists have recognized that it is no longer only a matter of working out what a child needs as treatment for medical problems but, also, how to enable a child to learn motor control and daily functional activities. A child, adolescent or adult is thus enabled to access education and to socialize more adequately with his/her peers.

Aims of physiotherapy, occupational therapy and speech therapy are:

(1) To develop forms of communication (gesture, speech, typing and alternative

forms of communication with signs or electronic aids).

(2) To develop independence in the daily activities of eating, drinking, dressing, washing, toileting and general self-care with and without aids.

(3) To develop abilities to play and achieve hobbies and recreational activities with or without adapted equipment.

(4) To develop some form of locomotion and independent mobility which may include wheelchairs, playthings, tricycles, or driving adapted motor vehicles.

All these aims need to be considered in terms of learning processes interacting with neurological and orthopaedic aspects. Therefore all therapists draw on the fields of education and psychology and gain much from close teamwork with teachers, psychologists, social workers and psychotherapists. The psychotherapists and social workers are important as learning is intimately involved with emotions. Many learning models do not give adequate attention to this fact. The role of social and cultural factors in learning needs to be understood by everyone.

The many adapted utensils, toys and other aids make learning of motor function easier. The child is more motivated to strive for independence and be rewarded by his own achievements.

Summary

Whilst it is difficult to summarize the principles of treatment concisely, the following guidelines may be useful provided they are studied after reading Chapters 1 and 3 and 'Motor Training', Chapter 8.

(1) The child should be seen as having primarily a motor impairment but may have individual associated impairments due to the brain damage. The motor and other functional disabilities are created by the impairments as well as by lack of many everyday learning experiences.

(2) There is an interaction between the communication, intellectual, perceptual and motor functions. Physiotherapists therefore consider the influence of other disabilities on the motor programmes.

(3) Treatment is aimed at problems of gross-motor and fine-motor function which consist of individual combinations of:

- Absent or abnormal postural mechanisms of balance
- Abnormal movement patterns (synergies) of voluntary movement
- Weakness of various kinds
- Hypertonicity, hypotonicity and involuntary movements
- Abnormal postural alignments
- Abnormalities of muscles, joints and soft tissues
- Abnormal reflexes or reactions.

Views differ on the significance of specific problems and also on the relationship between them.

(4) Therapy programmes should not have a strict adherence to specific diagnostic classifications and aetiology may not influence the treatment used by therapists.

(5) Emphasis needs to be given to the daily functional activities which are priorities of a child or an adult with disabilities and of their families.

(6) The various impairments need to be treated *in the context of* total daily functions as well as in specific treatments for individuals.

(7) The therapist also needs to recognize the impairments and emerging functional *abilities* within each child's developmental pattern. Normal developmental schedules are only guides and need to be carefully adapted.

(8) Management and therapy is planned from infancy throughout an individual's lifespan to take account of clinical change and different circumstances in an individual's home, schools and community.

(9) Physiotherapists need to integrate motor learning principles in their treatments of impairments and disabilities. Motor learning models need to encompass emotional, cultural and social issues.

(10) Treatment and management need to commence as early as possible for parental support and to minimize musculo-skeletal problems.

2 Outline of Treatment Approaches

There are many systems of treatment for cerebral palsy (Levitt 1962, 1976; Scrutton 1984; Tecklin 1999). Although these therapeutic approaches were devised for the cerebral palsies, many of them are also used for treatment of children with other conditions of developmental delay and for adults with neurological defects. It is not the purpose of this chapter to describe each system in full detail and reference should be made to the literature and study observations of each system in practice. The author presents the essence of each system after many personal observations, discussions, practical work and reading of the work of the originators.

MUSCLE EDUCATION AND BRACES

W.M. Phelps, an orthopaedic surgeon in Baltimore, was one of the pioneers in the treatment of cerebral palsy who encouraged physiotherapists, occupational therapists and speech therapists to form themselves into cerebral palsy habilitation teams (Phelps 1949, 1952; Slominski 1984). The main points in his treatment approach were:

Specific diagnostic classification of each child as a basis for specific treatment methods. He diagnosed five types of cerebral palsy and many sub-classifications.

Fifteen modalities were described and specific combinations of these modalities were used for the specific type of cerebral palsy.

The modalities (methods) were:

(1) Massage for hypotonic muscles, but contraindicated in children with spasticity and athetoids.
(2) Passive motion through joint range for mobilizing joints and demonstrating to the child the movement required. Speed of movement is slower for children with spasticity, increased for rigidity.
(3) Active assisted motion.
(4) Active motion.
(5) Resisted motion followed according to the child's capability.

The above modalities were used for obtaining modalities 6, 8, 10 and 12.

(6) Conditioned motion is recommended for babies, young children and mentally retarded children.
(7) Confused motion or synergistic motion which involves resistance to a muscle group in order to contract an inactive muscle group in the same synergy. Mass movements such as the extensor thrust or the flexion withdrawal reflex are usually used. For example, using the hip-knee flexion dorsiflexion synergy, inactive dorsiflexors are stimulated by resistance given to hip flexors. Confused motion is further discussed in the next chapter.
(8) Combined motion is training motion of more than one joint, such as a shoulder and elbow flexion using modalities 2, 3, 4 and 5.
(9) Relaxation techniques used are those of conscious 'letting go' of the body and its parts (Levitt 1962), tensing and relaxing parts of the body. These methods are

mainly used with athetoids. They attempt to lie still or relaxed or use contract-relax relaxation for grimacing and other involuntary motion.

(10) Movement from relaxation is conscious control of movements once relaxation has been achieved. It is mainly used for children to control involuntary movements.

(11) Rest – periods of rest are suggested for athetoids and children with spasticity.

(12) Reciprocation is training movement of one leg after the other in a bicycling pattern in lying, crawling, knee walking and stepping.

(13) Balance – training of sitting balance and standing in braces.

(14) Reach and grasp and release used for training of hand function.

(15) Skills of daily living such as feeding, dressing, washing and toileting. Many aids were devised by the occupational therapists.

Braces or calipers. The appliances were designed and developed by Phelps. He prescribed special braces to correct deformity, to obtain the upright position and to control athetosis. The bracing is extensive and worn for many years. The children are taught to stand and step in long leg braces with pelvic bands and back supports, or sometimes spinal brace. As they progress, the back supports are removed, then the pelvic band and finally they wear below-knee irons. The full-length brace has locking joints at hip and knee so that control can be taught with them locked or unlocked.

Muscle education. Children with spasticity are given muscle education based on an analysis of whether muscles are spastic, weak, normal or *zero cerebral*, or atonic. Muscles antagonistic to spastic muscles are activated. This is to obtain muscle balance between spastic muscles and their weak antagonists. Athetoids are trained to control simple joint motion and do not have

muscle education. Ataxics may be given strengthening exercises for weak muscle groups.

Others, including Rood (1962) and Tardieu *et al.* (1982), have developed ideas on bracing and muscle education. Plum and Molhave (1956) advocated strengthening spastic muscles as well as their antagonists. However, he exercised the spastic muscles in their outer ranges as the muscles are usually shortened, whereas the antagonists are exercised in their middle and inner ranges. Tabary *et al.* (1981), in a 'factorial analysis' identifies the specific problem in the muscles which gives rise to abnormal movements or deformities. According to this careful analysis, treatment is given where indicated. Alcohol injections were used to diminish spasticity; muscle education, specific bracing and a preference for early orthopaedic surgery were recommended. Unlike most of the other orthopaedic approaches, Tardieu's includes neurodevelopmental studies. Tabary *et al.* (1972), Tardieu *et al.* (1982) and Dietz (1992) have shown specific changes in muscle length which warrant treatment.

PROGRESSIVE PATTERN MOVEMENTS

Temple Fay, a neurosurgeon in Philadelphia, recommended that the cerebral palsied be taught motion according to its development in evolution. He regarded ontogenetic development (in humans) as a recapitulation of phylogenetic development (in the evolution of the species). In general, he suggested building up motion from reptilian squirming to amphibian creeping, through mammalian reciprocal motion 'on all fours' to the primate erect walking. As lower animals carried out these early movements of progression with a simple nervous system, they can similarly be carried out in the human in the absence of a normal cerebral cortex. The midbrain, pons and medulla could be involved in the stimulation of primitive patterns of movement and primitive reflexes which activate the handicapped parts of the body. Fay also described 'unlocking reflexes' which reduce hypertonus. Based on these ideas, he developed *progressive pattern movements* which consist of five stages (Fay 1954a,b):

Stage 1. Prone lying. Head and trunk rotation from side to side.

Stage 2. Homolateral stage. Prone lying, head turned to side. Arm on the face side in abduction-external-rotation, elbow semiflexed, hand open thumb out towards the mouth. Leg on face side in abduction, knee flexion opposite stomach, foot dorsiflexion. Arm on the occiput side is extended, internally rotated, hand open at the side of the child or on the lumbar area of his back. Leg on the occiput side is extended. Movement involves head turning from side to side with the face, arm and leg sweeping down to the extended position and the opposite occiput arm and leg flexing up to the position near the face as the head turns round.

Stage 3. Contralateral stage. Prone lying. Head turned to side, arm on the face side as in stage 2. The leg on the face side is, however, extended. The other leg on the side of the occiput is flexed. As the head turns this contralateral pattern changes from side to side.

Stage 4. On hands and knees. Reciprocal crawling and on hands and feet stepping in the *bear walk* or *elephant walk*.

Stage 5. Walking pattern. This is a *sailor's walk* called by Fay 'reciprocal progression on lower extremities synchronized with the contralateral swing of the arms and trunk'. A wide base is used and the child flexes one hip and knee into external rotation and then places his foot on the ground, still in external rotation. As the foot is being placed on the ground, the opposite arm and shoulder are rotating towards it. As weight is taken on the straight leg, the other leg flexes up.

The Doman-Delacato system (Doman & Doman 1960) which follows the basic tenets postulated by Fay, also recommends periods of inhalations of CO_2 from a breathing sack, restriction of fluid intake and development of cerebral hemispheric dominance. Cerebral dominance is attempted by principal use of dominant eye, hand, foot and arm and other methods. Children are also hung upside down and whirled around to stimulate the vestibular apparatus. They are also asked to hang and 'walk' their hands along a horizontal ladder as observed in apes.

The progressive pattern movements are first practised passively for 5 minute periods at least five times daily. One person turns the head, another person moves the arms and leg on one side, and another person the arm and leg on the other side. Locomotion beyond the stage of the child's patterning level is not permitted. A child who is not proficient in cross pattern creeping is prevented from walking. 'Neurological organization' is considered possible if each developmental level is established before going to the next level. This approach restricts itself to prone development and expects demanding daily regimes of treatment, amounting to 8–10 hours a day in many cases.

SYNERGISTIC MOVEMENT PATTERNS

Signe Brunnstrom, a physical therapist, produces motion by provoking primitive movement patterns or synergistic movement patterns which are observed in foetal life or immediately after pyramidal tract damage. The main features of her work are as follows (Brunnstrom 1970).

Reflex responses are used initially and later voluntary control of these reflex patterns is trained. Most of Brunnstrom's therapy has been on adult hemiplegia – in relation to the studies on the stages of recovery of flexion and extension limb synergies leading ultimately to isolated motion.

Control of head and trunk is attempted with stimulation of attitudinal reflexes such as tonic neck reflexes, tonic lumbar reflexes, and tonic labyrinthine reflexes. This is followed by stimulation of righting reflexes and later balance training.

Associated reactions are used as well as *hand reactions*, e.g. hyperextension of the thumb produces relaxation of the finger flexors. The training of a patient's voluntary control is developed later in the therapy programme.

Brunnstrom uses proprioceptive and other *sensory stimulation* in her training programmes for adult hemiplegia.

PROPRIOCEPTIVE NEUROMUSCULAR FACILITATIONS

Herman Kabat, a neurophysiologist and psychiatrist in the USA, has discussed various neurophysiological mechanisms which could be used in therapeutic exercises. With Margaret Knott and Dorothy Voss, he developed a system of movement facilitation techniques and methods for the inhibition of hypertonus (Kabat *et al.* 1959; Knott & Voss 1968; Voss 1972; Voss *et al.* 1985). The main features of these methods are the use of:

Movement patterns (called mass movement patterns) based on patterns observed with functional activities such as feeding, walking, playing tennis, golf or football. These patterns are spiral (rotational) and diagonal with a synergy of muscle groups. The movement patterns consist of the following components:

(1) Flexion or extension.
(2) Abduction or adduction.
(3) Internal or external rotation.

Sensory (afferent) stimuli are skilfully applied to facilitate movement. Stimuli used are touch and pressure, traction and compression, stretch, the proprioceptive effect of muscles contracting against resistance and auditory and visual stimuli.

Resistance to motion is used to facilitate the action of the muscles which form the components of the movement patterns.

Special techniques

(1) *Irradiation* – this is the predictable overflow of action from one muscle group to another within a synergy or movement pattern or by *reinforcement* of action of one part of the body stimulating action in another part of the body.
(2) *Rhythmic* stabilizations which use stimuli alternating from the agonist to its antagonist in isometric muscle work.
(3) *Stimulation of reflexes* such as the mass flexion or extension.
(4) *Repeated contractions* of one pattern using any joint as a pivot.
(5) *Reversals* from one pattern to its antagonist and other reversals based on the physiological principle of successive induction.
(6) *Relaxation* techniques such as contract-relax and hold-relax. Ice treatments are used for relaxation of hypertonus.

There are various combinations of techniques.

Functional work or *mat work* involves the use of various methods mentioned above in training rolling, creeping, crawling, walking and various balance positions of sitting, kneeling and standing (Levitt 1969, 1970b).

NEUROMOTOR DEVELOPMENT

Eirene Collis, a therapist and pioneer in cerebral palsy in Britain, stressed neuromotor development as a basis for assessment and treatment (Collis 1947; Collis *et al.* 1956). Her main points were:

The mental capacity of the child would determine the results.

Early treatment was advocated.

Management – the word 'treatment' was considered misleading in that beside the physiotherapy session there should be 'management' of the child throughout the day. The feeding, dressing, toileting and other activities of the day should be planned.

Strict developmental sequence – the child was not permitted to use motor skills beyond his level of development. If the child was, say, learning to roll he was not allowed to crawl, or if crawling he was not allowed to walk. At all times the child was given a 'picture of normal movement' and, as posture and tone are interwoven, Collis placed the child in 'normal postures' in order to stimulate 'normal tone'. Once postural security was obtained, achievements were facilitated and developmental sequences were followed throughout this training.

The CP therapist. Collis disliked the separation of treatment into physiotherapy, occupational therapy and speech therapy. She established the idea of the *cerebral palsy therapist*.

NEURODEVELOPMENTAL TREATMENT WITH REFLEX INHIBITION AND FACILITATION

Karl Bobath, a neuropsychiatrist, and Berta Bobath, a physiotherapist, base assessment and treatment on the premise that the fundamental difficulty in cerebral palsy is lack of inhibition of reflex patterns of posture and movement (Bobath, B. 1965, 1971; Bobath, K. 1971, 1980; Bobath & Bobath 1972, 1975, 1984). The Bobaths associate these abnormal patterns with abnormal tone due to overaction of tonic reflex activity. These tonic reflexes, such as the tonic labyrinthine reflex, symmetrical tonic neck reflexes and asymmetrical tonic neck reflexes, have to be inhibited. They are not used in a reflex chart today, but are fundamental in treatment which 'counteracts the abnormal patterns

of released postural reflex activity, and at the same time facilitates normal reactions by special techniques of handling'. Once the reflex patterns of abnormal tone are inhibited the child is said to have been prepared for movement. In addition, various primitive reflexes of infancy should also be inhibited. The main features of their work are currently being modified, but the focus on treatment of tone continues (Mayston 1992).

Features of the approach are:

Reflex inhibitory patterns specifically selected to inhibit abnormal tone associated with abnormal movement patterns and abnormal posture.

Sensory motor experience. The reversal or 'break down' of these abnormalities gives the child the sensation of more normal tone and movements. This sensory experience is believed to 'feedback' and guide more normal motion. Sensory stimuli are also used for inhibition and facilitation and voluntary movement.

Facilitation techniques for mature postural reflexes.

Keypoints of control are used by the therapist to attempt to change the patterns of spasticity so that a child *is prepared for movement* and more mature postural reactions. The *keypoints* are usually head and neck, shoulder and pelvic girdles, but there is also work from distal keypoints. Abnormal tone is the cornerstone of this approach, which tries to 'normalize' it.

Developmental sequences were more strictly followed in the past, but are now greatly modified according to each child (Mayston 1992).

All-day management should supplement treatment sessions. Parents and others are advised on daily management and trained to treat the children. Nancie Finnie (1997) has written a book for parents on this all-day handling of the child in the home.

SENSORY STIMULATION FOR ACTIVATION AND INHIBITION

Margaret Rood, a physiotherapist and occupational therapist, bases her approach on many neurophysiological theories and experiments (Rood 1962; Stockmeyer 1967, 1972; Goff 1969, 1972). The main features of her approach are:

Afferent stimuli. The various nerves and sensory receptors are described and classified into types, location, effect, response, distribution and indication. Techniques of stimulation, such as stroking, brushing (tactile); icing, heating (temperature); pressure, bone pounding, slow and quick muscle stretch, joint retraction and approximation, muscle contractions (proprioception) are used to activate, facilitate or inhibit motor response.

Muscles are classified according to various physiological data, including whether they are for 'light work muscle action' or 'heavy work muscle action'. The appropriate stimuli for their actions are suggested.

Reflexes other than the above are used in therapy, e.g. tonic labyrinthine reflexes, tonic neck, vestibular reflexes, withdrawal patterns.

Ontogenetic developmental sequence is outlined and strictly followed in the application of stimuli.

(1) Total flexion or withdrawal pattern (in spine).
(2) Roll over (flexion of arm and leg on the same side and roll over).
(3) Pivot prone (prone with hyperextension of head, trunk and legs).
(4) Co-contraction neck (prone head over edge for co-contraction of vertebral muscles).
(5) On elbows (prone and push backwards).
(6) All fours (static, weight shift and crawl).
(7) Standing upright (static, weight shifts).
(8) Walking (stance, push off, pick up, heel strike).

Vital functions. A developmental sequence of respiration, sucking, swallowing, phonation, chewing and speech is followed. Techniques of brushing, icing and pressure are used.

REFLEX CREEPING AND OTHER REFLEX REACTIONS

Vaclav Vojta, a neurologist working in Czechoslovakia and in Germany, developed his approach from the work of Temple Fay and Kabat (Vojta 1984, 1989; Von Aufschnaiter 1992). The main features are:

Reflex creeping. The creeping patterns involving head, trunk and limbs are facilitated at various *trigger* points or *reflex zones*. The creeping is an active response to the appropriate triggering from the zones with sensory stimuli. The muscle work used in the normal creeping patterns or *creeping complex* have been carefully analysed. The therapist must be skilful in the facilitation of these normal patterns and not provoke pathological patterns. There are nine zones for triggering reflex locomotion.

Reflex rollings are also used with special methods of triggering.

Sensory stimulation. Touch, pressure, stretch and muscle action against resistance are used in many of the triggering mechanisms or in facilitation of creeping.

Resistance is recommended for action of muscles. Various specific techniques are used to apply the resistance so that either a tonic or a phasic muscle action is provoked. The phasic action (through range) may be provoked on, say, a movement of a limb creeping up or downwards. The tonic action, or stabilizing action, is obtained if a phasic movement is prevented by full resistance given by the therapist. Therefore the static muscle action of stability occurs if resistance is applied so that it prevents any movement through range. *Rising reactions* are also provoked using resistance and all the methods above.

CONDUCTIVE EDUCATION

Andras Petö in Budapest, Hungary, originated *conductive education*. Since Professor Petö's death, the work has been continued by Dr M. Hari (Cotton 1965, 1970, 1974, 1975a,b; Hari *et al.* 1984, 1990; Beach 1988; Cottam & Sutton 1988). The main feature is the integration of therapy and education by having:

A conductor acting as mother, nurse, teacher and therapist. She is specially trained in the habilitation of motor disabled children in a four-year course. She may have one or two assistants.

The group of children, about fifteen to twenty, work together. Groups are fundamental in this training system.

An all-day programme. A fixed time-table is planned to include getting out of bed in the morning, dressing, feeding, toileting, movement training, speech, reading, writing and other schoolwork.

The movements. Sessions of movements take place mainly on and beside slatted plinths (table/beds) and with ladder-backed chairs. The movements are devised in such a way that they form the elements of a task or motor skill. The tasks are carefully analysed for each group of children. The tasks are the activities of daily living, motor skills including hand function, balance and locomotion. The purpose of each movement is explained to the children. The movements are repeated, not only in the movement sessions of, say, the *hand class* or *plinth work*, but also in various contexts throughout the day. The children are shown in practice how their 'exercises' contribute to daily activities.

Rhythmic intention. The technique used for training the elements or movements is rhythmic intention. The conductor and the children state the intended motion: 'I touch my mouth with my hands'. This motion is then attempted together with their slow, rhythmic counts of one to five. Motion is also carried out to an operative word, such as 'up, up, up' repeated in a rhythm slow enough for the children's active movement ability. Speech and active motion reinforce each other.

Individual sessions may be used for some children to help them to participate more adequately in the work of the group.

Learning principles are basic to the programme. Conditioning techniques and group dynamics are among the mechanisms of training discussed. *Cortical* or conscious participation is stressed, as opposed to involuntary and unconscious reflex therapy. They feel reactions to handling cannot create active learning by a child.

ADJUNCTS TO THERAPY

Targeted training

This option in physiotherapy for spastic cerebral palsy has been developed by Butler and Major (1992) using a biomechanical study for motor learning. In the training of sitting and standing balance, targeted training reduces the number of joints at which motor learning of control must occur. A specially designed equipment stabilizes the joints below the targeted joint so that stability, weight shift and tilt is segmentally sequenced from the head downwards in the upright posture. This uses the cephalo-caudal development more precisely than say in the Chailey Levels of sitting and standing development (Pountney *et al.* 2000). These levels are from no balance in sitting (level 2) to maintain balance of head to pelvis (without moving) in the next level 3. In standing level 2 with axilla support to standing level 3 without trunk or pelvic support with load bearing through child's feet and hands. The MOVE assessment, below, also progresses sitting with full support (prompts) to the next level of sitting without any support. In severely involved children an interim stage of spinal joint control in these upright postures would be developmentally and biomechanically advisable and encourage parents and child to see progress no matter how slow.

Targeted training selects children who are potentially able to gain control of relevant joints and results have shown sitting achievement in a shorter time, even gaining sitting in a child for the first time at age 7 years. Intellectual ability is not necessary but epilepsy should not be present. Research continues in targeted training (Butler & Major 1992; Farmer *et al.* 1999).

Neuromuscular electrical stimulation or functional electrical stimulation

This is used for muscle re-education, strengthening, decreasing spasticity or as a biofeedback for training function such as gait pattern or wrist with hand function. The desirable action of a muscle within function is used to provide sensory feedback (Carmick 1993; Hazlewood *et al.* 1994). Shumway-Cook and Woollacott (2001) and others have used electrical stimulation with biofeedback in adults and its use with children is relatively new. The evidence in children is still controversial and poor, especially for Carmick's studies (Siebes *et al.* 2002), but there is increasing interest in this therapy option. The child with multiple disabilities and the young child cannot give reliable reports on discomfort nor comprehend the purpose so that motor learning can be transferred to function without electrical stimulation. Improved strength of a muscle group does not necessarily lead to its use in function.

Low-intensity electrical stimulation which does not produce muscle contraction, has slight sensory effects and is tolerated during sleep, is used in Canada (Reiner *et al.* 1996) to promote muscle growth associated with an increase in growth hormone assumed to be stimulated during sleep. This must be accompanied by functional physiotherapy treatments over a year. This electrical treatment is called Therapeutic Electrical Stimulation and only used for children over 2 years of age.

Lycra suits and splinting

The UPsuit (Blair *et al.* 1995) cerebral palsy pressure suit and others on the market, as well as the compression Lycra bracing (Hylton & Allen 1997), are flexible supports for stabilizing trunk and proximal joints so that movements can be controlled by a child. Sensory input is provided by splinting a body part or the whole body and limbs, whole body and shoulder and pelvic girdle. Each child needs to be assessed before appropriate splintage is planned. Reliable evidence of results is still being researched, but parents and children as well as clinical therapists give anecdotal reports of more postural stability allowing better hand function or better sitting, walking and gait. Disadvantages range from difficulties in putting on Lycra garments, discomfort when hot, and toileting problems among other practicalities affecting compliance. There is no adequate evidence of postural control without the Lycra splinting following its use at the moment and studies continue. (See Fig. 8.211 of arm splint used in a child with hemiplegia.)

Specialized medical treatments

Drugs to reduce spasticity, manage epilepsy and general health problems, particularly chest infections, are used for individual children and adults. The therapist will obtain information from the medical consultants responsible and find out from them if there are any side-effects. Drugs to reduce spasticity (Albright & Neville 2000) are usually baclofen (McKinlay *et al.* 1980) as an oral medication or as intrathecal infusions into the spine (Albright & Neville

2000). Localized injections of botulinum toxin A to reduce spasticity and allow muscle lengthening are also used (See Deformities). Treatment of spasticity with any drugs is planned together with therapists, parents and carers, as therapists' programmes are essential for best results.

Selective Dorsal Rhizotomies or Selective Posterior Rhizotomies to reduce spasticity are used mainly in the United States and Canada (Peacock & Staudt 1991; Oppenheim *et al.* 1992; Steinbok *et al.* 1997; McLaughlin *et al.* 1998; Wright *et al.* 1998; Neville 2000). Selective dorsal rootlets most responsible for spasticity at the spinal levels across L2–S2 are divided. Patient selection includes children with spasticity who have underlying voluntary power, who are ambulant, intelligent and motivated and another non-ambulant group whose spasticity prevents bathing, perineal care and positioning for daily care and classroom activities. Intensive follow-up physiotherapy for 6–12 months is needed for the post-operative weakness and to training new motor patterns as well as stretching for range (Giuliani 1992).

SYSTEMS-BASED TASK-ORIENTED APPROACH

This approach is proposed by Shumway-Cook and Woollacott (2001) for the assessment and training of posture and movement in people with neurological disabilities and motor problems in the elderly population. Most of the discussion considers therapy for adults but theoretical studies in children are given.

The main aspects of this approach are:

(1) Constraints on a motor task are hypothesized as

- motor impairment and inefficient movement strategies
- cognitive impairment
- sensory impairment

(2) The demands of a motor task include the person's interaction with relevant features of the environment in which the task is performed. For example, the task may demand motor, cognitive and visual abilities to manage locomotion on rough, slippery surfaces, the moment when terrain changes or whether the surface is moving, unstable or stationary. Movement solutions need to be adaptable and efficient for changes in direction and at different speeds.

(3) Motor learning strategies are used to train motor behaviour. The specific task or intended goal will have a number of possible 'goal-directed' movement strategies or a variety of potentially useful solutions. The same task performed in different environments demands different movement strategies. Therefore motor tasks need to be learnt and practised in a variety of environments and situations.

(4) Augmented feedback is given to assist the achievement of the task.

(5) Treatment mitigates impairment or the environment is structured for achievement of the task despite the person's impairments. For example this involves adapting the home and providing appropriate equipment for function.

Therapists using this approach are influenced by dynamic systems theory on motor control proposed by Thelen *et al.* (1987, 1989) among others. For example, they state that 'Development of a particular motor pattern depends on a combination of mechanical, neurologic, cognitive and perceptual factors in addition to environmental contributions specific to both the task and the context of the infant's action.'

Shumway-Cook and Woollacott mention that methods for their approach are still developing and they include selected neurofacilitation methods for adults.

Shumway-Cook and Woollacott's Motor Control and Motor Learning approach has many similarities with the movement science-based model of Shepherd (1995), Horak (1992), Gentile (1987) as well as with elements in Conductive Education and in Learning Motor Function in Chapter 4 of this book.

MOVEMENT OPPORTUNITIES VIA EDUCATION (MOVE)

This is a mobility programme from California which was composed by a teacher in special education and a physiotherapist (Bidabe & Lollar 1990). A Move Europe (2001) has been published. The motor tasks are broken down into components well-known to cerebral palsy physiotherapists. It uses 'prompts' for guiding movement which are decreased as the child achieves each component after repetition. Decreasing support and guidance not termed 'prompts' with the repetition of function are also traditional in physiotherapy but not as systematically structured as in this approach. What physiotherapists may find useful are the systematic teaching methods used to develop motor control. The programme is best used for older children with severe and profound learning problems who have poor mobility. Results state that older children and adolescents have achieved sitting, standing and walking, although this was not expected and not enthusiastically pursued in the past. Teachers are expected to give an hour practice daily and integrate motor control within the teaching day and in the community of the person with cerebral palsy.

Developmental stages are arbritarily changed with many neurological omissions in the belief that there is no time for the child to follow developmental stages of motor functions other than sitting, standing and stepping. 'Treatment' appears to relate to treatment of the impairments so that the MOVE programme is not called a therapy. Supportive equipment is linked with the training programme, and is usually selected from the Rifton catalogue.

3 Synthesis of Treatment Systems

All the various treatment systems claim good results. It is difficult to decide which system is superior, whether on theoretical grounds or on the basis of a scientific study. Clinical experience of many therapists, as well as my own, has not confirmed the superiority of any one approach. Perhaps this is not a worthy aim to pursue on theoretical grounds or research studies.

THEORETICAL GROUNDS

Every therapist wishes to understand 'why we do what we do' and unfortunately may accept a therapy system because it offers a ready explanation. However, there is no all-encompassing theory which fully explains all the abnormal motor behaviour presented by people with the different cerebral palsies. In addition, theories may not adequately explain the effects of various treatment systems or, in some cases, for specific procedures. Theories also do not fully clarify mechanisms underlying motor behaviour from infancy to adulthood. Each therapy approach is based on scientific evidence available at the time and the neuro-facilitation systems are based on a number of controversial neurophysiological hypotheses. There are currently newer theories on motor learning and motor control. However, controversies exist so that current neuroscience and behavioural psychology do not favour a single model for motor behaviour. Therapists continue to work with an underlying theoretical framework with some scientific evidence but also with assumptions about motor control, motor development or motor learning. Increasing scientific understanding of brain function and motor behaviour

will contribute to therapy and its knowledge base. Therapists will need to judge the relevance of such studies and advances and apply them to clinical work. It is still unwise to be dogmatic about a theoretical framework or about procedures which arise from that. Therapy techniques cannot fully rest on different and more current theories underlying motor control or motor learning. We still have to learn to live with these doubts.

Although the therapist should continue to ask herself why she is using a particular method, this enquiry should focus more on the careful observations of motor behaviour and any changes in behaviour after treatment procedures. Increasing clinical studies and research together with clinical experience will offer scientific evidence underpinning treatment procedures. Therapists need to draw on those studies which are relevant to their particular patients.

RESEARCH STUDIES

These are fraught with many problems and to date no study to compare the value of different treatment systems has convincingly dealt with all the problems. Firstly, the results of treatment are not only influenced by the methods dictated by the concept of an approach but by the severity of motor function and impairments, age and sex of an individual. Secondly, results are influenced by possible associated impairments and disabilities of vision, hearing, communication, perception, cognition as well as by the presence of epilepsy and poor health. A child's personality and 'drive' as well as his home background contribute to the results of therapy. One must also recognize that the therapist's enthusiasm, personality and her abilities to make positive professional relationships as well as her technical skill may have a strong effect on the results of treatment with any methods.

There are other problems. The results of a scientific study would have to be obtained over a long period of time as progress is slow. At least a 6-months follow-up is now generally recommended. Crothers pointed out many years ago that one would really need a follow-up to adulthood to establish the ultimate effects of treatment methods in childhood (Paine 1962; Levitt 1962). However, this view needs to be reassessed with more current information on the deterioration related to specific physiological and psychological factors in older persons with cerebral palsy.

REVIEWS OF RESEARCH STUDIES

The research studies that have been carried out have been reviewed by Parette and Hourcade (1984) for the period 1952–82, by Tirosh and Rabino (1989) for the period 1973–88 and by Siebes et al. (2002) from 1990–2001. They all found in their reviews that the research designs were not rigorous enough and they discuss the problems facing researchers. Siebes et al. (2002) point out that although the methodology in research studies had clearly improved, this did not lead 'to a substantial improvement in the scientific foundation' of the motor interventions for children with or at risk for cerebral palsy.

Tirosh and Rabino (1989) suggest that a much larger number of subjects in a multi-centre study should iron out many variables and that more reliable data might be obtained. They pointed out the importance of psychosocial influences. Bower and McLellan (1992) found pitfalls in eight major studies, most of which are included in Tirosh and Rabino's review except for Palmer et al. (1988) and Bairstow et al. (1993), which took place after the earlier

reviews. A review of studies specifically on the Neurodevelopmental Treatment (Bobath) approach by Butler and Darrah (2001), like Siebes et al., classifies levels of evidence from I down to V. Both these reviews find that two-thirds of the studies are below levels I and II. Furthermore, each of these reviews shows that the more scientific the study the fewer the number of statistically significant results due to therapy.

Single-case studies to evaluate specific treatment procedures together with more sensitive and more specific measures for cerebral palsy are suggested by Siebes et al. (2002). Katz et al. (1995) recommend the single-case experimental design in rehabilitation as it can show treatment efficacy without the difficulties associated with obtaining large homogeneous sample size. Single-case studies have increased and are useful for evaluation of procedures such as training postural control (balance), use of below-knee plaster casts (inhibitory casts), ankle foot orthoses and similar procedures. Single-subject studies, carefully designed, offers more for clinical studies in therapy. (See below for appraisal of research.) Nevertheless, Siebes et al. note an unfortunate decrease in single-case studies from 50% to 30% in their review. Single-case study design is discussed by Kazdin (1982), Wilson (1987), Edwards et al. (1990) and Riddoch and Lennon (1991).

STUDIES OF SPECIFIC TREATMENT SYSTEMS

The NDT review by Butler and Darrah, approved by the American Academy for Cerebral Palsy and Developmental Medicine Treatment Outcomes Committee Review Panel, has been mentioned above. They state that the 'preponderance of results did not confer any advantage to NDT over the alternatives to which it was compared'. The Doman-Delacato system was found unproven in results by Sparrow and Zigler (1978) and by Cummins (1988). Vojta's approach received criticism by Jones (1975), Bleck (1987) and Forssberg and Hirschfeld

(1992). Vojta's list of postural reflexes is not accepted by Norén and Franzén (1982) as a reliable measure of diagnosis and results. The results of Vojta's very early therapy for babies at risk as well as any other early intervention such as that of Kong (1987) cannot show that it was the intervention that obtained results and not the fact that babies 'at risk' might have become normal anyway. Nelson and Ellenberg (1982) and Touwen (1987) point out how unreliable early diagnoses can be. Nelson and Ellenberg found in their large sample of infants suspected of cerebral palsy there was a high rate of these infants becoming normal. However, neonatal studies by paediatric therapists continue and show positive value for intervention. Carlsen (1975) showed improvement using methods from Rood, Ayres, proprioceptive neuromuscular facilitation and NDT compared to a functional occupational therapy approach. She had a small sample of 12 children. Bairstow et al. (1991, 1993) carried out studies on conductive education compared with a neurophysiological and developmental approach in a selected group necessary for conductive education. No difference was found between these two groups. However, the assessors were not masked to the intervention and control groups. Titchener (1983) describes an evaluation of conductive education.

OTHER RESEARCH

A series of research studies in cerebral palsy have been carried out by E. Bower and D.L. McLellan, investigating the effect of intensive physiotherapy with specific measurable goals. All the studies use the Gross Motor Function Measure (GMFM – Russell et al. 1989, 1993). The first pilot study (Bower & McLellan 1992) used a controlled series of single-case studies with only seven children. The trend was that increased intensity for 3 weeks with goal-setting generally improved the rate of progress as compared to routine physiotherapy.

The intensive treatment was carried out by the researcher.

In a subsequent randomized controlled study of 44 children (Bower et al. 1996), the subjects were assigned to four different groups of 11, with careful checks being made that each group was similar. Intensive physiotherapy was given for 2 weeks to two of the groups, one with general aims and the other with specific goals for physiotherapy. The other two groups received routine physiotherapy for 2 weeks, again one with general aims and the other with specific goals. The study showed that intensive therapy together with specific goals can accelerate the acquisition of motor function. There was no follow-up to see whether these gains were subsequently maintained.

A further study of 56 children (Bower et al. 2001) used four groups as before. However, the period of routine or intensive therapy lasted 6 months and, unlike the 1996 study, there was a period of 6 months routine therapy (about half an hour a week) with aims (baseline observation period) before the treatment period and a similar (follow-up) period afterwards. In the baseline period, there was some progress which accelerated with intensive therapy (average $3^{1}/_{2}$ hours a week). The mean total score on the GMFM improved by 5.9 percentage points on intensive therapy whereas by only 3.1 percentage points on routine therapy. There was no difference as to whether aims or goals were used in the intensive or routine treatment period. The follow-up 6 months later showed that the average child did not maintain the lead gained during the intensive therapy. However, despite this obvious difference, Bower reports that the lead during the treatment period was not statistically significant.

Studies of rhizotomy by Steinbok et al. (1997), McLaughlin et al. (1998) and Wright et al. (1998) provide data on rates of progress on the GMFM during intensive physiotherapy alone. These show a range of average gains of 4.2 to 5.2 percentage points over a period of 9 to 12 months. This is less than the gain of 5.9 points from 6 months intensive therapy found by Bower *et al.* (2001).

RESEARCH AND CLINICAL STUDIES

Whenever possible, these are quoted throughout this book in relation to experts' experiences, ideas and methods.

It is important to understand that absence of evidence of effectiveness is not proof or evidence of ineffective treatment. Future research is needed for more information so that better evidence for practice is gained. Meanwhile, clinicians need to critically appraise their work with careful observation and good records. Research and academic therapists communicate current scientific studies in a dialogue with clinicians so that relevant rationale for practice is developed. (See *Paediatric Physiotherapy Guidance for Good Practice* by Association of Paediatric Chartered Physiotherapists – APCP 2002.)

CLINICAL EXPERIENCE AND EVIDENCE-BASED PRACTICE

Every paediatric physiotherapist or occupational therapist wants to know that her intervention or treatment produces benefit to a child and his family. Good practice has therefore used evaluations for the records of therapists and medical consultants throughout the history of management of cerebral palsy. Today, what evidence of the evaluation of therapy is available to the clinician?

(1) *Professional experience* We still use findings from long experience of our own and of acknowledged experts in the field. Careful observations, evaluations and clinical judgments from practical experience and from related studies remain important and many references to such studies from a number of disciplines are quoted throughout this book.

(2) *Measures of outcome* Current practice continues to develop objective evaluations of outcomes (results) of motor training or treatment which are not biased by a school of thought or therapy system. There are methods of assessment and reassessment which are often self-validating in terms of the theories of a system. Because the theories or concepts are controversial, such evaluation measures of progress are not objective enough. Furthermore, measures need to be devised to avoid the risk of subjective views of any senior colleague or expert. Measures for evaluation of therapy outcomes are discussed in Chapter 7 on Assessment.

(3) *Research studies* These are an increasingly valuable source of evidence for therapy. They offer quantitative or qualitative evidence for the value and effectiveness of physiotherapy and occupational therapy.

Quantitative research aims to measure effects and present the results as numerical data.

Qualitative research aims to identify and describe the common experiences and relationships of all those involved in treatments, including the therapists (Patton 1980). It is often called 'client-centred' and is then concerned with the meaning that treatments and outcomes have for the patient (client) and their family. Studies also interpret how therapy affects the individual's thoughts and feelings about their quality of life. The collection of data uses methods such as semi-structured interviews or open-ended questionnaires.

The different research styles of quantitative and qualitative studies provide different kinds of useful information and are complementary. They are each scientific in that their different methods are systematic and disciplined (Stone 1991). Some issues such as quality of life and empathy can be studied by quantitative methods using scales derived from counselling, psychology

Vojta treatment under 6 months obtained better results than the same treatment after 9 months, but the younger group were less severe than the older group.

(b) The therapists carrying out the treatment should be independent of the research because therapists are expected to be highly motivated, to be helpful and see results of their work. It is wise to have a number of therapists carrying out a procedure to be tested, in case the research is really a test of one therapist's skill. All therapists should be of professionally acknowledged skill.

(c) The assessors measuring the effects should not know (be 'blind' to) which child has received which treatment, otherwise they may unwittingly bias their measurements.

(7) *Analysis of results* Graphs need to be clear when giving results to the clinician. They are useful for ABA research designs, as they can show trends during each of these three periods. For example, an upward trend in the first A period may be markedly increased in period B. The trend in the second A period shows whether any gains made during period B are *maintained*, once the bout of intervention has stopped.

Research studies differ from routine clinical measures and assessments in that statistical methods are used. Statistics are needed because people are variable and cerebral palsy is a heterogeneous condition. These statistics should be explained and not be so obscure that the clinician cannot decide on the value of the study.

Results are given as differences between the groups of children studied. These differences or changes in outcome may be positive, non-existent or even negative! However, the change may be a fluke or due to unknown factors which give a chance result, and the purpose of statistical analy-sis is to show whether the change is genuinely due to the intervention. This is what the phrase 'statistically significant' means. This is stated as a p-value. A p-value less than 0.05 is taken to show that the results are statistically significant. Remember, a statistically significant result is no guarantee that the research is worthwhile unless all the elements of the research are satisfactory. Clinicians and research workers are more knowledgeable about those elements than are statisticians. But even if the change is statistically significant, it could be quite small and may not be 'humanly significant'. Is it worth people making the effort in time, energy and money? Is it great enough to warrant a change to clinical practice?

Quality of life can matter more than a large, statistically significant increase in, say, active ranges of movement.

Studies which use large numbers of children are more likely to give statistically significant results, as they can average out the variability. However, if a study is focused on one well-defined treatment procedure aimed at a specific impairment and if the effect is quite a marked change post-treatment, then a small number of children is acceptable. Even a control group is not absolutely necessary. Clinicians know the usual history of such cases in the short term.

Statistical significance cannot be calculated for only one or two cases. In addition, one cannot generalize from one or two cases to all children with the same condition. Certainly a marked improvement in a clinical case encourages the therapist to try out the treatment with other similar children. It may well serve as an idea for a research study, with more children.

The clinical practitioner needs to consult colleagues who are research therapists for further discussion. Useful references on research methods are:

Ottenbacher 1986; Kazdin (1982); Hicks (1995), notably Chapter 12; Whalley Hammell *et al.* (2000).

THE ECLECTIC VIEWPOINT IN THERAPY

As it is difficult to confine oneself to any particular system and as each has made valuable contributions, an eclectic approach is recommended (Levitt 1970a, 1974, 1976).

The eclectic viewpoint has become increasingly accepted. Hagbarth and Eklund (1969), McLellan (1984), Griffiths and Clegg (1988), Dietz (1992) and Burns and MacDonald (1996) recognize elements of value in many different approaches and that selection of methods for an individual child is advisable. In the USA Umphred (1984) and Farber (1982) suggest integrated approaches, quoting other colleagues who support this. In Britain, studies by Bower and McLellan *et al.* (1992, 1996, 2001) point out that most physiotherapists use an eclectic approach. In *Paediatric Physiotherapy Guidelines for Good Practice* (Dunn *et al.* 1990) and in the revised edition (APCP 2002) by the Association of Paediatric Chartered Physiotherapists there are recommendations 'to select appropriately from the various approaches for each individual child'.

Different varieties of eclectic practice are used by individual practitioners (Horn *et al.* 1995). To some it is selecting different neuro-facilitation methods from Rood, Ayres, Bobath, Knott and Voss for an individual, but without active motor learning principles. In this chapter both an historical and current review is given of how to draw on both traditional neuro-facilitation and developmental systems, orthopaedics and motor learning models. Synthesis is based on consideration of postural mechanisms, voluntary motion and perceptual-motor function intrinsic to function, and it is particularly function that must draw on learning.

In developing the eclectic approach, it has been necessary to try to understand the rationale underlying the methods in various systems of treatment.

At first, the systems appear different and even contradictory to one another. However, this is not really the case. Although there are differences, there is also common ground. The following discoveries emerged in my comparative study of the theory and practice of various treatment approaches – neurophysiological, developmental, motor control and motor learning:

(1) Different rationale are given by different systems for the same or similar methods. The common ground is the method, but the reasons offered differ.
(2) In some instances, the rationale are not really different, but only couched in different terminologies. The common ground is both the method and the reason for it.
(3) In other instances, the rationale are the same, only couched in different terminologies, but the methods suggested differ from system to system. The common ground is the rationale but methods differ.
(4) There are still differences in methods and rationale.
(5) Although methods may differ they are sometimes given the same name.

I have attempted to analyse and clarify this complicated field in order to bring together isolated but valuable pockets of knowledge. During these studies, it has also been difficult to know which methods and ideas in any particular system are the ones which are responsible for the results achieved. In any system there are methods and ideas which are superfluous. It is not correct that 'everything in a system depends on everything else'.

Methods and ideas have been selected rather more according to the problems of the children than according to the theories underlying the methods. In this way a synthesis of treatment can be made. This has now developed further and study continues in drawing on different models of motor learning to synthesize with therapy. (See Chapters 4 and 5.)

SYNTHESIS OF TREATMENT SYSTEMS

Despite different terminologies and methods the following aspects are fundamental to the various systems of treatment and motor learning models:

(1) The postural mechanisms.
(2) Voluntary motion.
(3) Perceptual motor function.

THE POSTURAL MECHANISMS

The postural mechanisms are neurological mechanisms which maintain posture and equilibrium and are involved in locomotion. They have been described by various neurological workers (Belenkii *et al.* 1967; Martin 1965, 1967; Roberts 1978; Foley 1977a, 1998; Marsden *et al.* 1981; Cordo & Nashner 1982; Shumway-Cook & Woollacott 2001).

Paediatric neurologists have studied ages in babies when certain postural reactions called *automatisms* normally appear with maturation. Terminology varies and Milani-Comparetti and Gidoni (1967) grouped them into *righting reactions*, *parachute reactions* and *tilt reactions*. Physiotherapists first focus on postural stability and postural adjustment needed for motor function and add training of these righting, parachute and tilt reactions in both active as well as reactive methods.

Purdon Martin's presentation (Martin 1967) has drawn on many neurological studies with his own observations. His clear functional scheme provided me with a practical observational framework for clarifying terminologies and methods in different treatment approaches. In this book it has been slightly modified and related to children with cerebral palsies and other motor delays.

Whatever the terminologies and different viewpoints, postural mechanisms are stimulated or trained within most treatment approaches. However, particular systems have emphasized some, but not all of these postural mechanisms. Some assessments for therapy such as Chailey Levels of Ability (Pountney *et al.* 1999), Gross Motor Function Measure (Russell *et al.* 1989) omit examination of the tilt and the saving postural mechanisms as their therapy focuses on other aspects. Children with cerebral palsy with severe visual impairments are among those individuals who cannot function safely and fully independently without these postural mechanisms (Shumway-Cook & Woollacott 2001; Hirschfeld 1992; Foley 1998; Butler & Major 1992; Levitt 1984, Chapter 9).

It is important to draw on all treatment approaches to make sure that none of an individual's potential postural mechanisms are omitted. In addition, those therapy approaches that have given attention to all the problems of postural mechanisms have not necessarily suggested methods to cover the needs of all children and older people. Therefore methods need to be selected from different systems or clinicians so that dormant responses can be activated in individuals.

The postural mechanisms are given and illustrated in the practical chapters. In outline they consist of:

The antigravity mechanism or the mechanism which helps to support the weight of the body against gravity. This provides a pillar of the limb for support against gravity. This rigid pillar is decreased with development of the postural mechanisms below.

This is also known as the *supporting reaction* in infants, *leg straightening reflex* or *positive statzreaktion*.

The postural fixation (stabilization) of parts of the body, i.e. head on trunk, trunk on pelvis and fixation of the shoulder girdles and pelvic girdles and the lower jaw, pharynx and tongue. Postural stabilization of the body as a whole. Although quiet stability results, there are subtle adjustments called 'postural sway'.

Terminologies also used for this are *stability, heavy work, tonic activity.*

Counterpoising mechanisms are closely associated with postural fixation. They are adjustments of the trunk and other parts of the body so that a movement can be made whilst the person maintains posture or equilibrium. Movements of the limbs or head provoke these adjustments of equilibrium. Weight shift precedes limb movements and is minimal before any movement is started. Anticipatory postural adjustment is discussed with voluntary motion.

Terminologies also used are *balance during motion, load shift, weight shifts,* and various *balance exercises* and *movement superimposed on co-contraction.*

Righting or rising reactions make it possible for the person to rise from lying to standing, or sitting to standing or many other changes of position. Rising into position as well as returning to the original position are both part of these reactions. Rising involves a sequence of motor actions which is pro-active as well as reactive. For example, body-on-body righting reaction precedes active rising. Other terminologies used are *assumption of posture, moving into position* and *movement patterns.* The latter is confusing as there are also movement patterns which are voluntary movements and different to these automatic changes of posture. *Righting* is also used meaning either *postural adjustment* or *tilt* reactions and is not the sense in which I use it.

Tilt reactions occur when a person is tilted well off the horizontal plane and adjusts his trunk so that he preserves his balance. Tilt adjustments are antero-posterior or lateral to each side with equal response.

Reactions to falling or saving from falling. These are various reactions in the limbs which prevent the person from falling over, if the tilt reactions cannot preserve balance. These reactions do not, on their own, stop falling over completely. For example, the arms may be thrown out to save the person from falling forward, sideways, backwards and in more complicated patterns. If the person is falling over from the standing position he may stagger, hop or quickly place a foot out to stop the fall. In sitting, kneeling and other positions the legs also move in order to save him from falling from these positions.

Another terminology for these reactions is *protective responses.* Particular arm saving reactions are also called *parachute reactions, saving and propping on the hands, protective extension, arm balance responses, precipitation reaction* or *head protective response.*

Equilibrium reactions or *balance reactions* are also terms used which mean a combination of tilt and the limb reactions. These terms are confusing as all the postural reactions above are involved with equilibrium or balance. Maintaining a posture is synonymous with maintaining balance. Also, lack of tilt reaction seems to augment limb saving reactions and vice versa. This is seen in ataxic and athetoid children.

Besides the six main postural reactions above, there are also:

Locomotive reactions which serve to initiate stepping, continue stepping and stop stepping. They are also known as the mechanisms for propulsion or progression. They need stability and adaptation for human gait.

Ocular postural reflexes and control of facial musculature are also interwoven with the postural mechanisms.

All these reactions can be stimulated within developmental training, using methods drawn from different systems of treatment. It is helpful to follow motor developmental levels, for as the child acquires functional motor control he is acquiring these neurological mechanisms. However, the developmental sequences may vary in normal and abnormal children. This is discussed below in the section on developmental training.

VOLUNTARY MOTION

Voluntary motion which is purposeful, conscious, willed motion is sometimes confused with the active automatic movements which occur in the postural mechanisms such as rising or saving from falling. Although some of the automatic movement synergies are also seen in voluntary movement, stimulation of the automatic patterns only corrects abnormal postures and movements but does not contribute enough to the training of voluntary motion. Voluntary motion uses many different synergies and there may be a great variety of synergies in any one child for the same task. Therapy needs to offer a variety of patterns so a child can have a choice for a task. In time he chooses the most effective pattern.

Voluntary motion is, however, far more complex, in that it is involved with perceptual, praxic and cognitive function. Physiotherapists contribute neuromuscular and musculo-skeletal techniques which need to include more than the stimulation of automatic arm and leg patterns of postural reactions. These patterns are drawn from many systems of treatment and are discussed in particular reference to arm and hand function in Chapter 8. Additional advice must be obtained from other disciplines working on the learning of motor skills, i.e. psychology, special education and physical education.

Voluntary motion and postural control

Voluntary motion is intertwined with the postural mechanisms. Postural mechanisms allow voluntary movement to take place and any voluntary motion itself activates the relevant postural mechanisms. When a child makes a voluntary movement he has to maintain his balance as he does so. If his postural stability and counterpoising is inadequate the child may not be able to initiate or carry out the move-

ment. Should he manage to carry out an active movement on a background of unstable posture, the movement can be either imprecise, clumsy, incoordinated or weak. Clinicians need to avoid over-emphasizing training of voluntary movement of arms, hands and legs in isolation from the postural control. In addition, isolated training of postural stability and adjustment without a variety of hand and limb actions is not sufficient.

Since Martin's work (1967) there have been many research studies to show that his postural fixation and counterpoising are anticipatory postural responses (Marsden *et al.* 1981; Cordo & Nashner 1982). Useful reviews by Hirschfeld (1992), Mulder (1991), Shumway-Cook and Woollacott (2001) and others quote many studies including their own, showing an anticipatory postural response before an intended voluntary movement is begun. This is a 'feedforward' mechanism among others which are activated before voluntary initiation of movement. For example von Hofsten (1992) in his many research studies of infants' visually directed reaching had his infants fully supported as they did not have stability and antipatory counterpoising under the age of 4 months. Amiel-Tison and Grenier (1986) manually stabilized an infant's head on his trunk to reveal pre-reaching arm movements. von Hofsten's studies also showed that an infant's reaching became more successful as his postural control developed from 4 months of age. Anticipatory postural responses of their trunks were observed at the normal age of 9 months.

Postural control of the head and trunk helps eye-hand co-ordination in voluntary movement. Oro-facial muscles function better with head control (Winstock 2003). The use of vision promotes development of postural mechanisms. Younger children until about age 3 years find vision more important than proprioception for postural control, whereas adults depend more on the proprioceptive input for postural control (Lee & Aronson 1974). Sugden (1992) and Van Vliet (1992) review vision, postural control and movement. (See section on motor development and the visually impaired child in Chapter 8.)

PERCEPTUAL MOTOR FUNCTION

The therapy systems explored in this book touch on the role of the physiotherapist, occupational therapist and speech therapist's contributions to stimulation of all the senses, linking of sensations, sensory discrimination, developing body image, body scheme, spatial relationships and direction and other aspects which are related to perceptual motor function. The psychologist, occupational therapist, teacher and other specialists make specific structured contributions to these aspects. The neuromuscular techniques in the various therapy systems may be integrated with the perceptual motor training, usually part of occupational therapy (Ayres 1979; Fisher *et al.* 1991).

TREATMENT PRINCIPLES FOR A SYNTHESIS OF THERAPY SYSTEMS

The common ground between the different systems forms the principles of treatment. These common denominators will be discussed so that the therapist can understand where they exist and where differences are apparent or real.

General principles of treatment which are commonly accepted by various schools of thought are:

(1) Team work. (Chapters 1, 5 and 11)
(2) Early treatment. (Chapter 1)
(3) Repetition of a motor activity. (Chapters 4, 8 and 9)
(4) Education of family member, parent or carer either for home treatments or practical management.
(5) Motivation and support of child and parent (Chapters 4 and 5) or older person with or without carer.

Specific principles of treatment. Common factors detected in the various systems of treatment are:

(1) Developmental training.
(2) Treatment of abnormal tone.
(3) Training of movement patterns.
(4) Use of afferent stimuli.
(5) Use of active movement.
(6) Facilitation.
(7) Prevention of deformity.

DEVELOPMENTAL TRAINING

Viewpoints differ as to whether to strictly follow normal developmental sequences, or modify them. Viewpoints also differ as to whether to train a total motor function such as rolling, crawling, standing or walking or whether to break each function down into elements for training (Rood 1962; Cotton 1975a; Bobath & Bobath 1975; Levitt 1986, 1991; Vojta 1989; Levitt & Goldschmied 1990). Most therapists prefer to train elements or *bricks* which build up the motor function as well as train the total function. However, views differ as to what these elements are. Some talk of different types of muscle tone, different reflexes, different muscle work and biomechanical ideas. In addition, *basic motor patterns* are recommended as the basic abilities which underlie many motor functions on the developmental scales. For example, Bobath & Bobath (1975) suggest training the fundamental motor patterns of head and trunk control, symmetry, extensor activity, rotation, arm support and equilibrium reactions; Rood (1962) suggests muscle work in main stages on an *Ontogenetic developmental sequence*; Vojta (1989) uses the basic creeping complex and reflex rolling from which stabilization and rising are facilitated. Fay (1954a,b) and Doman *et al.* (1960) use levels of creeping, crawling and only prone development; Cotton (1975a) recommends symmetry, grasp, elbow extension, hip flexion and mobility as fundamental in cerebral palsy. Green *et al.* (1995) emphasize loadbearing on body parts, pelvic and shoulder girdle position, and head posture. It is possible to contain all these viewpoints in recognizing that:

(1) Elements of tone, strength and reflexes are impairments. Basic motor patterns and biomechanics are abilities underlying whole function.

(2) Training postural reactions and locomotive reactions described above, as well as voluntary motion, includes symmetry, grasp, head and trunk control, rotation, and other abilities and impairments according to the assessment of individuals. It is important to look at the postural reactions in each *part* of the body, i.e. head, shoulder girdles, trunk, pelvic girdle, and check their pattern.

(3) Developmental sequences are only relevant to the sequence of development of these postural mechanisms and voluntary motion and *not* to the sequence of milestones or *total* motor function. For example, it is easier for the child to acquire postural stability of the head in a motor function at say 3 months normal developmental level than at say the more demanding functions at 6 and 9 months levels. Control of the head in supporting sitting (3 months) is easier than head and trunk control in unsupported sitting (7–9 months). Tilt reactions are easier in lying (6–9 months) than in sitting (9–12 months). Rising on to all fours (6–9 months) is easier than rising on to two feet (18 months). These are natural biomechanics.

(4) Modifications of sequences are also needed for individual children and older persons to find their own pattern of development of the various postural reactions. For example, shoulder postural stability and postural stability of the head may be acquired not only when the child is in prone, leaning on forearms (at about the 3 months normal level) but also when he is sitting leaning on forearms supporting his body against a low table, or standing leaning on forearms with body supported against a table. There are many examples of total motor functions at apparently higher levels on the developmental sequences that are useful in obtaining the same postural reactions which also occur in total motor functions at stages in earlier developmental milestones (Fig. 8.33).

(5) The infantile reflexes are not all modified in a strict sequence by the later sequence of equilibrium reactions as previously thought by workers such as Barnes *et al.* (1978). Function of a child may use other strategies and in severe cases infantile reflexes are even selected for independent function.

(6) Postural reactions of one part of the body may be more advanced than another part, e.g. the head may be better than pelvis and vice versa; shoulder girdle may be better than pelvis and vice versa. The developmental sequence may be atypical due to the impairments.

(7) Modifications of the developmental sequences may also be required if a child has a preference for particular abnormal postures of the head, trunk or limbs. For example, repeated use of flexor postures and movements must be corrected by selection of motor functions which use more extension and any patterns *other* than the preferred flexion patterns.

(8) Modifications of sequence are also indicated if a child strongly dislikes prone or other positions. Prone is commonly disliked in a few children who bottom shuffle rather than crawl before they walk, or in children with breathing problems. In addition, the full list of motor functions in prone development (or any other channel), may be impossible in hemiplegics or in others with severe involvement of both arms. It may still be possible to walk, to sit and to achieve the postural mechanisms and voluntary motion through other developmental motor functions (Robson 1970). Solomons and Solomons (1975), among others, have observed different sequences in *different cultures* or different environments.

Development Assumptions

The developmental training of the past trained first head control and only then rolling, next sitting, then crawling and, only after all these, standing and walking. This view of one developmental ladder may have arisen because these motor skills *appear* more or less in this sequence. However, in normal children all these skills are developing simultaneously but are not fully achieved until different milestones (*motor ages*; development levels) are reached. At birth, the child is able to take weight on his feet and momentarily hold his head upright. These are the elements of standing, but it will take many months before the full achievement of standing alone. The same occurs for crawling, for rolling and for sitting. The therapist should work on developmental sequences for each motor function of 'stages for crawl', 'stages for sitting' and so on, in supine, prone, sitting and standing positions. Parallel motor developmental channels are more relevant to therapy and are more task-specific biomechanically, for muscle groups and joint ranges (see Chapter 8) (Levitt 1970a, 1987; Bobath & Bobath 1975; Green *et al.* 1995).

The use of parallel developmental channels by some therapists has also generated unproven views. There are many examples such as: back extensors must first be trained in lying or use of the Landau reaction before upright standing; reciprocal leg movements must first be trained in lying and crawling before stepping in walking; rolling is necessary for the rotation component of sitting and reaching across or behind the body or for the gait pattern. Biomechanical views such as load-bearing and load shift in lying must be trained to precede sitting and standing. Yet, the influence of gravity is quite different in lying on a surface from upright positions. These examples are all clinical observations which appear to correlate motor components in different positions. But correlation is not causation. Therapists need more research to confirm the beliefs of what are the prerequisites of motor function. We need to avoid confusion of sequence with consequence.

In this book there are sequences in each channel in say, lying to rolling to getting out of bed, prone to crawling, sitting to bottom-shuffling or lying, sitting and standing associated with counterpoising for hand function. The supported infantile stepping, weight-bearing to independent standing and walking as a sequence has been used since the first edition of this book in 1977. This seems to be supported by research (Forssberg 1985) to show the effect of postural mechanisms on the development of walking and the muscle actions involved.

The postural mechanisms in lying, sitting or standing positions need to be activated in the positions in which they underlie particular motor functions and their levels of development. The activation of the rising reactions so that a child can change position or assume a posture depends on its own sequence and inevitably overlaps from one channel to another. Therapists can achieve results of treatments for strengthening, stretching short muscles, decreasing spasticity and mobilizing joints in motor functions in lying positions of children and adults. However, transfer to other positions is not likely unless all these aspects are trained within motor functions in sitting and standing.

To summarize. This book uses parallel developmental sequences with selected motor activities which activate fundamental postural reactions. In the practical chapters ideas are selected from various approaches to train the motor activities in the developmental sequences. Modifications of developmental sequences are recommended when necessary.

TREATMENT OF ABNORMAL TONE

Hypertonicity

Cerebral palsied children were often called 'spastics' and to this day spasticity is given particular prominence, for diagnosis and orthopaedic procedures by many workers. Physiotherapists may take their lead from such workers. However, spasticity is not of great significance for function. If spasticity is reduced or even removed by, say, alcohol or phenol injections, the child will still be disabled (Nathan 1969). Pederson (1969) remarks on the lack of correlation of spasticity with voluntary motion in his review of alcohol and phenol injections. After removal of spasticity, the voluntary motion may be stronger, weaker or absent. Increasing research showed that spasticity has been overemphasized and too little attention given to the absence or delay of motor function (Sahrmann & Norton 1977; Dietz & Berger 1983; Carr *et al.* 1987; Dietz 1992). Young and Wiegner (1987) state that 'spasticity may be partially responsible for joint contractures, it does not produce most of the functional disability . . .' and Giuliani (1992) in her many assessments of the results of dorsal rhizotomy to remove spasticity states that '. . . assumptions that spasticity is the underlying cause of disordered movement and that reducing or eliminating the spasticity will improve movement are unfounded. . . . Reducing spasticity may increase range of motion, but may unmask underlying weakness rather than underlying control'. Almeida *et al.* (1997) also do not relate spasticity to abnormal function.

Martin (1967) also found that his patients with Parkinson's disease showed no correlation between their rigidity and the presence of postural reactions. The reason children do not develop motor functions is not because of their spasticity. After all, at first babies are often not spastic. However, they are motor disabled as they do not have motor functions which depend on postural reactions (Foley 1977a, 1998). Paine's studies (1964) of the evolution of postural reflexes show no correlation between them and increases or decreases of tone.

There are situations when spasticity is relevant to function. This is when spasticity contributes to abnormal postures and shortens muscles, creating deformities which offer a mechanical block to function. As any experienced therapist knows, many deformities do not equal disability, or in other words do not always block function. Examples of blocking of function are plantarflexed feet which prevent the achievement of plantigrade feet needed for standing or in many cases as two extra props for helping to overcome insecure sitting; flexed hips and knees in standing prevent the postural fixation of the pelvis in the vertical position and the counterpoising mechanisms from operating efficiently for walking and for arm motion in standing; adductor spasticity which prevents a wide sitting base for the development of sitting and severe scoliosis with severe *windswept* legs blocks function.

Treatment of the spasticity varies from system to system. The neurophysiologists Hagbarth and Eklund (1969) were not able to accept any of the theories as the 'answer' and support my suggestion that one should draw on different systems of treatment. This eclectic view is also held by McLellan (1984) and Dietz (1992). Lin (2000) points out that there are various mechanisms causing spasticity which affects medical decisions.

In all systems of treatment motor developmental levels of posture and movement are being trained. Thus the child is being helped to move with a greater variety of actions as possible and this will *include* the treatment of the effects of spasticity or other hypertonus. Treatment of the patterns of abnormal performance discussed in the practical chapters will counteract short spastic muscles in dynamic and to some degree in fixed deformities and help the child 'look better' as well as avoid any mechanical blocks to function.

See Chapter 10 for further discussion of short (hypo-extensible) spastic muscles in relation to deformity. Chapter 10 shows that direct treatment of spasticity may be helpful, but in some cases removal of spasticity may even remove function if there are no normal postural reactions. Spasticity and contracture increase to compensate for no postural control so the person can be propped up against gravity.

Hypotonicity

Hypotonicity is also not correlated with strength of voluntary motion but seems more associated with the postural reactions. Improvement of the postural reactions seems to coincide with improvement of the hypotonic muscles. 'Floppy babies' or Downs' hypotonia improve as the postural mechanisms are activated. Tactile stimulation and other techniques aimed at increasing tone are useless unless accompanied by training of the motor functions or postural mechanisms, or in fact replaced by this training.

Fluctuating Tone

Fluctuating tone or severe sudden spasms and involuntary motion seems to 'throw the child off balance', but may not prevent the development of the postural reactions. The association of these athetoid symptoms and postural reactions is not clear yet. Severe dyskinesia has disrupting spasms or tone fluctuations and severe disability in function. Nevertheless in some children voluntary motion can be trained, despite disturbance by the involuntary movements. Improvement of postural mechanisms seems to *decrease* the disrupting effect and sometimes the degree of involuntary motion.

To summarize. The therapist should not collect techniques for abnormal tone *as such* but rather:

(1) Emphasize training the motor functions composed of postural mechanisms and voluntary motion.
(2) Enlarge the amount and variety of motor abilities.
(3) Train the best pattern of performance so that deformity is prevented or decreased.

(4) Concentrate on threatening and established deformities which may block function, e.g. spastic plantarflexors which contribute to toe standing and increase difficulty in sitting. A secure base is needed for function and short spastic muscles may narrow the base needed, making stability difficult. (See Chapter 10.)

TRAINING OF MOVEMENT PATTERNS

Some therapy systems assess and treat individual muscle groups (Phelps 1952; Plum & Molhave 1956; Slominski 1984) and this muscle education is associated with orthopaedics (Sharrard 1971; Samilson 1975). Apparently contradictory views are held in the neurological approaches, which strongly recommend assessing and training movement patterns, and patterns of posture. There is no total contradiction for the following reasons:

(1) Movement patterns are made up of muscle groups. In fact a synergy or a *movement pattern* is a vague term as movement patterns may look the same, but be composed of different muscle actions in different children. Holt (1966) demonstrates with electromyography that the muscles acting in the same pattern of posture are different in different children. In orthopaedics, particular joints may be more deformed than others so that presumably some muscle groups are more troublesome than others *within* any abnormal patterns. It is therefore helpful to analyse the muscle work in abnormal patterns of movements and posture with electromyography and clinical observation as for example in gait analyses (Leonard *et al.* 1988, 1991).
(2) Although individual muscle groups may be assessed *in isolation* as is usual in orthopaedic physiotherapy, there is no need to limit treatment to isolated muscle education. Muscle education can be obtained *in*

pattern as well. At early levels of development the child cannot easily isolate his movements. More severely brain damaged children and adults can only use mass movements or stereotyped synergies of muscle action and cannot respond to localized muscle education. Damiano *et al.* (1995) strengthened muscles individually in older children who were also less severely affected and were walking.

(3) Besides the level of function of any particular child, there is also the fact that training a muscle group, or relaxing a spastic muscle group, does not guarantee that the particular muscle group will work correctly within a function. Muscles are activated as prime movers, synergists or fixators when they contract, as well as being inhibited (relaxing, 'letting go') as antagonists, during motion. Muscles have to shorten and contract (concentric work or isotonic), keep the same length and contract (isometric work) or lengthen and contract (eccentric work) in different movements. These various muscle actions are best trained in the movement in which they will be used in motor function. For example, during dressing in supine, bridging hips is used. Bridging hips and 'hold' involves concentric followed by isometric muscle work (see Task analysis in Chapter 4; The therapist's specialized assessment in Chapter 5 and Function and ranges of motion in Chapter 7).

Movements are presented as various movement patterns by different treatment systems. Movement patterns are often considered separately from a motor function and are:

Movement patterns seen in the infant's spontaneous motility and in the infantile reflex reactions (Table 7.2) such as the Moro, the tonic neck, the withdrawal and crossed extension reactions and many others (Capute *et al.* 1984). There are also the spontaneous movements seen in normal infancy, which are now considered of

special importance for study (Prechtl 1981; Prechtl *et al.* 1997, 2001; Cioni *et al.* 1992; de Groot 1993; Aniel-Tison & Grenier 1986).

Movement patterns preferred by brain damaged patients which include some infantile primitive synergies such as the flexor synergy of hip flexion-knee flexion-dorsiflexion (the withdrawal reflex, mass flexion reflex, von Bechterew reflex or Strumpel's phenomena) or the extensor synergy of hip extension-knee extension-plantarflexion (extensor thrust), and crossed extensor reflex which is the flexor synergy in one leg with the extensor synergy in the other leg. There are also various abnormal patterns which may not be seen in normal infants, but which are only seen in neurological cases with damage to the central nervous system. These are being studied in ongoing research in pre-term, full-term and older babies. Examples already known are opisthotonus, severe asymmetries and dystonias in older children. (See Table 7.2.) Shumway-Cook and Woollacott (2001) refer to their work on postural perturbations resulting in abnormal synergies in the legs of children with cerebral palsy. Those synergies were useful to a child in his balance control.

Infantile or abnormal synergies will not be used by some therapists in any children over 6 months developmental stages. There are, however, children who are immobile and severely impaired who remain for long periods below the 6-month normal stages. The reflex or active primitive patterns are the only ones which are possible. The reflex creeping complex, reflex rolling, withdrawal reactions or automatic stepping may be used to provoke movement. Such movement is also selected to counteract persisting abnormal postures. A severely impaired child may lie stiffly with his legs in extension-adduction-internal rotation. The legs will move into flexion-abduction-external rotation if reflex forward creeping is provoked. Fay (1954a,b) called the reflex flexion and other reflex motion *unlocking reflexes* as they unlocked a spastic position or pattern. Brunnstrom (1970) and Slominski (1984) are some workers who found they could only achieve action of an inactive muscle group if this muscle group could be activated within these primitive synergies. Lack of action in particular muscle groups contributes to deformity.

It is, however, desirable to attempt more mature patterns if they are possible. These are for example the patterns of Kabat's *mass movement patterns* seen in functional activities (Knott & Voss 1968), and Bobath's mature patterns in the developing child (Bobath 1971; Bobath & Bobath 1975, 1984).

Mature patterns of movement are patterns with more rotation and a variety of combinations of flexion and extension within any one synergy.

To summarize. Considering the many different methods used for muscle education and movement pattern training, it is *generally* advisable to 'Stimulate movements initially through primitive mass patterns, reflexes (Fay, Kabat), confused motion (Phelps) or through early patterns seen in infancy of the severely impaired children. Whenever possible it is best to modify these early combinations of movements into more controlled and advanced patterns (Kabat, Bobath) and finally into selective or isolated movements (Phelps, among others)' (Levitt 1962).

Motor learning, discussed in Chapters 4 and 5, emphasizes a person's use of movements adapted to a task rather than separate movement patterns devised to reduce muscle tightness, mobilize joints and obtain motion. But practising them in isolation does not lead to their use in function. A child/adult may use different movement strategies to carry out a task. Impairment may be treated at the same time using the desirable therapeutic patterns as well as patterns spontaneously activated by an individual. The therapist enables and teaches an individual to select movement patterns that are desirable for minimizing impairments

and for adapting to a task. Therefore, when possible, take the lead from a child's initiation of motion to solve motor problems in his daily life.

USE OF AFFERENT STIMULI: AUTOMATIC AND CONSCIOUS MOTOR ACTIVITY

Most treatment systems use afferent stimuli of touch, temperature (cutaneous) or pressure, stretch, resisted motion, joint compression or retraction (proprioceptive stimuli) as well as visual and auditory stimuli. With various methods, therapists use their hands on the child to elicit muscle actions, reduction of abnormal postural alignments and stimulate movement patterns. These motor activities are often on an automatic level. The child 'reacts to the stimuli' and feels a movement or posture he cannot achieve himself. In time this sensory-motor experience helps him acquire the motion or posture on his own. The action of the muscles within the response of automatic movement or muscle action is *active* as opposed to *passive* motion. What is not active is the child's initiation of the motion or the child's active concentration or participation in carrying out the patterns of movement and postures. His active efforts are considered to increase spasticity or abnormal patterns of function (Bobath & Bobath 1984; Vojta 1989). Rood is quoted as saying 'let us use our heads to do other things than run our muscles' (Goff 1969). When we move and balance, we do not think of these actions.

It is important to recognize that movements and postures are automatic *after* they have been achieved. In the process of training motor function as, say, in learning to drive a car, play tennis or ice skate, concentration on the movement and equilibrium is needed. Children should concentrate on, say, movements for rising from the floor, on maintaining balance, on putting their hands out to save themselves, to stop themselves from falling during training. For example, children with severe visual impairments have been taught to save themselves with verbal instructions to 'put out your arms'. Later this becomes automatic. Automatic reactions may be possible in some procedures and should also be actively learnt as well as reactive to a therapist's handling.

The child should also have his conscious attention on the afferent stimuli used by the therapist, as they are often cues to direction or to parts of his body and convey what movement is required. In addition, the child can be asked to 'pull', 'push', 'stretch up', 'try to sit alone' and so on. Some children, especially younger and mentally disabled children, respond better to concentration on an incentive for a particular motion, 'touch this', 'catch this', and on the motivation of toys and play. Neurophysiological techniques to facilitate automatic motion and counteract abnormal motor activity have obviously to be interwoven with the child's conscious or active attention and participation (see Chapters 4 and 5).

The Petö approach is particularly careful to use the child's *cortical* or conscious control of motion (Cotton 1970, 1974, 1975b). However, this approach does not carry out every aspect of motion consciously. The active efforts may focus on, say, voluntary arm motion whilst automatic head and trunk control are simultaneously activated. Conscious actions that are selected do not aggravate spasticity as these active motor activities are not too far ahead of the child, so that he is *pushed* to make abnormal efforts to achieve a movement. The afferent stimuli are contained in the auditory and visual stimuli in the instructions the children use. *Fixation* or manual holding of a part of the child's body is also used, but not in the same way as in neuro-facilitation, as little of the training of motion is based on afferent stimuli by the therapist handling the child. Current motor learning models may sometimes avoid manual handling so that active learning is assisted.

To summarize. It is advisable to show the child how and where to move by the therapist's af-

ferent stimuli for movements and postures. However, as soon as possible and even in the same therapy session, check whether the child can carry out the motor activity on his own even though it will be partial or unreliable. He should then concentrate and practise the motor activity without being handled or touched by the therapist. The motor activity selected should be at his level of development so that he can achieve something on his own. The child gains more from any corrective motor activity that he does himself. If, however, the child is so severely disabled that there is no activity possible on his own, facilitation with afferent stimuli or handling may be the only way to begin motor activity. Taub (1980), Rothwell *et al.* (1982), Gordon (1987) and others have drawn attention to research that shows that movements can be achieved without afferent input. However, Rosblad and von Hofsten (1992) demonstrated that sensory input is essential for fine coordination. There is a central motor programme in a child's central nervous system which can be used without afferent stimuli. Afferent stimuli are, however, needed to modify the child's actions and achieve accuracy of motor control. 'Hands on' sensory stimuli are therefore not always necessary. Vision and cognition with language may assist a child's acquisition of motor function.

PASSIVE OR ACTIVE MOTION

Most physiotherapists consider that active movement offers more progress than passive procedures of passive motion and splints. Passive *patterning* of children or a *full range of passive motion* cannot contribute much, if anything, to training motion. They only keep the joints mobile, and help to prevent deformity.

Passive correction by splintage, equipment for lying, sitting and standing, plasters or orthopaedic surgery passively changes the child's positions so that he obtains a better proprioceptive experience or position from which to develop active motor function. Passive correction of, say, the child's feet in plasters makes his active correction of knees and hips and balance possible.

Passive motion may be used to show the child what motion is required, but afferent stimuli are more effective if there is an active response to these stimuli giving a better proprioceptive as well as visual-auditory demonstration of what is required. Active or active resisted motion provides better proprioceptive information than passive motion (Kabat 1961; Held 1965).

The previous section on automatic and conscious movement should also be read to obtain the whole picture of active and passive therapy. The chapter on learning motor function emphasizes the need for *active* motor function but with *active* learning on the part of the child.

FACILITATION

Many systems of treatment have used the activation of one part of the body to facilitate action in another part of the body, e.g. arm elevation simultaneously activates head elevation and back extension, creeping techniques triggered at the legs facilitate activity in the whole child. Stimulation of one part of a synergic movement pattern activates the other muscle groups within the same synergy. These facilitation techniques involve normal *overflow* of activity from one area of the body to another. Feldenkrais (1980) has made an intensive study of such interactions in the whole normal body.

It is, however, possible to activate undesirable actions in other parts of the body, e.g. grasping may increase flexion in the elbows and shoulders in a child already round-shouldered and flexed, use of the arms may increase abnormal postures in the legs and grasping with one

hand may be associated with clenching of the other hand. There are other abnormal *associated reactions* observed by Bobath and Bobath (1984). Facilitation techniques, including afferent stimuli and the use of resisted motion, must be used in such a way that the rest of the body does not become abnormal (Levitt 1966, 1969, 1970).

In this context it is important to combine the ideas of Bobath with those of Knott in facilitating motion. Knott facilitates motion in one part of the body with afferent stimuli and resistance. The rest of the body must be *positioned* so that abnormal overflow does not occur. Vojta's techniques use resistance to creeping but, as the whole body is moving in a corrective pattern, positioning is unnecessary. Also much rotation within facilitation patterns in people with spasticity prevents associated abnormal motor activity in other parts of the body.

To summarize. Any patterns facilitated in one part of the body should be accompanied by careful observation of the whole child and not only of the part being activated. Normal or abnormal overflow of motor activity should be observed when using techniques in one part of the body to facilitate activity in other parts of the body. Physiotherapists can learn more about normal interactions of body parts in their own experience in 'Feldenkrais classes' (Feldenkrais 1980).

PREVENTION OF DEFORMITY

Every system aims to prevent or correct deformity. There are many methods to counteract deformity as well as many viewpoints as to the genesis of deformity. Chapter 10 is devoted to this aspect.

4   Learning Motor Function

Some therapists point out that most learning processes are dependent on the ability to move. Therefore motor function is stimulated and developed drawing on one or more systems. Once the ability to move is achieved, this is then applied to learning self-care, classroom activities, play and hobbies, household chores and, later, work. It is important to consider that a child does not move by neurophysiology alone:

- A child with brain damage *learns* motor functions such as sitting, standing, changing postures, using hands and the various forms of locomotion.
- A child *learns how* to use equipment such as walking aids, wheelchairs and playthings.
- A child *learns to* use his motor functions to achieve self-care, play and interaction with people and objects in most daily tasks.

Studies and clinical experience now show that activation of muscles or motor patterns on their own can show an improvement, but this is a performance in a therapy session and is not necessarily learnt. The improved motor performance does not transfer into the actions of daily life (Goldkamp 1984; Gordon 1987; Mulder & Hulstijn 1988). In the next chapter I have been starting with motor patterns in the context of the daily lives of children and their parents based on the need to translate my technical knowledge into what has meaning for them (Levitt 1986, 1991, 1994). This is followed by specific practice of any motor patterns which are inefficient and by activation of motor actions which are dormant but necessary for any daily life activity. Any improvement in

motor pattern is immediately used within the daily task at the same session.

LEARNING METHODS

Many experienced paediatric physiotherapists and occupational therapists do intuitively select training methods which suit an individual's learning style. This art and common sense of therapists can be supported by some of the knowledge and research presented by experts in the behavioural sciences. It is nevertheless of much value to learn from such experts so that a therapist comes to understand more deeply and analytically what she is already doing so that she can be more precise in the way that she works. These studies also offer theories for our work and new ideas are likely to be developed (Carr *et al.* 1987; Mulder 1991; Forssberg & Hirschfeld 1992; Shumway-Cook & Woollacott 2001).

A BEHAVIOUR

This is a term used by psychologists and teachers to convey any action of a child that can be observed. When behaviours are troublesome for therapists and parents in that a child refuses to cooperate, dislikes handling or having splints applied then these are discussed with team members. A clear description of what a child does, when he does it and people's responses to his behaviour is discussed so that a constructive approach can be worked out.

The behaviours which are more directly the concern of physiotherapists are motor acts. A description of what a child does with the criteria for success of a motor act is called *behavioural objective* for therapy (Presland 1982; Steel 1993). For example, 'Sitting on a potty for one minute independently without extending backward or falling to the right' (Bower & McLellan 1992). This gives the motor act, how it is done and for how long. We need to go further and state a carer's or a therapist's response to a child's motor achievement as is done with other behaviours. This will affect a child's learning of any motor function. A carer may comment or quietly look approvingly at his achievement or calmly ignore it when he does not succeed. 'Feedback' by a therapist on subsequent trials by a child helps the child learn a motor function (see below).

THE DEVELOPMENT OF A CHILD'S ATTENTION

Cerebral palsies may create apathy, hyperactivity and fleeting attention in children. Besides the brain damage which causes these difficult behaviours, they may be due to some drugs, exhaustion and emotional stress of a child. Fatigue and fears of falling are common. His refusal to cooperate and concentrate also has a number of other explanations. Parents find their child's poor concentration and restlessness very demanding (French & Patterson 1992). They are enabled to understand that therapy depends on concentration by a child on a number of tasks at his level of development which will therefore improve not only the tasks but his attention span. Therapy needs concentration and is not necessarily only a set of automatic movement responses or specialized neuromuscular procedures during which a child 'receives treatment'.

IDEAS TO PROMOTE ATTENTION AND LEARNING

(1) The programme is at each child's stages of motor, sensory, perceptual and cognitive development.

(2) Use small steps within each stage or modify a task so that achievement is possible. Successful achievement maintains attention. (See 'feedback'.)

(3) Impairments are known so that the influences of other disabilities are appreciated.

(4) Difficult and new motor tasks need to be interspersed with easier ones. Rest periods may need to be interspersed.

(5) Ensure that the therapy session does not have too many activities and that priorities are chosen.

(6) The time of day must be considered. A child may be better in the morning or some time after a meal or rest. Clearly, concentration of a child is not enhanced if he is taken away for therapy from his favourite lesson in school or from a special hobby or play activity.

(7) The length of a therapy session must relate to the child's attention span.

(8) Avoid distractions of too many people moving around, too much noise or nonstop television or radio during sessions. Later, *following achievement*, train the motor function grading the distractions in his natural environment.

(9) Keep a child looking at an object or task and not at the therapist. He learns to attend and solve problems for himself.

(10) A child's attention is best appreciated in terms of his stage in the usual sequence of development of attention, so that too much is not expected of him. Infants normally attend to more of their internal activities and to stimulation very close to them. Around 6 to 12 months their attention can be focused on stimuli of sight and sound further away from them. Fleeting attention in infants becomes longer in duration until they focus rigidly on one thing at a time. Later they will allow an adult to shift their attention and become more flexible in use of their attention (Cooper *et al.* 1978).

LEARNING A MOTOR FUNCTION

When a child focuses his attention on a motor task, he is more likely to learn it. The therapist clarifies for him where he needs to concentrate. In the first stage a child focuses his attention on the purpose for moving. This is his *intention* to move or the *action goal*. This may be a child's daily living activity of, say, eating, washing, dressing or interacting with his mother or other family member. It may be exploring an object or getting to a place where he wants to be.

Once focused on the goal, the child uses what are called *goal-directed movements* together with postural mechanisms. His attention is kept on the task as he learns which motor actions are used to achieve this goal. Therapists need to avoid *goal confusion* by their emphasis on the *best motor pattern* rather than maintaining a child's attention on the goal (Gentile 1987). Once some understanding of what to do is shown by a child, then his attention shifts more to how to do it. The action of movement and posture is therefore not separated from the purpose of that action. Van der Weel *et al.* (1991) showed how using pronation and supination in order to bang a drum obtained better action than pronation and supination as an exercise in a cerebral palsy study.

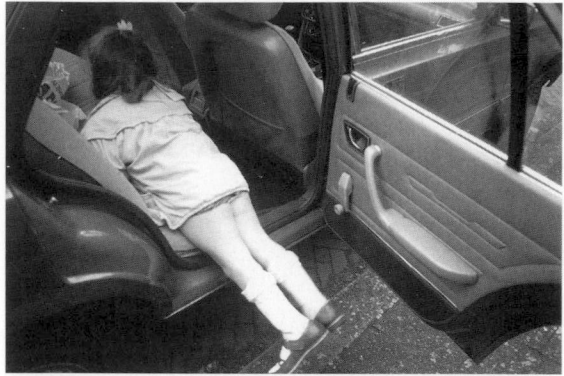

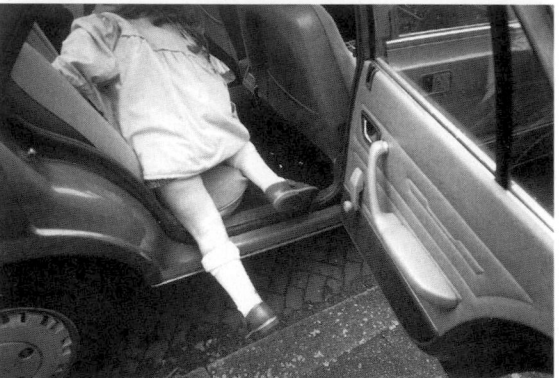

Fig. 4.1 a, b Child finding her own strategy of getting into a car; b is more desirable as she herself corrects spastic adduction of her legs.

A CHILD'S OWN GOALS AND STRATEGIES

A learning model often involves an adult explaining what a child is going to do, showing him how to do it and keeping his attention on these aspects. However, if one precedes this approach with discoveries of what a child himself wants to achieve, he may not need to have explanations of what he is going to do. If a therapist also observes how he goes about trying to achieve his own goal *she* learns about his motivation and what he can already do using his choice of postural controls and movement patterns (see Fig. 4.1). These may be:

- An approximation of the whole task.
- An initiation of the task without completion.
- An unusual way of doing the task.

The therapist can then show that child how to develop or modify the task if his approximation of a task is at a *lower developmental stage* of performance, *uses symptoms* of his type of cerebral palsy, *increases deformity* or shows *disuse* of any part of his body or muscle groups. Once a task is initiated by a child the therapist assists him to complete it. When unusual ways of performing a task are seen, then careful consideration is needed as these patterns do not always cause deformities or disuse and may be a variation of performance, much like normal variations of motor function are acceptable in able-bodied people. When a child uses immature, pathological or biomechanically compensatory patterns which do cause deformity, blocking of further development or demand excessive energy then they are corrected and discouraged. However, these motor patterns may be the only ones possible for a child to achieve independence in a particular skill. It is then important to plan other motor activities in his day which use motor patterns to counteract the choice of his abnormal patterns for independence. Additional splinting and treatments are also added to counter undesirable motor patterns. Accepting abnormal motor patterns for independence in a skill depends on the age of a child as younger children have more potential for correction. The severity of the physical condition, the degree of intellectual impairment and the degree of visual disability lead to some compromise on the use of abnormal motor patterns for selected motor tasks.

TASK ANALYSIS

In order to assess which movements and postures to improve, develop or discourage, a task analysis is made. The child's actions are compared with those in his age group and with those at an earlier stage of normal development. Task analyses include:

- A sequence of actions such as getting up from the floor through various postures (see Fig. 8.179). There is a sequence of actions for eating, drinking, washing and other daily tasks. There is a sequence of actions in using walking aids, wheelchairs and transfers or play equipment.
- The postural mechanisms at a particular developmental stage together with patterns of voluntary movements (synergies).
- The motor action and its related sensory, perceptual and cognitive areas. This involves analysing where a child looks and what he hears, smells, tastes and touches during the motor action. At the same time, he senses

what he is doing in both movement and postural control (vestibular input and proprioception). Finally, what he understands as the purpose of his action and all the senses which inform him of this.

When analysing a motor function for an individual, consider the feedback by a therapist to augment the residual or established abilities of sensations, perceptions and level of a child's cognition and motivation.

The physiotherapist also contributes to the motor components of a task by considering how the following affect the quality of motor function:

- Ranges of joint motion.
- Muscle lengths and strength.
- Postural alignments including asymmetries.
- Deformities both fixed and unfixed.
- Involuntary movements, spasms or reflex reactions which interfere with motor function.

These aspects are discussed in Chapter 7 which covers assessment.

There are different viewpoints on the analyses of tasks not only among physiotherapists but also between professionals. It is therefore necessary for members of a team to share their views on a child they all know. Common ground between physiotherapists has been discussed in Chapter 3, in the sections on Synthesis of treatment systems and Treatment principles. Research on motor analyses progresses and therapists need to continue their studies so that better task analyses are developed in the future. Interdisciplinary studies and experience also add to better task analyses involving sensory, perceptual, cognitive and motor interactions.

CUES FOR LEARNING

Cues for learning need to be clearly given in therapy. Each child will respond to different cues according to his stages of development and the presence of specific impairments. Cues are given for the starting position, during the action and for the final result of the action. A child needs to detect or be informed of any errors in his performance as well as his success (Winstein & Schmidt 1989; Winstein *et al.* 1989).

Therapists may use sensory input, verbal guidance and rewards to help a child learn motor control. Experts in motor learning call such cues *feedback*; they are not only given by a therapist but are intrinsic to the child's own experience in actively performing any task. Feedback by a therapist needs to be skilfully minimal. Winstein and Schmidt's research (1990) shows that too frequent feedback makes a learner too dependent on an instructor and dependency can be demotivating.

An example of an approach which may be adapted to different individuals is:

(1) *Set the scene so that a child can actively manage* what he can on his own. This means modifying the environment by having non-slip mats, place mats, appropriate toys, sturdy furniture and equipment according to the child's size and providing adequate light and colour to encourage achievement. Placing toys or objects in different areas activates and provides success in the training of movements. In this way a child's own action gives him feedback for learning. He senses errors so that he can correct them through his motivation and understanding of the task and how to move. The use of motor patterns *he* discovers is best for learning, provided they do not seriously increase his symptoms.

(2) *A therapist's hands can physically guide* a child through a whole task to demonstrate what is to be done and how to do it. She must then immediately remove her hands at any time that a child takes over this action from her. This may be at the beginning, middle or in finishing the task.

(3) *A therapist gives minimal support* to a child's body, shoulders or hips so that a task can be actively attempted and practised by a child. She may use equipment to support a child, allowing active movement of the body or limbs that he can begin to control. (See Fig. 4.2.)

(4) *Appropriate manual assistance or resistance* to a child's movements or stabilization of his head, body, hips and shoulders allows him to sense what to do and how to do it. Joint compression also alerts his sensory understanding of postural stabilization (fixation). Once correct postural alignment is manually given by a therapist, the child is encouraged to hold the posture. Starting positions are first assisted so that a child's action on his own is more effective for his purpose. The therapist's appropriate manual resistance also conveys to a child which body part to move and in which direction to move it. Other neuromuscular facilitation methods offer this as well.

(5) *Visual feedback* can inform a child of what he is to do and how he is doing it. Encourage him to look at his own body. Mirrors may help, though the reversed image may sometimes cause difficulties. His own observation of another child with cerebral palsy similar to him is most helpful. He may observe the therapist or his parent carrying out a task which he needs to learn. Observing others directly or on video can only be used for children who are able to imitate others. Thus severe visual impairment or severe learning impairments may make this impossible. Videos of themselves may be used by some children if they are not upset by seeing their inadequate performances. A child's best performance or desired behaviour should be videoed for feedback.

(6) *Feedback with sounds, visual displays or vibration* can inform a child on the results of his actions. These biofeedback techniques may also be arranged to augment the most desirable motor patterns of posture and movement. However, like therapy 'exercises' they do not transfer to daily

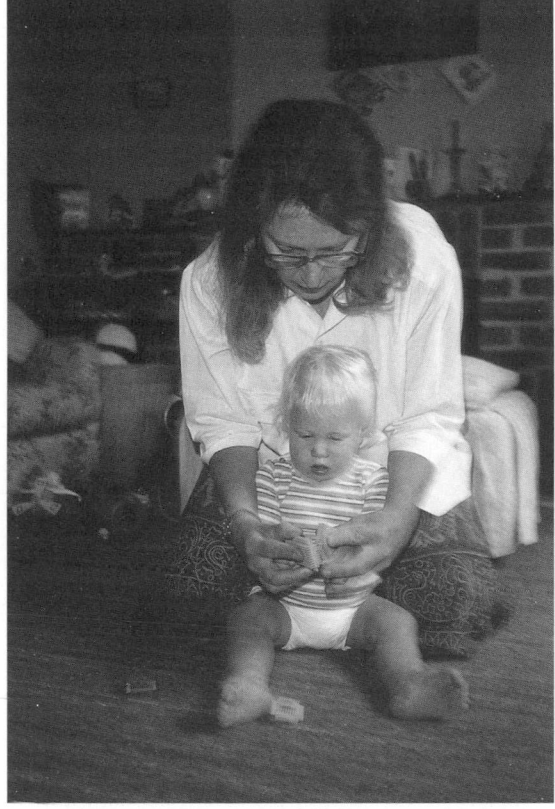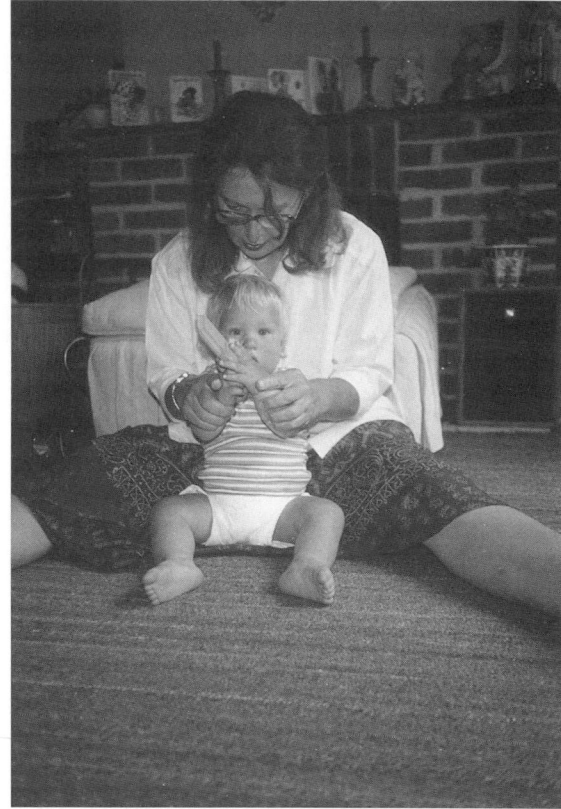

a   b

Fig. 4.2 Physical guidance for learning arm and hand function.

living if feedback on isolated actions is given (Mulder 1985). Babies and severely intellectually impaired children who cannot understand *cause and effect* are not able to use feedback. They have to be enabled to learn that their movement created a sound or switched on a light.

VERBAL GUIDANCE

This is only possible when a child understands words. It includes all or some of the following verbal instructions:

(1) Informing a child what is going to happen or the purpose of the motor patterns, for example 'You are going to . . .'.
(2) Suggesting the starting position, the movement or balance and commenting on the

results of these motor patterns. This may be done together with physical guidance. For example when showing a child how to stand up from a chair, verbalize the skill by saying 'Keep your feet flat, go forward over your feet and stand up'.

However, it is usually best if minimal verbal guidance is used with young children. Sometimes an operative word like 'step, step, step' or 'push, push, push' can be helpful. For many children, especially those who are multiply disabled, it is advisable to set the scene and physically guide or use clear gestures for communicating what is expected in a task. Also, use specialized (adaptive) equipment and toys. It is then best to be quiet and attentive as a child learns from his own experience. Quiet encouraging looks at the task and glances towards a child avoid distractions from the task to what a therapist is saying. Such an approach encourages better focusing of that child's attention on the task.

Comments on the results of a child's efforts may not always be necessary if he clearly understands that he has achieved what he has set out to do. Motivation can be maintained by phrases such as 'you sat nice and straight' or 'you stretched your elbows well'. This provides the feedback of information and praise so that the task can be learnt. Praise for the achievement of a component ability within a task is as important as the completion of the whole task. However, a child needs to learn the component within the whole task and not on its own. Unless well understood 'in context' of a task, components can be less motivating.

Remember: care needs to be taken that physical guidance and words do not themselves distract a child. A child with visual impairment or multiple disabilities may become attracted to a therapist's touch or speech rather than keep his attention on the task to be learnt. One needs to avoid a child becoming passive and dependent on your physical guidance or *facilitation method*. It is wise to remove your hands as soon as possible.

REWARDS

Although children can gain intrinsic reward in their own achievement or a task there are those who have such profound impairments that they warrant additional rewards which are extrinsic. Many teachers recommend giving a child with profound intellectual impairment a reward *immediately after* he has completed a task or even *the intention* to try to do it. Smiles, words of approval and of information may not be understood. Very basic rewards which do not depend on language or social development are suggested. There are many possibilities and each child is observed to discover what he prizes most as satisfaction. This may be food, juice, music or lights. A variety of tactile stimuli such

as stroking, patting, cuddling, blowing on his face and vibration may please him particularly. The goals for a child must be tangible so that he can be rewarded, rather than fail to achieve goals well out of his range of abilities. It is important to observe when a child has had too much of the same reward and become bored with it. This applies to all children who enjoy the incentives of a variety of toys and play during daily tasks. We continually use our imagination to find satisfying rewards for children.

Apparent rewards of 'good boy', a hug and other social praise should not be used indiscriminately as, for example, when a child is not doing anything constructive such as slumped in a chair or carrying out undesirable movements or mannerisms. This does not help learning and confuses a child as to what adults expect from him.

Natural rewards of enthusiasm and delight, together with clear information on what a child has struggled to achieve or tried to initiate, are recommended. When basic rewards need to be used these are decreased as a child with profound learning disabilities learns and retains the achievement of a motor task (Levitt 1982, 1984 Chapter 8; Presland 1982).

Older children and young children who can appreciate it may be given a progress chart with ticks for abilities gained, or collect stars or tokens for achievement. They are also rewarded when their friends, classmates and their family members approve their hard work and specific achievements.

PRACTICE AND EXPERIENCE

In the next chapter the collaborative learning outlines ways of sharing the practice of a motor task with others assisting a child's development. Practice of a motor task incorporated into activities used by teachers, playgroup workers and family members is planned with them. A motor function is also practised on its own. The stages of learning are as follows:

(1) A consistent way in which postural control, postural alignment and movements are first practised so that some ability can be initiated and developed.

(2) In the therapy session a child may have tried out various different motor patterns to accomplish his goal and improved on them with a therapist's suggestions. When his own strategies were unsuccessful he will have been shown alternative patterns by his therapist. The successful patterns are those that will be practised so that they are consolidated. Whenever possible, the motor patterns discovered as successful for a child's purpose by that child are used. They may be unusual but not deforming nor increasing symptoms of motor dysfunction.

(3) Once consistency of practice has led to abilities, these are used in a variety of situations. A child is encouraged to use his motor function to explore inside and outside his home and school. He rolls, crawls or walks on different surfaces indoors and outdoors. Surfaces may be stationary at first, but moving for later motor control. This may happen when a child is taken on visits to shops, the zoo, the countryside and other places for his education as well as for his motor experiences. During these visits, time and patience need to be given so that he can use his movements and balance as he acquires sensory, perceptual and cognitive experiences. Various play experiences with sand, water, snow and many other materials are at first presented so that he uses his motor abilities or emerging abilities in play. Control of posture, movements and the use of his hands develops further during his own spontaneous exploration.

(4) It is best to develop and practise a task in a child's familiar environment. This offers him well-known clues for learning motor function. When home visits or school visits are difficult, then a clinic or centre needs to create situations similar to those known by a child so that transfer of motor function learning can be achieved.

(5) The training of the motor components of posture and movement needs to happen at home either following or preceding their use in the whole motor function or daily living activity. In this way training motor components is not reserved for a clinical session in one venue and use of these components in their meaningful context in another venue. Training and practice of components are only necessary if these need to be separated due to the complexity of particular tasks. To help learning, a child needs to understand the relevance of components to the whole task, as outlined in Chapter 5.

A word of caution: a child should not be made to feel that unless he is achieving a motor skill he will not be loved. He needs to feel loved and appreciated for the person he is whether he is working hard or not and whether he is successfully achieving or not. There are many ways of building this attitude into relationships with a child.

SUMMARY

Learning motor function needs to be integrated with the purpose or meaning of such motor function to a child. Consideration needs to be given to the following aspects of learning a motor function, either on its own or within a daily activity:

(1) Developing a child's attention.
(2) Discovering a child's own goals and strategies and following this lead.
(3) Analysing the task for learning for each child.
(4) Giving cues for learning what a child is going to do, how he performs and the results of what he does.
(5) A child's own actions and results of them provide him with sensory information for learning a task.

(6) Sensory-motor experiences need to be understood by a child. The clear links with an individual's choice of task needs to be given in therapy.

(7) Verbal intructions are usually minimal but are useful in working with children who understand them.

(8) There is intrinsic reward in achieving the task itself. However, external rewards may also be incentives for individuals.

(9) Practice is necessary to develop motor function. It needs first to be consistent and then within a variety of situations. A variety of movement experiences helps to reinforce motor learning.

5 A Collaborative Learning Approach

WORKING WITH PARENTS

Today, therapists recognize the importance of working with the mother of each child. Yet mothers become both physically and emotionally exhausted with caring for their children with disabilities, the rest of the family and possibly their own work outside the home. Many therapists have therefore also shared their programmes with fathers and other adults in a child's family. Not only are they a ready-made team, but their participation helps them feel of value to a child with a disability.

Rosenbaum *et al.* (1992), in their studies of components of care for children with disabilities, found that 'parental involvement' in decisions about their child 'reduces stress and personal worries'. This was stated at the top of the parents' list of components of care. I believe this applies to parent participation in therapy programmes.

In the last years I have been developing a style of working which involves a child along with his parents in a collaborative learning experience with a physiotherapist. All take responsibility in assessments, therapy and evaluations (Levitt & Goldschmied 1990). It is a creative learning process, not only for a child and his parents but also for any therapist. The therapist learns what the hopes and expectations of a child and his parents are and what they already know and can do. Using these resources, therapists are better able to draw on their technical expertise for a more relevant programme. The respect and trust given to what parents and child already understand and can manage develops their confidence. More posi-

tive relationships grow between parents, child and therapist. There is more motivation as parents and child respond positively to a therapist who appreciates their desires and their ideas for solving some of their own problems.

COLLABORATION WITH OTHER ADULTS

When considering parents as adult learners, I feel supported by the studies of workers such as Rogers (1983) and Knowles (1984) in adult education. It is useful to draw on their ideas, not only for parents but for other adults such as family members, other professionals and carers assisting a child's development. A physiotherapist or occupational therapist will grow both professionally and personally as she learns about the priorities and knowledge of these adults. She becomes better able to select and devise methods to suit individual adults involved with a child. She also gains information about various environments and cultures in which a child needs to function.

THE COLLABORATIVE LEARNING APPROACH

A child and his parents are offered:

- Opportunities to discover what they want to achieve.
- Opportunities to clarify what is needed for these achievements.
- Opportunities to recognize what they already know and can do.

- Opportunities to find out what they still need to learn and do.
- Participation in the selection and use of methods.
- Participation in the evaluation of progress.

Genuine participation in all these aspects by child and parents helps them feel more committed to the programme of work. It gives them some sense of control which decreases many of their anxieties and builds their confidence. They become more able and more willing to absorb ideas, information and practical suggestions from therapists.

This style of work with parents coincidentally tunes in with the views of Bailey and Simeonsson (1988) in the field of developmental disabilities. My focus is more on the neuromotor aspects and on a person with neurological conditions and his/her family. Bailey and Simmeonsson found in their many studies that parents and families want:

- Education and information.
- Parental training in skills to help their child.
- Emotional support.

This collaborative learning approach takes account of all these aspects. The studies of Sluys *et al.* (1993) call for more education of patients by their physiotherapists and my 'family-centred physiotherapy' approach offers a response to this (Levitt 1991b).

OPPORTUNITIES TO DISCOVER WHAT PARENTS AND CHILD WANT TO ACHIEVE

Many parents are quick to say what their expectations from therapy are. Others want time to discuss this with their families. Some parents are unaccustomed to asserting what they want as they have anxieties and 'learned helplessness' (Greer & Wethered 1984; Seligman 1992). They may also sense that their therapist might be upset if they choose what therapy might focus on for *their* lives.

The therapist invites them to talk about a typical day in their lives by saying which daily activities they would like to improve further and which daily activities are most stressful or time consuming. These may be the same or different activities such as feeding, washing, dressing, toileting and getting from place to place. The therapist prompts parents and child to think about these activities as they are familiar to them. She explains that if she knows about their daily activities then she can plan a more relevant therapy programme with them. If a child cannot communicate what he would like to achieve or do better, then he is observed to see what interests him. He may enjoy bath time, meal time or special times for play with his parent. In a more specific situation, a baby or an individual at an early stage of development can easily be observed as wanting to touch or grasp a person they like or a toy of interest.

It is essential to start with the priorities of child and parents rather than set goals for them. Even if we set goals and then ask for their agreement, *we* are really setting the goals. This does not enable them to discover their own aims and their ability to make decisions.

In their study on the values of activities of daily living in stroke patients with hemiplegia, Chiou and Burnett (1985) compared the choices of these patients with the choices made by their therapists. It was found that in 29 therapist–patient pairs, only one pair showed similar views regarding specific values placed on the daily activities. As in the study by Rosenbaum *et al.* (1992), professionals with clinical wisdom and experience do know what is needed for parents or patients, but do not really know what is needed for particular parents or patients at specific times. This leads to frustration on the part of both therapists and their recipients. Physiotherapists often say 'they do not really understand our aims' (Levitt 1986, 1991). This is despite technical explanations clearly given by a therapist. It is the connection of a therapist's 'goals' with an individual's 'goals' that matters.

OPPORTUNITIES TO CLARIFY WHAT IS NEEDED FOR THESE ACHIEVEMENTS, TO RECOGNIZE WHAT THEY ALREADY KNOW AND CAN DO, AND TO FIND OUT WHAT THEY STILL NEED TO LEARN AND DO

These opportunities are given in the following ways:

(1) The parents themselves carry out the daily task on their own. This is the task they have selected, but they first need to learn what that task involves. As a parent enacts the task, he or she is prompted to observe which *main* movements and postures are being used. They notice where they look, what they may hear and other sensations relevant to a task. Comments from a parent are encouraged so that a therapist learns something about their knowledge of, say, their own body movements and balance. She then only adds to their knowledge according to their stage of understanding.

(2) The therapist herself may demonstrate their chosen daily task, drawing attention to the general aspects of balance, movement and some sensations. Some parents may prefer this before they carry out the task themselves.

In both points above, attention is drawn to the fact that observation is being made of able-bodied and adult actions. However, their child may then be observed to have achieved some of these, such as looking, listening, head control, hand-to-mouth movement, grasp or other components normally retained from infancy and the early years. Any 'normal' components already achieved by their child boosts both the parents' and child's confidence. Parents begin to feel that their child is not 'all wrong'.

(3) A mother or father can then apply these educational experiences by actually doing the task together with their child. This can also be used to learn what is needed to achieve a task. However, it especially demonstrates what a child and parent can do already and what they still need to learn to do. The therapist first underlines what they can do before saying what is still needed for successful achievement of their task.

(4) The same procedure is used with a child who is invited to try and carry out his chosen activity as best he can. He experiences what he can do – which he often may not yet have recognized – and then what he still needs to achieve. The therapist emphasizes what he can do in simple words such as 'you can keep your head up' or 'you started to pull your sleeve down', according to the task. Even if not all words are understood, the parents appreciate what is being said as their child is reassured by the therapist's tone of voice and approving facial expression.

A therapist needs to continue her studies on task analyses in different paediatric conditions so that she draws attention to the most appropriate components in each child. Although medical symptoms such as problems of hypertonus, involuntary motion or deformities are not stated they are being observed by the therapist. Her comments on such problems relate to 'what needs to be learnt' such as 'you still need to stretch your elbow more' or 'you still need to learn how to sit more steadily'. This is a more motivating style.

Once child and parents show what they can do the therapist can suggest additional positioning, modification of the physical environment, appropriate manual support or physical guidance to reveal more of their abilities.

Small achievable steps. The task analyses have already been outlined in the last chapter. By stating the components of a motor function or daily task to parents and child, the therapists show what has been achieved no matter how minimal. This is a particularly encouraging way of looking at tasks to be learnt and counters feelings in parents or child of 'I'll never do this!'

Once parents and child have their priorities accepted by a therapist they are more willing to listen to what this therapist adds to the ultimate aims of the habilitation programme.

The therapist's specialized assessment. Once the motor and sensory components of a task have been observed by a therapist within a whole task, she decides how much more she needs to assess. She can then carry out more detailed assessments of impairments of muscle work, joint ranges and tone, postural mechanisms in all positions and other sensori-motor details. However, the advantage of first seeing all these separate aspects within a whole task reveals many ideas which challenge the accuracy of only using separate examinations of impairments or motor components (motor abilities, prerequisites).

The tasks have been chosen by the parent or child and are being performed by a motivated person. Results of such an assessment tend to be more positive. There is interaction between all aspects of a task so that ability in one component activates any residual ability in another component. In my experience tests of reflexes may be abnormal if carried out in isolation, but if observed within the context of parent–child interactions during daily activities the assessment shows a more positive result. For example, a grasp reflex becomes immediately modified as a baby places her hand on her mother's breast during feeding; an asymmetrical tonic neck response or a Moro reaction may be overcome as a child puts both her arms around her father's neck or holds her head up in eye-to-eye contact during activities (Levitt 1986).

Therapists will also discover the *task specificity* (Carr & Shepherd 1987) of muscle work and postural control. Assessments on the couch may or may not transfer into other positions or motor functions. For example, shoulder girdle muscles may work well in crawl position but

not in a muscle test on the couch. Back extensors may be well activated in prone but not in sitting or standing. Extension of the elbow is greater when a child reaches out for a desired object than when tested with the conventional 'stretch your elbow' in muscle tests. Kerr (1992) refers to recent developments in physiology where activation of an isolated muscle depends on the mechanical actions of other muscles acting around a joint. Thus, isolated muscle training is neither physiological nor functional.

Records are being made, in a collaborative style, of:

- The priorities of parents and of a child: *ultimate aims.*
- What parents and child can already do: *initial abilities* (baseline).
- What parents and child still need to achieve: *immediate aims* (learning components and minimizing impairments).

It may be easier to record the function of parent with his/her child in a video. A framework is devised so that the same scenes are checked when evaluations are made. A set time for evaluation may be arranged so that the immediate aims or *behavioural objectives* are fully defined (see Chapter 7). This arrangement is also called a *contract* of long-term and short-term aims planned between parents, child and therapist.

PARTICIPATION IN THE SELECTION AND USE OF METHODS

There is no sharp division between the assessments just described and methods. Many of the assessment methods become methods for training function. A therapist's addition of positioning, physical guidance and manual support become extended to include selection of equipment, orthoses and furniture, shoes and playthings.

As parent and child develop their confidence, they will share their own ideas with their therapist (Fig. 5.1). She always welcomes their ideas as they are showing an eagerness to take some responsibility in the programme and not become totally dependent on her. The therapist considers their suggestions and if inappropriate modifies them or shelves them for a later stage in a child's development. With any validation of the ideas of parents or child they become more able to cope with times when some of their ideas are incorrect. Clearly a therapist needs to become more flexible so she can be open to what parents and child offer. This means that she cannot stick rigidly to any system of therapy.

As with a child, a parent is first observed practising a method of training her/his child, then guided physically or verbally by the therapist to improve that method. Details are added according to what each parent can absorb and manage. Each parent also has their own pace of learning and some need many more repetitions of a method than others. We avoid overwhelming a parent with a 'mountain of knowledge and tasks'. This may exhaust them and disrupt family life creating additional feelings of inadequacy (Featherstone 1981; Hinojusa 1990; Ross & Thomson 1993).

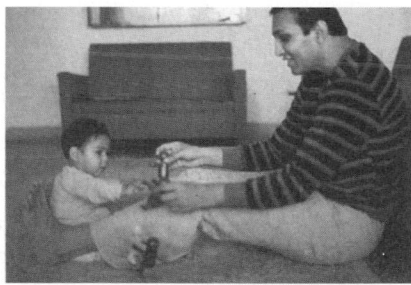

Fig. 5.1 There is pleasurable interaction between this father and his child as the child's postural control with hand function is being developed. Father chose to use his feet to assist his child in symmetrical weight bearing on hips and weight shifting from side to side or forwards and backwards during play.

Special physiotherapy techniques. Once a parent has some confidence in methods for the familiar, everyday tasks in child care, they can add selected physiotherapy techniques. Some parents are intimidated by unusual techniques whereas others overdo them. They believe or want to believe that these strange techniques are 'magical treatments' and overdo them at the expense of developing their natural parenting abilities and positive relationships with their child. It is these relationships which are fundamental to real progress. Exercises such as ranges of motion, stretchings, specific balance training and strengthening exercises may be carried out in a didactic style which parents may have observed in a physiotherapist treating their child or perhaps treating some other person with another medical condition. A study by Kogan *et al.* (1974) found that mothers acting as therapists interacted negatively with their children. This was not the experience of von Wendt *et al.* (1984), who found positive interactions by well-supported parents.

Any negative behaviour need not happen if we first set the scene as described above and we find methods within play activities. For example, a child's postural mechanisms and movements are developed on his parent's lap, when being carried and handled during all daily activities and play (Figs 5.2–5.4). A child's spine and limbs can be stretched and moved within positioning for daily tasks as well as in water and during musical rhythms and action songs. When a mother also assists a child to enjoy his body parts which are being kissed, tickled and touched by her as well as moved to her song, then she also develops a more positive view of her child's body. This pleasure in both mother and child contributes to their developing relationship in a creative way. It is important to develop parenting abilities at the same time as promoting a child's function, and methods can be found to do this (Figs 5.1–5.5). This also avoids an increased dependency and excessive demands on a therapist for 'magical treatments'. Parents need to recognize that their handling of

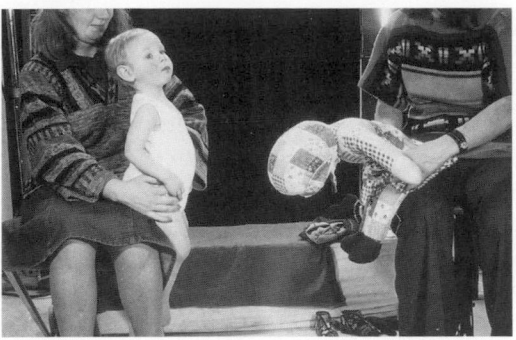

Fig. 5.2 Therapist showing tilt reaction facilitation on a doll so that this mother can interact with her child on her lap playing a 'see-saw' game. The position of the adult's hands on the child's hips rather than on the trunk is important.

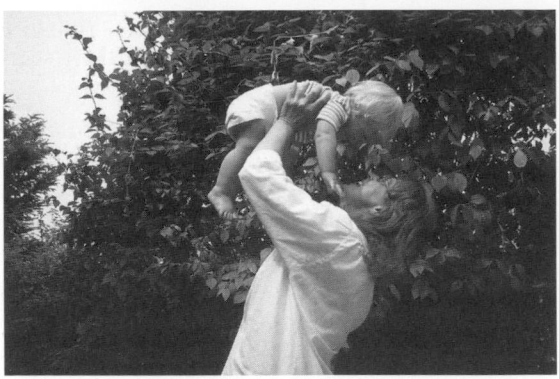

Fig. 5.4 Stimulating head control in parent/child interaction.

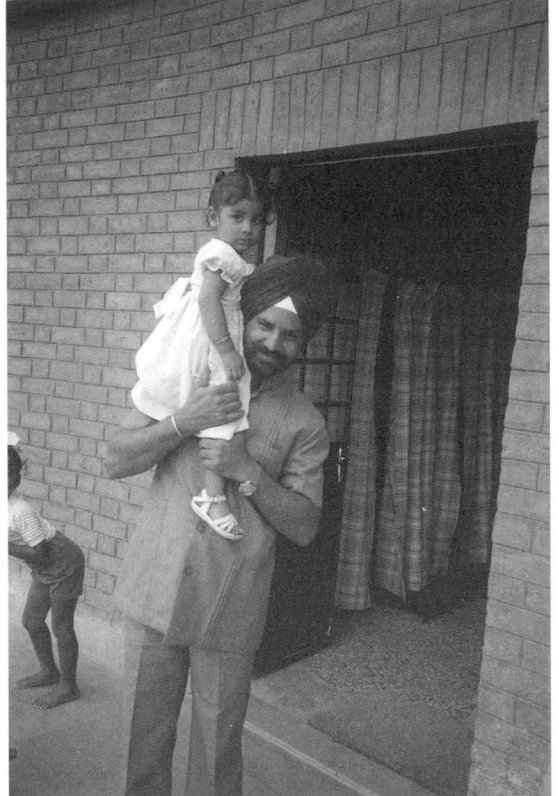

Fig. 5.3 A child developing postural control on her father's shoulders in playful activity.

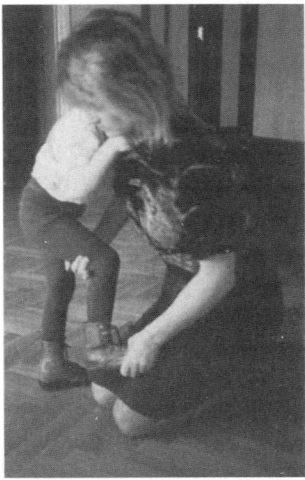

Fig. 5.5 Learning early balance on one foot during dressing and undressing, washing or drying with body closeness between mother and child.

their children is as important as special treatment sessions.

PARTICIPATION IN THE EVALUATION OF PROGRESS

Throughout the therapy sessions it is reasuring for all to know how well they are progressing. Parent and child are asked to report on any new achievements based on the original assessments. They may have gained more of the steps in a sequence of actions in a daily activity or more postural control, more postural alignment or more hand use in their child.

Improvements from a child's baseline abilities can be recorded on video, with graphs or in written records. Professionals use their own recording techniques discussed in Chapter 7. These special methods as well as results of consultants' special tests need to be explained to parents and, when understanding is available, to a child.

Modifications of methods may then be made or new methods added for future progress. Equipment is checked together with parents to confirm correct size and function. The relevance of equipment to a child's home and lifestyle as well as acceptance of their aesthetic aspects is a continuing assessment with parents and child.

Behavioural progress

It is essential to comment on the progress of child and parent in their development of confidence, motivation, communication skills and personal relationships. It is after all not only functional gains that are important, but how much more viable life becomes for parents and child as a result. More qualitative research and parent satisfaction studies are being undertaken to evaluate these aspects (see Chapter 3 – research).

PARENT–CHILD INTERACTION

When familiar daily activities are used in the programme, a therapist is able to see a parent and child functioning together. As Winnicott (1964) points out, 'there is no such thing as a baby, only a baby with someone else'. During these daily activities there is normally mutual pleasure between mother or father and child. However, a child with disabilities gives unusual communications as clues for a parent to know how to parent such a child. If a child has a floppy head, a visual problem or hypertonus this is not only a worry from a functional viewpoint but interferes with a child's response to a parent. Such a child cannot initiate communication with his head and eyes, hands or body to indicate his wants. Without head or trunk control a child cannot turn away from his parents to show when he has had too much stimulation and may become irritable. Parents may find their child hypersensitive to touch, difficult to cuddle or exhibiting unexpected startles of distress. It is easy for parents already unsure of their parenting abilities to feel rejected and anxious. The natural expertise of a therapist may make them feel more inadequate. There are, of course, other parents who are especially responsive to their child and discover many subtle cues of communication from their child. They can clarify for a therapist what their child's body communications and sounds mean.

It is essential that during the joint assessments of feeding, dressing, bathing, playing and other tasks, the therapist points out that:

- A child's unusual body actions, hypersensitivity or increase in stiffness is due to the cerebral palsy and not to poor parenting.
- A child's fears, apathy, hyperactivity or poor concentration are due to the cerebral palsy and not to poor parenting.

Enabling a parent to position a child well, to handle him and modify his neurological symptoms will improve not only motor function and daily activity but also communication and relationships. It is not just correct handling but a positive reciprocal interaction between parent and child that is being promoted (Figs 5.6 and 5.7a,b; see also Figs 5.1–5.5 for parent–child interaction and Fig. 9.3).

HELPING A CHILD TO LEARN MOTOR CONTROL

This is discussed in Chapter 4. The therapist makes sure that a parent develops these behaviours to reinforce a child's learning. Points to note are:

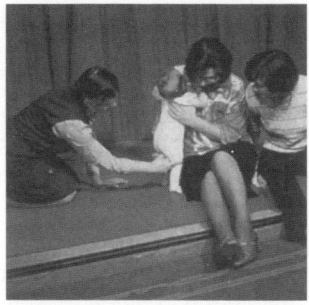

Fig. 5.6 Physiotherapist enabling a mother and her key worker to learn how to activate early standing with close body contact as support.

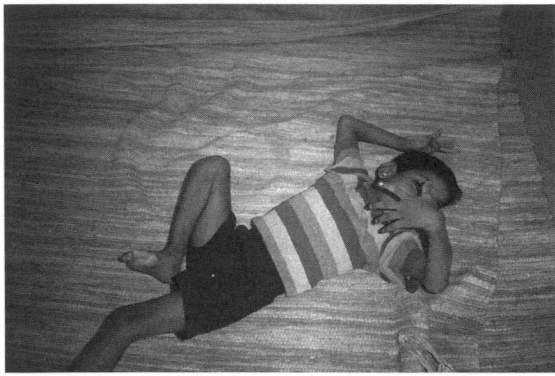

Fig. 5.7a Child with athetoid quadriplegia in supine.

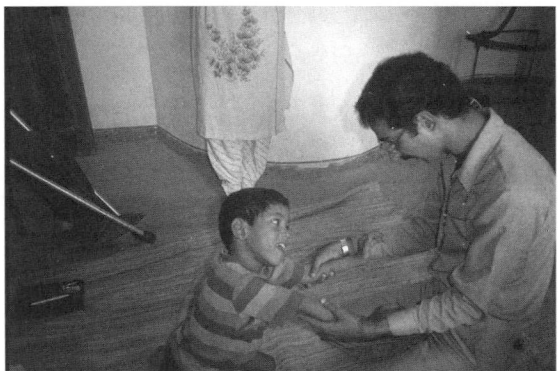

Fig. 5.7b Parent and child interact, enabling the child to master his symptoms.

- Wait for a child's initiation for a motor action and follow his lead.
- Wait for a child's response to the parent's initiation of an activity.

- Adjust a task so that a child can experience some success.
- Find ways to alert and maintain a child's attention.
- Show appreciation for a child's small and large achievements.
- Grade sensory input so that a child is not overstimulated.
- Make appropriate demands on a child so he needs to make some effort to achieve a task without excessive increase in hypertonus, athetoid motion, tremors or startles and spasms.
- Give time for the gradual development of parent–child relationships and be patient with oneself as a parent learning to interact with an unusual child. Many parents have *their own ways of managing* which therapists must acknowledge, especially when cultural differences also exist.
- Learn from family members what their cultural and customary practices are in child rearing. They may have their own individual modifications and views (Levitt 1999).

OBSERVATION OF PARENT AND CHILD INTERACTION

There are psychologists and psychotherapists who are specialized in observing mother and baby interactions and the building of optimal relationships for a child's positive development (Stern 1985). There is increasing research effort on interactive styles of mothers with children with disabilities, some of which shows such mothers as being more directive as their children take fewer interactive turns with a parent (Hanzlik 1990). When a physiotherapist or occupational therapist assesses a child together with his parent, she can draw on the studies of psychologists or work closely with such a specialist on the team.

The therapist therefore observes not only the movements and postures which form the daily activities but also those that speak of the relationship between parent and child, and between child and therapist. She informally notices the body language of how a mother and child look at each other, touch and move together. She notices how their bodies mould towards or away from each other. A child may initiate taking turns or need encouragement to do so in movement, eye contact or sounds and speech. The upright posture not only develops postural control but better communication and alertness. The way a parent supports and especially removes manual support demonstrates his/her anxiety and ability to trust a child to function alone. The parent's willingness to follow their child's lead and wait for their child's slow achievement can be very difficult for them. The therapist's support and confidence in the parent's developing skills in parenting is essential.

The therapist needs to include such interactions in the therapy methods and may have to avoid methods which decrease positive interplay between parent and child. The therapist herself also models how to play, feed, dress, enable a child to move and enjoy these and other activities. However, care is always taken to make parents feel as competent as possible at their stage of learning. Information is regularly given on the neurological symptoms which can be modified to enhance nonverbal and verbal communication and speech therapists can offer much in these areas. As a child is enabled to make a choice to communicate his interests and his specific wishes to function he will be more participant in this collaborative therapy approach (see Chapter 4).

EMOTIONAL SUPPORT

It is clear that therapy is not just 'a bag of tricks' to increase a child's motor function or independent daily skills. A therapist is not only showing practical ideas but needs to give time for listening to the worries of a parent. However, she is always balancing her time for the parent and for the child. Listening and observing a child's facial expressions and body language tells her not only about the appropriate pace of work with a child but his emotional needs in general. When listening to a parent's or child's anxieties, a therapist need not immediately reassure them. It is a therapist's empathetic and attentive listening which serves them best. She needs to repeat back to each of them what she has heard them say and only later clarifies what she can do to help.

Therapists become aware of a variety of underlying anxieties in individual parents. A parent may be experiencing a complex mixture of emotions such as despair, anger, disappointment, frustration or guilt. This not only varies from parent to parent but in the same parent at different periods in their life with their child. Hall (1984), among others, perceives such emotions as part of the grieving process related to loss of the expected normal baby. There is hardly time for parents to work through this grief as they feel pressure to accept the very different child who is alive and may be making great demands on them physically and emotionally.

Therapists face a difficult situation in which their offer of help can make a parent feel more helpless. Some parents may then become more dependent on a therapist and burden her with excessive demands. Others resent their dependency, becoming angry that they should need professionals to show them how to parent their child. This anger can also be directed at the very professionals who are doing their best for such parents. Either way, a therapist needs to grow in maturity and they become the 'patient ones' rather than the patients. To do this therapists benefit from their own support groups and sensitive support from others in a team. This support is essential to maintain therapists' energy, understanding and motivation (Greer & Wethered 1984; Chapter 1 in Levitt 1984, 1991a; Price *et al.* 1991).

When a parent is particularly stressed, taking excessive time and energy from a physiotherapist or other professional, then this needs to be discussed with the team or with a qualified psychotherapist, family therapist or specialized counsellor. The therapist will gain guidance on how best to manage such a parent and if *and* how to refer such parents for professional help from psychotherapy.

The collaborative approach described changes the situation of a professional being the helper and the parent the helpless one to that of more equal partnership. The therapist therefore is not placed in any position where her help is rejected which may understandably upset her, possibly inviting anger. The parent learns to ask for help instead of just receiving it. Parents who find it difficult to accept help may be able to do so in a more collaborative situation with therapists.

TEAMWORK WITH PARENTS

The example of the collaborative learning approach can be carried out best with the therapist as the key person or primary interventionist. This has the advantage of developing an ongoing relationship between therapist and child along with his parents and other members of the family. Parents find that visits from one professional is more desirable than from a stream of experts. One person can coordinate the habilitation programme and avoid contradictory advice from different sources. This is particularly helpful in community work.

The key person will be designated by a team of professionals who will support her with their assessments and selection of ideas to suit the aims of parents and child. The key person will learn from the team when specialized assessments and advice are necessary and when any specialized 'hands-on' sessions are indicated. This applies to any other key worker designated by a team, who is also compatible with parents and child. He/she will judge the frequency of home visits so that dependency is not generated by them (McConachie 1986).

This type of teamwork is called the *transdisciplinary* model. There can also be an *interdisciplinary* model in which collaboration with parents can take place between each professional such as physiotherapist, occupational therapist, speech therapist and teacher. Each

professional will integrate the ideas of the others into her sessions with child and parents. When professionals work as a multidisciplinary team then such integration is rarely attempted as each professional carries out her own assessments and therapy or teaching sessions in the area of his or her discipline.

A support team may consist of medical consultants in paediatrics, neurology, ophthalmology, orthopaedics, audiology and psychiatry for psychologists, physiotherapists, occupational therapists, speech therapists, teachers, nurses and social workers. Excellent progress has nevertheless been made by children with a much smaller and well-integrated primary team including their parents and other family members, provided the whole child is considered.

The principle of teamwork varies from multidisciplinary, interdisciplinary and transdisciplinary approaches and is discussed in Chapters 4, 5, 9, and 11. Effective teamwork does not consist of separate assessments and isolated specialized treatments of specific disabilities by each team member as if they equal the 'whole' child. Although specialized work is important, attention must be given to the interplay that exists between all functional areas of a child. Assets in one function may be used to develop another different and inadequate ability. For example, speech may reinforce movement, motor activities stimulate speech, words and movement assist the training of perception and perceptuomotor programmes develop understanding and language. The work of Stroh and Robinson (1986, 1991) is an example of functional learning which integrates motor, perceptual and emotional needs in the development of understanding and language. Interplay between apparently different developmental aspects is outlined in a book for parents and carers (Levitt 1994).

An Integrated Approach

In both the transdisciplinary model and interdisciplinary model, or combinations of both, professionals working with a child and the parents need to carefully learn the following:

(1) Which postures and movements, including patterns of locomotion, to encourage so that a child develops them through practice in all environments.
(2) Which undesirable motor and other behaviours to discourage.
(3) Which positions make it easier for a child to see, hear, move and communicate.
(4) How to prevent and correct deformities.
(5) Which sensory, perceptual and cognitive experiences to encourage.
(6) Which aids, equipment or orthoses to use to facilitate a child's function.
(7) How to lift and carry a child so that he participates and corrects his neuromotor problems, and how this is done to protect the backs of the adults.
(8) Which toys, playthings and recreational activities are specially recommended.

These aspects are managed in both anticipatory guidance and ongoing guidance based on a therapist's knowledge and experience.

All these areas of specialized information for the individual child are interwoven by a team of collaborative adults so that a whole programme is shared with a child. In Chapter 10, such collaboration is outlined when a child is in a peer group.

Teamwork is facilitated in many ways. For example:

- Staff conferences in small or large meetings.
- Staff meetings may or may not include parents, depending on the agenda and parent's availability.
- Informal discussions with team members including parents.
- Visits to one another's workplace.
- Combined sessions with different therapists, with teachers, with health visitors or with social workers.
- Assessment by a number of professionals together with parents can be arranged using

a one-way window so that the key person and child are alone together in a room. A parent may be in the room or watching with other professionals to learn about their child's actions and behaviour. Parents can then talk easily as they are not in front of their child and their comments add to everyone's insight. It is important to know whether a child's behaviour with professionals is typical or different from that at home (Newson 1976).

PARENTS' HEALTH

Physiotherapists are well trained to advise parents on where to learn relaxation methods and to care for their backs and for mental and physical health. Information on parent support groups, special organizations and respite child care needs to be obtained for parents who want this. Financial advice may be needed by some parents and moments of crises of various kinds will be handled by social workers and the team. Unless the priorities of parents and families are appreciated, then attention to physiotherapy and occupational therapy advice and programmes may be difficult for parents to manage (Fox 1975; Tarran 1981). Parents need to have their worries appreciated and respected or they cannot give full attention to the suggestions of therapists.

SIBLINGS

Although a therapist is busy with a child she needs to acknowledge the feelings of his siblings as well. Their normal rivalries are difficult to handle, especially when their brother or sister with disabilities receives so much extra attention. It is wise not to shoulder them with responsibilities for any treatment of their sibling. Although they may respond to their mother's need 'for an extra pair of hands', this should not be overdone. Brothers and sisters may respond to play activities which are therapeutic for the child with disabilities. They

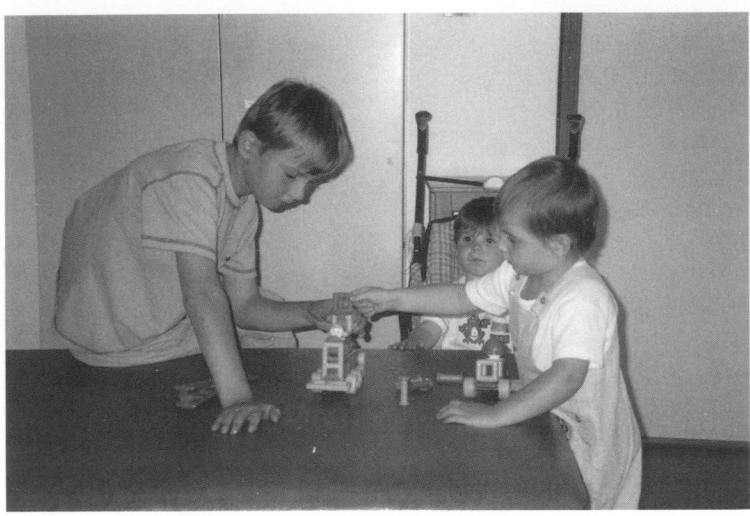

Fig. 5.8 Therapeutic actions within play between siblings.

may invent their own games together (Levitt 1994). (See Fig. 5.8.)

Simeonsson and McHale (1981) found many individual reactions in siblings which may be positive in many respects, especially if they are not overburdened and given their own lives to lead as well.

ALTERNATIVE AND COMPLEMENTARY TREATMENTS

Parents may wish to mention an interest in or need to obtain alternative and complementary treatments, and the therapist needs to respect their needs and inform herself about what is to be carried out on the person for whom she is responsible. It is important to make clear that such treatments are no more able to cure cerebral palsy than traditional methods in Western medicine and therapies. However, parents of children with cerebral palsy and older people with cerebral palsy report improvements and a sense of well-being following such treatments. A therapist needs to continue to hear what is being done for those people for whom she is responsible. She should show understanding about the need of parents and other individuals to 'do all they can' to help their child. Her compassionate interest encourages parents and

others to share what they need to explore so that discussion can take place. The theories underlying complementary medicine are very different from Western clinical medicine. There is always an extensive history and far-reaching information on the 'whole' person, including the individual's preferences for colours, odours, weather, seasons as well as as his fears and dislikes.

The physiotherapist or occupational therapist needs to observe any undesirable effects on an individual with cerebral palsy following alternative treatments and give an opinion on what she observes. She should draw on her knowledge and experience to say what she considers may be inadvisable for a child and his parents.

There are almost no research studies on the effects of alternative treatments in the field of cerebral palsy. Nevertheless some positive effects due to relaxation associated with many treatments as well as a patient's strong beliefs do provide additional support for parents and some individuals with cerebral palsy. Some complementary therapies are briefly outlined for information (Hurvite *et al.* 2003).

Acupuncture. This is conventionally used for pain, though other benefits are also claimed.

The technique involves partial insertion of a fine needle into the skin or the use of pressure (acupressure) using finger tips.

Homeopathy. A minute dose of a well-diluted preparation (similar to that which causes the condition) is given to the patient. The patient's body is believed to heal itself by responding to this increase in the condition. The homeopath advises how long the healing process will take.

Herbalism. Medicinal properties of herbs are claimed and used, being often gentle in action. The dosage is dependent on the age of the patient. Like homeopathy it aims to 'restore the healthy balance of the body and use its self-healing powers'. Herbal remedies are used for common health problems in all children such as colds, coughs, catarrh or sore throats as well as sleeplessness.

Cranial osteopathy. A qualified practitioner gently massages or moves the bones and skin of a child's skull. It is believed that this affects the brain function and improves relaxation throughout the body, although this does not cure the cerebral palsy.

Reflexology. The soles of a person's feet are massaged, which is found to be relaxing and appears to increase circulation in relatively immobile children. Pain and spasm are said to decrease in the limbs and body. It is claimed that areas of the sole relate to organs in the body so that reflexology improves their function. Therefore, constipation, congestion and dispersal of toxins in the body can also be treated.

Aromatherapy. Aromatic oils from plants and flowers and other substances are used and believed to have a variety of healing effects in conjunction with body and limb massage. Massage increases relaxation and improves circulation as well as helping to draw a child's attention to different body parts in a gentle and pleasant way.

Massage without aromatic oils is used in baby massage, which creates relaxation in both mother and child and helps mother–child bonding. The sensations of touch and smell are developed in a pleasant way for a young child.

Shiatsu massage does not use oils but massages certain meridia beneath the surface of the skin, which is believed to contribute in the healing of a number of ailments.

CONTRAINDICATIONS

Qualified practitioners must be used. A parent should not carry out any of the procedures from a lay person's guide. A therapist needs to have information from the practitioner as to what procedures will be used.

Any alternative treatment should not replace the drugs essential for controlling epilepsy. If this is attempted then there needs to be discussion with a child's medical consultant so that any drug is not suddenly stopped and parents are educated about the epilepsy.

Massage needs to be gentle and carried out by a qualified practitioner. A child may be hyperactive if the soles of his feet are touched or the palms of his hands receive pressure. Hypertonic muscles, especially those with spasticity, may be hyperactive or hypersensitive to touch and pressure. Massage is preferably applied to the antagonists.

Parents and child may spend a great deal of energy and time as well as expense in visiting practitioners of alternative and complementary medicine. This can result in fatigue or exhaustion and priorities need to be discussed. As with any therapy programme, parents need to avoid overwhelming themselves with too much to do. However, parental involvement in some of the therapies above could benefit the parents as well.

SUMMARY

A collaborative learning approach involves a therapist in a joint venture with a child and his parents. It can be used with other family members and with colleagues in a team. It is a radical departure from the traditional model in which a therapist takes full responsibility for assessments, treatment plans, use of methods and evaluation. Instead, all this is shared with parents and a child who can understand this. Their culture and values can also be directly learnt from them.

Emotional aspects are outlined in relation to parent–child interaction, as well as therapist–child and therapist–parent interactions. The education, and the needs of parents and their priorities are given attention as well as care for their health. Therapists also deserve support in their own groups and teams. The collaborative learning model enables a therapist to develop both professionally and personally and learn to knit together ideas from counselling, communication skills and the study of human relationships.

Brazelton (1976) suggested that

'the success of any intervention programme should be measured not only by the child's development but by increased family comfort, decrease in the divorce rate, lower incidence of behaviour problems in siblings . . . perhaps by pretty soft signs but they may be a lot more important as measures of effectiveness of intervention than is a rise in IQ or increased motor capacity on the part of the child'.

6 The Older Person with Cerebral Palsy

The aims of therapy stated in Chapter 1 remain as lifelong aims. These are:

(1) Communication, either verbal or non-verbal.
(2) Independence in activities of daily living.
(3) Recreational activities.
(4) Independent mobility and/or some form of locomotion.

The priorities of these aims depend on the individual's choices and, for the older person, are more focused in the context of social, educational and employment situations. It is particularly recommended that the Collaborative Learning Model outlined in Chapter 5 is used directly with an adolescent or adult with cerebral palsy.

The Collaborative Learning Model provides for fundamental emotional needs during the changes of puberty and for the autonomy of individual adolescents and adults. For example:

A sense of control, opportunities for individual choice and opportunity to use more of an individual's problem-solving skills. Collaboration makes new strategies and an individual's innovation possible, especially as educational progress increases an adolescent's understanding. Authoritarian behaviour in professionals and parents provokes rebelliousness and non-cooperation. Avoidance by therapists of negative patronizing comments is associated with their calm, firm manner and sense of humour. Therapists overcome any sense of intimidation by adolescents through negotiation, concessions and offering constructive professional knowledge without threats.

Sensitive listening to individuals and demonstrating action on what adolescents and adults discuss is essential in the collaborative approach. This respect and personal value is very much needed by an adolescent facing the consequences of long-term disability and experiencing biological changes at the same time.

Adolescent distancing from parents and preparation for adulthood is particularly difficult when physical independence is not fully achieved due to disabilities. The collaboration with an individual gives him support and respect so that independent views can be expressed and responsibility developed as far as possible. Parents and siblings also need support and encouragement so that their many years of help can be gradually withdrawn. Such anticipated withdrawal needs to be discussed in late childhood, around ages 10–11, to prepare the individual and his family for future changes.

The older individual can choose which activities he will practise and which motor skills need improving for daily life, and be given responsibility for carrying them out. Plans and methods are jointly discussed as to when, how often and where activities can be carried out. The older person is expected to say when he has time to practise a motor activity or exercise. Being specific about therapy programmes avoids feelings of doubt that physiotherapy is unrealistic and irrelevant in an older person's daily life.

The therapist focuses and negotiates short-term aims and methods which will demonstrate success. The adolescent's responsibility and related success is helpful to parents so that they can feel able to withdraw their help. At the same time successful independent achievements by an adolescent promote his confidence and self-esteem. If possible, differing views of parents and siblings are not given priority over that of the adolescent, but much tact will be needed.

More severely affected individuals who cannot make decisions can show their distancing from parents by carrying out enjoyable activities in peer groups. An adult facilitator of peer group exercises, discussions, games or other educational activities is often particularly useful. The therapist either works with groups or suggests functional positioning so that communication and social interactions are assisted. Self-help groups especially for adults are appreciated and also foster independendent decision-making, which some have not experienced for many years.

Confidentiality. When physiotherapists carry out slow stretches or ranges of motion to counteract deformities, there are opportunities for an adolescent or adult to have conversations about their anxieties, concerns or problems. What emerges needs to be kept in confidence so that trust is maintained with an individual. The therapist may sometimes be an advocate for an individual. Counselling sessions with a qualified professional are recommended if desired by an individual.

ROLE OF THE PHYSIOTHERAPIST

The role of a physiotherapist is valuable as increased motor control contributes to an individual's participation in social, educational and work activities. Environmental restrictions need to be discussed and problem-solving carried out with the individual and others involved.

Occupational therapists work together with physiotherapists in assessment and supply of equipment for different environments in which the individual finds himself. Specific aims of physiotherapy and occupational therapy are:

(1) To maintain motor abilities and reactivate abilities decreased by disuse.
(2) To prevent and decrease deformities wherever possible.
(3) To learn a healthy lifestyle including physical fitness.
(4) To develop appropriate community mobility.
(5) To continue the training of self-care skills.
(6) To teach the individual all he or she needs to know about the condition.

ISSUES OF CONCERN IN THE OLDER PERSON

There is a deterioration in adolescence and adults reported by a number of workers (Thomas *et al.* 1989; Wilner 1996).

Pain. This can be due to many factors. There are abnormal biomechanics causing joint and muscle pain. Excessive range of athetoid motion and muscular dystonia can cause spondylosis of the neck or arthritic changes in joints. Inability to change postures increases joint and muscle pains and skin pressure points. Abnormal shoulder girdle postures, especially if pulling in a downward direction, may cause nerve traction. New health problems related to aging such as urinary and bowel problems can cause severe discomfort.

Pain may not receive adequate medical attention or may not be reported by the individual owing to inexperience or due to communication difficulties of cerebral palsy. This also applies to many other health problems in cerebral palsy.

Fatigue. Many are functioning and moving at their peak of performance with little rest. Locomotion is at a high physiological cost for both health and neuromotor problems. The older person is unaccustomed to working out strategies to conserve their energy. For example the effort to speak need not accompany movement which makes greater energy demands. Distances may be better managed with wheelchairs rather than walking so that energy is conserved for any social or other activity desired by the person.

Early and minor deterioration. This is often not detected by the person and increasing compensatory motor patterns are therefore used to 'keep going'. These motor patterns can cause increased deformities, stiffness and pain which add to the person's fatigue. Speech and swallowing problems are also increased in some and they may need regular monitoring by a speech and language therapist and medical practitioner.

Urinary problems appear in older persons either because their locomotion has deteriorated and they cannot reach toilet facilities in time or there are bladder problems needing medical attention. Retention of urine is known to occur if adductor tightness has increased so that initiation of urination is prevented.

Increased musculo-skeletal deformities due to biomechanical changes, increased spasticity, weakness and disuse may occur as more time is being spent in sedentary academic or social activities. There is an increase in weight and height which makes more demand on the neuromotor and musculo-skeletal systems, leading to compensatory biomechanical response which can result in deformities and fatigue.

New environments of schools, homes and in the community offer new problems not easily overcome using familiar strategies. More help is needed due to a person's increased size. The older person needs to be educated in how he can let people know what assistance is appropriate for him. Therapists' communication skills need to be fine-tuned so they can let teachers, instructors, youth leaders and others know what the physical needs of older persons might be. Unless others are informed of what assistance is necessary, a person with cerebral palsy remains at home and cannot join in community activities, as aging parents are unlikely to have the capacity to help him do so.

Discrimination in society. Teachers and social workers and disabled people themselves do assist in dealing with discrimination against people with disabilities in society. Therapists are involved in pressing for access, environmental adjustments and other attention to physical needs of the person with disability with whom they are working.

Services for older people. These have been poor and a link-person is really helpful in knowing what is needed and how to obtain health, educational and leisure opportunities and services. This is particularly needed during a child's transition to adolescent and adult services.

MOTOR ABILITIES AND SELF-CARE ACTIVITIES

Recent research on the growth and development of brain structures and neural pathways (Paus *et al.* 1999; Sowell *et al.* 2002) suggest that potential for learning continues to mature. The Europe programme with teachers and therapists (MOVE 2001) reported successful teaching of sitting, standing and walking when others have considered that this was not expected or that walking was not essential for a person's lifelong rehabilitation.

As many paediatric physiotherapists have focused on children, and plateaus of motor achievement have been reached by adolescence, further potentials have not always been adequately explored. In addition, social and educational needs have correctly received emphasis and time for specialized treatments discouraged (Goldkamp 1984; Cantrell 1997). However, if motor learning approaches are used rather than only neurophysiological treatments, abilities and functions can be maintained or activated. Motor abilities in motor functions within daily life activities are recommended. As already discussed, these are based on the priorities of the individual and the context of his everyday activities.

The main motor functions needed in school, social situations and in the community are sitting, rising to standing, standing and walking as well as hand function. This book offers many practical suggestions for learning these functions independently, with assistance or with equipment such as special chairs, wheelchairs, walkers and walking aids. Although 'a child' is given in the text, this can often be an older person with modifications for his size and weight.

Some individuals may still want to re-learn or learn to walk with or without appropriate walkers. This may be possible in the home and in some other environments. An individual may feel more independent, participate more in transfers and manage to exercise with a walking frame rather than remain seated most of the time. Individuals with severe motor disabilities may actively participate in their care by 'bridging' hips for dressing, rolling over, using minimal arm and hand actions or grasping a support. Participation by an individual with disabilities, no matter how minimal, avoids passivity and a feeling of helplessness.

Carers may also find an individual's participation useful, especially if his abilities in sitting, standing and stepping are maintained or trained. Carers may well be able to make less effort and save time. If an individual's active participation is adequate this can minimize the carer's need to lift and carry. The use of two carers may then not always be necessary. A Manual Handling Assessment together with therapist and individuals is necessary to confirm this. Although hoists and equipment need to be selected, they may not always be manageable in all environments. It is always important to explore the views of both carer and the individual with disability to assess what is realistic in different situations and to assess what potential for assisted or independent function is present in an older person.

If an individual is interested in having specific training sessions, and if these sessions draw on motor learning models then they need to be supplied by neurological therapists together with teachers, carers or others involved with the individual (Umphred 2000).

Motor developmental assumptions

Some professionals consider that in older children, adolescents and adults, only training in sitting, standing and stepping functions is worthwhile because the individual no longer needs the child developmental sequences observed in prone or supine lying. Depending on the energy of an individual this may be appropriate. However, the analysis of tasks needed by the older person involves the selected functional abilities observed in early child development but they should nevertheless be age-appropriate.

All people need to turn in bed, get out of and into bed and get up to sitting or standing from lying. All assisted or independent transfers involve selected elements of head control, reach and grasp, support on arms, half-roll or full roll-over, push up from lying to sitting with legs over the edge of the bed, lying change to four-point kneeling, supported upright kneeling and finally supported standing. Instead of a maintained use of early postures, it is especially valuable to have the ability to use them in a transitional phase in any sequences of rising to sitting or standing. The series of rising observed in prone or supine developmental stages in this book are sequences seen in early childhood. Such early childhood patterns are the easier motor patterns and therefore may be more useful for an adolescent or adult with disabilities. Naturally there will be adaptations of postural stability, counterpoising and rising or changing of positions and the developmental sequences modified according to an individual's condition in specific environments. Generally, creeping, crawling, knee-stepping and use of arms and hands in lying and floor-sitting with and without equipment on the floor is not usually age-appropriate. Use of hands in lying in bed is naturally useful if an individual can pull up his blankets or use hand grasps to get into and out of bed or to switch off his alarm clock!

DEFORMITIES

These are discussed in Chapter 10. The physiotherapist plays an important role in preventing secondary musculo-skeletal problems and correcting as many as possible of those that are inevitable. Plaster casts are also used for the older person (Bertoti 1986; Mosely 1997). The tightness of spastic muscles appears to increase with age, especially as muscles become bulkier and do not grow as fast as bones. Botulinum toxin and other muscle relaxants are used and need to be associated with a physiotherapy programme (see Chapter 10 on botulinum toxin injections).

Scolioses, pelvic obliquities and hip dislocations are more common in older people than in children. Orthopaedic surgery is often indicated and surgeons have different approaches and post-operative physiotherapy regimes. Bony operations are often delayed until after growth spurts have ceased in adolescents.

Physiotherapy methods continue to be important, and prolonged stretching, positioning equipment, orthoses, range of motion exercises and position change are particularly recommended in the older age group. Active exercises, strengthening and actions within daily life activities need special attention. Rhythmic stabilization and other methods from Proprioceptive Neuromuscular Facilitation appeal to teenagers and adults as part of their strengthening and balance training. Stretching with manual methods for trunk and hips used in the Bobath Centre, London, are followed by the individual's active maintenance of the new alignment in sitting and standing as well as by specific facilitated walking patterns

(Christine Barber 2001). Conductive Education groups for adults focus more on function than on deformities, though there are corrective movement synergies (Kinsman et al. 1988).

Young people who can understand are motivated by measurements of increased range, strength and enjoy biofeedback training on force plates with video visual feedback of symmetrical weight bearing and weight shift, and other records (Winstein et al. 1989; Hartveldt & Hegarty 1996).

Explanations are given to educate an individual about why motor activities are necessary to minimize the effect of growth spurts, disuse, increasing weight with immobility. Deterioration of motor functions may decrease confidence in physiotherapy. Young people need explanations such as that shorter spastic muscles are bulkier and tighter in older people, that growth spurts lead to bone growing faster than muscles and cause deformities, and that deterioration is not due to poor physiotherapy or their lack of practice. Unwitting habits of prolonged sitting in one posture or repetition of movements in only a few patterns may lead to deformities.

Physiotherapy treatment for aches and pains need to be offered and responsibilities for attending treatment appointments are given to those who need them.

If possible, adolescents should be shown how to apply orthoses and given responsibility for doing so (Fig. 6.1). If hand function or balance does not allow independence, then the individual instructs someone in such applications. If speech is poor, then hand-out sheets can be prepared by therapist with an individual. These are examples of developing autonomy in growing adolescents and adults.

HEALTHY LIFESTYLE

The quality of life for an older and especially aging person with cerebral palsy is improved if the following are available:

(1) An understanding general practitioner who makes community resources available when an individual has pain, ordinary health problems or depressions. Blaming the cerebral palsy condition is not addressing the quality-of-life needs of the person.

(2) Communication problems due to speech and language disabilities result in a person not conveying their needs well enough and thus not receiving health care as any other citizen would. Advocates and education of hospital nurses and others in the community about the communication aids or methods used by a person with cerebral palsy will assist everyone.

(3) Adolescents and adults with disabilities need to have had education since late childhood about healthy lifestyles. However, this is even more important in adolescence and adulthood. Care with regard to nutrition, weight control, keeping fit and positive mental attitudes or stress management improves quality of life. Counselling or peer group discussions as well as health education in groups are valuable for different individuals. Others may prefer health workers or therapists in one-to-one sessions. This preference may be relevant when sexual and bodily functions are to be discussed.

Exercising on stationary bicycles, rowing machines or treadmills is useful for keeping fit (Fig. 6.2). The person with disabilities needs supervision by a therapist in case deformities are threatened by the movement patterns and efforts of the person. Fatigue needs to be avoided when such activities are overdone by enthusiastic people.

Respiratory problems may arise in later years due to immobility, scolioses and lack of ordi-

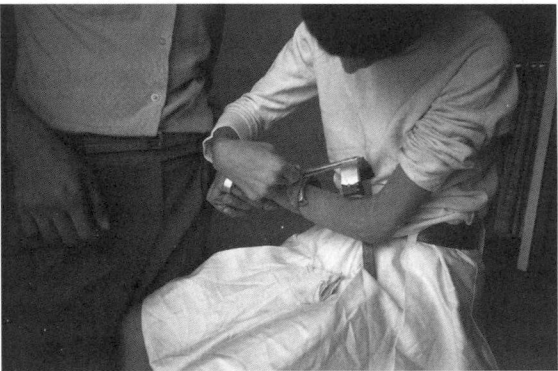

Fig. 6.1 An individual applying her own orthosis.

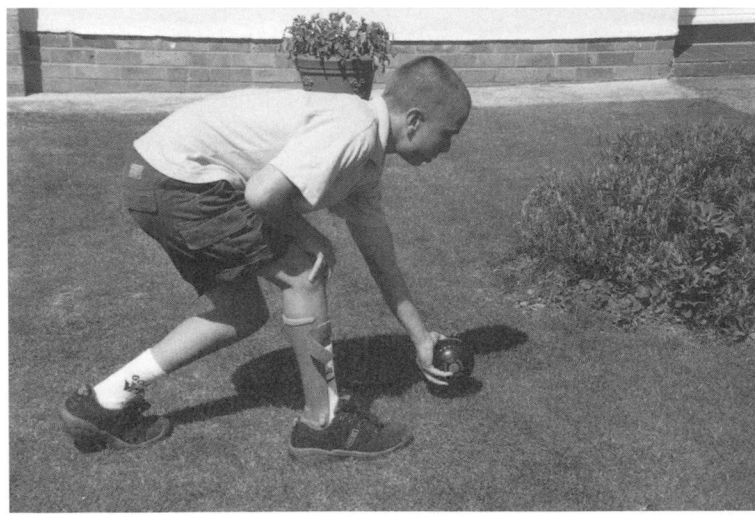

Fig. 6.2 Keeping fit with bowling and other motor activities. A hinged ankle–foot orthosis is worn on his right leg, allowing ankle motion.

nary health care. General exercises, aerobics and respiratory physiotherapy may be needed.

DEVELOP APPROPRIATE COMMUNITY MOBILITY

In order to access social clubs, meet friends or participate in education and work it is essential that appropriate wheelchairs and transport are considered. Electric wheelchairs and correct seating have improved considerably through seating clinics and technological advances. Occupational therapists often provide assessments and, together with a physiotherapist, an individual needs to learn to use a wheelchair correctly. In severe conditions the therapist assesses which part of the body an individual can reliably control or learn to control for using joysticks or switches.

Using a wheelchair does not automatically deter a person with cerebral palsy from learning to walk with a walker, with the help of a friend or carer or independently. The energy and motivation of an individual is crucial and realistically he may often only wish to walk within the home or in school rather than in the community. The distance, roughness or smoothness of the ground and weather determine the decision to walk outdoors. Once again discussions with the individual and comments by his family and friends contribute to planning. The physiotherapist considers the individual's weight-bearing abilities, stepping and adequate hand function for walkers (see Chapter 8 section on development of standing and walking).

TRAINING OF SELF-CARE AND COSMETIC APPEARANCE

This is discussed in Chapter 9 on motor function in daily care. The speech, occupational and physio- therapists are all involved with eating, dressing, washing, bathing, toileting and hygiene (Fig. 6.3).

Age-appropriate activities such as hair setting, hair cuts, use of cosmetics, clothes and

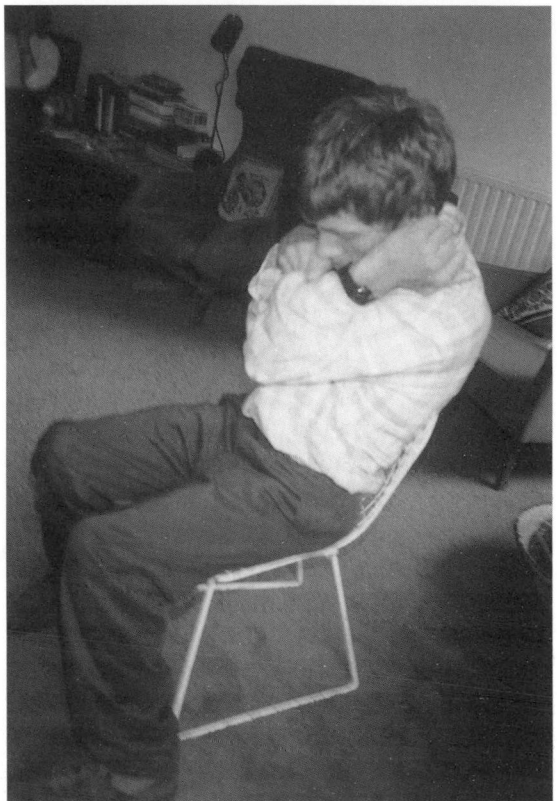

Fig. 6.3 An individual using his own strategies for independence in fastening sleeve buttons. No resultant deformities.

the interests of any normal adolescent are important parts of the programme. An interest in one's appearance has motivated some adolescents to practise good posture and keep-fit exercises. Sadness about appearance due to the cerebral palsy is not uncommon. Counselling and emphasis of all assets of a person need consideration. Skill with a hobby such as bird-watching, photography, or social assets give confidence to people and all need to find out what these assets are.

KNOWLEDGE ABOUT THE CONDITION

Teach the individual all he needs to know about his condition. This is implicit in the Collaborative Learning Model. If parents have already received this information over the years, they also convey this to their adolescent son or daughter. However, this needs additional education from a professional who explains aspects in a different style. In addition, adolescents who are feeling anxious or depressed may not have absorbed medical information. They are more 'grown-up' and need direct education for themselves and answers to their own questions.

Sex education is important and there are organizations and groups that offer information in this area.

THERAPEUTIC MOTOR ACTIVITIES

There is an increasing number of activities for people with all levels of disabilities. They not only keep an individual fit but maintain motor abilities and opportunities for treating deformities. Swimming is particularly useful for maintaining ranges of motion as it includes stretches. Horse-riding for the Disabled have a number of clubs and the sport helps individuals in maintaining balance, abduction and use of hand grasp. Sailing, angling and skiing for the disabled are some of the many activities which are beneficial. In Britain there are adventure holidays and imaginative activities designed for people with disabilities.

Social skills and friendships develop in the clubs which often have able-bodied with disabled persons present.

MEASURES

Reports by the individuals themselves are important. The decrease in falls, increase in any daily function, distance walked, wheelchair control and bed mobility and transfers are usually well reported and recorded.

There are a number of tests of balance, arm reach with postural control, spasticity and weakness that are used in adults with neurological conditions. These can also be adapted or used in cerebral palsy (Shumway-Cook & Woollacott 2000; Bower & Ashburn 1998; Umphred 2000).

7 Assessment for Therapy and Daily Function

APPROACH TO ASSESSMENT

The framework for all assessments is outlined to synthesize various approaches. This avoids use of assessment methods from any one therapy system.

The framework consists of the following assessments:

(1) The task(s) individuals want to achieve. Their choice may be a daily activity in self-care, play, social interaction or during recreation.

(2) The motor functions for the individual's chosen task, e.g. sitting, standing, using a form of locomotion and use of hands.

(3) The component abilities of each motor function needed for the chosen task. This includes specific postural mechanisms, relevant voluntary movements and perceptual motor abilities which may be present but abnormal or absent.

(4) The impairments which may be preventing achievement or causing abnormal performance such as limited range of motion, weakness, abnormal reflex reactions, abnormal movement patterns or limited repertoire of movements for the task.

(5) The constraints on motor functions and their components by other impairments and disabilities of vision, hearing, perception, understanding and communication.

(6) The abilities or residual abilities of these components of vision, hearing, perception, cognition and communication which can reinforce the learning of motor functions.

This process of assessment is discussed in Chapters 4, 5 and 6 to show how specific assessments of posture, movements and use of sensations are observed in the context of whole daily functions. Furthermore, whenever possible, these daily functions are best observed in an individual's natural environment most relevant to the tasks chosen by him and those involved with him. This chapter addresses the specific assessments and objective measures by a physiotherapist and occupational therapist which grow out of the Collaborative Learning models in the previous chapters. Separate motor functions, their specific components and impairments, often take place in physiotherapy rooms in hospital units and special centres. Therefore, depending on a therapist's workplace, appropriate organization is made to include the important observations of an individual in his own environment. The therapist is then enabled to complement her specific examinations and to assess:

- Which abilities are actually used and which are not being activated.
- Which physical obstacles in the environment prevent use of his abilities or block further development. Assessment both indoors and outdoors show, for example, whether access is available, ground is uneven or slippery, furniture is inappropriate or there are no stable objects or bars to grasp.
- Which attitudes and behaviours of people in the individual's environments may influence his motor or whole daily functions.

Occupational therapists in different places have expertise in environmental assessments and

share their information with centre-based physiotherapists. Simultaneous visits of physiotherapists with occupational therapists to a child's
or older person's environment are desirable
whenever possible. Community paediatric
therapists are well placed to obtain the broad
perspective of a child's function.

Purpose of assessments

(1) *To respond to the reason for referral*, which
    may be for additional medical information,
    for educational placements, for parental
    needs or for social or legal considerations.
    Some adolescents or adults with cerebral
    palsy refer themselves and state their
    reasons. People paying for therapy will
    want assessments indicating the need
    for physiotherapy and reassessments of
    outcomes.

      Therefore the type of assessment varies
    according to the referral. Physiotherapy
    assessments need to relate to what
    information is wanted and how it will
    be used.

(2) *To add to medical diagnostic* information as
    specific assessments before *and* during
    therapy involve long periods of time and
    close contact with a child and his family.
    Information may be revealed to a therapist
    which is not obvious in shorter consulta-
    tions with different medical consultants.
    A therapist will also detect any unusual
    deterioration which needs referral to a
    neurologist in case a progressive neurologi-
    cal condition rather than cerebral palsy is
    becoming obvious.

(3) *To participate in screening and follow-up* of
    children 'at risk' of developing cerebral
    palsy and to decide whether specialized
    physiotherapy or monitoring is indicated.

(4) *To plan a specific physiotherapy pro-
    gramme* of specialized treatment methods,
    equipment and with information and prac-
    tical ideas for all involved with a child or
    older person.

(5) *To evaluate progress* in reassessments which
    may lead to continuation, modification,
    changes or periodical stopping of specific
    therapy methods and sometimes of specific
    therapy sessions. The evaluation also
    changes practical suggestions for others.
    Any deterioration in a child's function due
    to neurological or increase in behavioural
    problems will be detected in reassessments
    so that referral to other professionals can be
    made.

(6) *To contribute to research into the effective-
    ness of therapy* by using standardized
    measures within a research study. Clinical
    assessments and measures also detect ques-
    tions for research (see Chapter 3, Appraisal
    of Research).

Review of a therapist's observations

Reviews are made during assessments together
with the child and parent or with an older
person with or without carers. They are
continued during 'hands-on' assessment and
evaluation and during ongoing therapy.

(1) *Behaviour*   Observe whether a child is
    alert, apathetic, irritable or fearful in a
    session or during particular activities.
    A child may become fatigued easily,
    make undue effort or show discomfort
    during an activity. Find out what motivates
    his actions. Is it a particular situation, a
    person or special plaything?

(2) *Communication*   Observe how child and
    parent interact. Find out whether a child
    initiates or responds with gestures, sounds,
    hand or finger pointing, eye pointing or
    uses words and speech.

(3) *Attention span*   What catches a child's
    attention? How does a parent assist him
    to maintain attention and what distracts
    him?

(4) *Understanding*   Does a child follow sug-
    gestions to move or promptings to act?
    What does he appear to understand?

(5) *Position*   Which position does he choose
    to be in and can he get into that position

on his own or with help? Observe if a parent can place him in position and if he participates in any way. His limbs and head may move more easily in some positions than in others. Involuntary movements may be decreased in some positions.

(6) *Postural control and alignment*   Observe how much parental support is given and check a child's own ability in postural stabilization and counterpoising in all postures. Parental support may be excessive or reasonable. Check whether a child bears more weight on one side of his body, or on one hand or foot. A child may collapse to one side, twist to one side or tilt and turn his head to one side. Observe any fears of falling in a child due to poor balance experience. Parental anxiety about falling may increase a child's fears.

(7) *Use of limbs and hands*   Observe limb patterns in changing or going into a position as well as using them in a position. There may be excessive flexion, extension or rotation in one part of the range. Observe whether one or both hands are used, type of grasp and release. Accuracy of reach and hand actions also indicates a possible visual problem. Observe any involuntary movements, tremors or spasms which interfere with actions.

(8) *Sensory aspects*   Observe a child's use of vision, hearing, of touch, smell and temperature in relevant tasks. Does he enjoy particular sensations? Notice whether he enjoys being moved or having his position changed. He may show an increase in tension and apprehension on being touched and handled.

(9) *Form of locomotion*   On entering the room observe how a child is carried, uses a wheelchair or uses walking aids. During the session create interest which motivates him to roll, creep, crawl, bottom shuffle or walk to where a daily activity is to be carried out. A child may have unusual

ways of getting about such as dragging himself along his stomach, along his back, *bunny hopping* on both knees, *running headlong* and other gaits.

(10) *Deformities*   Observe any recurring positions of the whole child as well as of parts of his body in all postures and in the movements he uses. This observation is checked with ranges of motion.

Note in Chapter 8 the details of motor assessment are given at each developmental stage under the headings of common problems in gross motor and basic arm and hand patterns. The parent and child interactions are informally observed as outlined in Chapter 5. Behaviour of child or older person is outlined in Chapters 4, 5 and 6.

Teamwork and the Influence of Other Disabilities

The therapist will need a comprehensive assessment from a team (see Chapter 1). She will learn from the different professionals what modifications to make for specific visual, hearing and sensory impairments. She will adjust her communication with a child in relation to any speech and language difficulties and find out what communication systems are being used, for example Paget, Makaton or Bliss. If a child has perceptual problems then adaptations will be advised for these difficulties during activities.

General points to remember for assessments

- Assessments need to be playful, interesting and non-threatening.
- Assess a young child as much as possible on his parent's lap.
- Observe a child among his familiar toys as well as with selected toys to activate interest as well as reveal dormant abilities.
- Keep sessions within the bounds of a child's concentration.
- Have an unhurried atmosphere.

- Have easy, successful actions of a child interspersed with difficult tasks.
- Avoid undressing a child, especially an adolescent, until he is happy about this.
- Time is needed for a child who is unhappy about a new environment, new professional or new experience of being assessed in a different style.
- An individual needs time to attempt new abilities in the assessment.
- Consider a child's state of health and energy.

Assessments take from one to four sessions, depending on each child's severity, mood, level of energy and cooperation. Observations, particularly when unobtrusive, must precede 'hands-on' examinations and measurements to gain rapport with child and parents.

In the Collaborative Learning model in Chapter 5, abilities are emphasized and assessments merge into therapy methods and evaluations so that parents appreciate the relevance of specific professional assessments.

ASSESSMENT AND MEASUREMENTS

Clinical assessment includes both careful observations and measurements. There is a growing importance of measurements for evidence-based practice. However, in cerebral palsy there are still observations of unique abilities and difficulties discovered in a clinical assessment of an individual. These are significant for therapy and for a child's own strategies. The observations for clinical assessment cannot always be easily measured using current measurement tools (Measures).

It is also recommended that a physiotherapist does not limit her assessments to existing Measures. Although Measures are important, they should not reduce her own innovative observations. In addition, current Measures are based on values which may change in the light of research.

Chapter 8 presents clinical assessments of function in prone, supine, sitting and standing positions and use of hands. A developmental sequence is used to show how the components of motor functions are normally developed and how an abnormal performance may be normal at an earlier age. For example, asymmetry is normal in a number of early actions and postures, so that weight-bearing on one side of the body in lying is expected at the 0–3 months developmental stages. A developmental framework also shows a therapist the degree of motor delay which has an effect on other areas of child development.

The examination of the individual in channels of prone development, supine development, sitting, standing and walking development, and hand function also shows the influence of impairments in the functions. Impairments which create deformities are discussed in these functional developmental channels as well as in an additional chapter on deformity.

The clinical assessment findings using the developmental channels are given in Chapter 8 so that the motor functions, components and impairments can be immediately related to treatment suggestions (sometimes called 'tactics and strategies') and equipment.

Green et al. (1995) and Pountney et al. (1999) also present a similar assessment of motor functions with their motor components in a sequence of functional levels. These levels in prone, supine, sitting and standing positions are based on normal child development. Biomechanical items are emphasized so that appropriate equipment is selected for prone, supine, sitting and standing positions.

Current Measures Used in Cerebral Palsy

The Gross Motor Function Measure (GMFM) (Russell et al. 1989, 1993). This assesses and measures changes over time in gross motor function in children from birth to 16 years. The motor skills are in the normal age range from birth to 5 years. This covers older individuals with cerebral palsy who are developmentally delayed and still functioning at these earlier normal developmental stages. However the GMFM is not suitable for individuals who are very severely disabled and unable to achieve any of the test items. Other individuals who are mildly disabled or become so, will be achieving skills beyond 5 years of normal development. The GMFM has 88 test items arranged in five sections or dimensions of lying and rolling, sitting, crawling and kneeling, standing and walking, running and jumping. Change in each dimension as well as a total score is calculated in percentage scores. The therapist can therefore use items as targets/goals for therapy from the dimensions which have the lowest scores or where change is expected from intervention. Results (outcomes) of therapy are measured on reassessment. The GMFM measures achievement of motor function but not the quality of performance and does not assess hand function.

A GMFM with 66 test items (GMFM-66) exists (Russell *et al.* 2000) but it is complicated, needing more analytical skill and special software. It is not suitable for children whose only abilities are in lying, rolling and some sitting.

Gross Motor Function Classification System (GMFCS) (Palisano *et al.* 1997). This describes the severity of disability, emphasizing sitting and walking (with aids if needed) and using age-dependent criteria. The quality of movement is not an important factor. This gives a shorthand description of a person with cerebral palsy.

Gross Motor Performance Measure (GMPM) (Boyce *et al.* 1995). This is a companion to the GMFM. It measures changes in quality of movement or performance of 20 items. Five components of weight-shift, alignment, coordination, dissociated movement and stability are addressed. There are other components which are not considered and only 20 items have been included.

The Pediatric Evaluation of Disability Inventory (PEDI) (Haley *et al.* 1992). This measures adaptive functions from 6 months to 7.5 years. These functions are measured in three domains:

self-care, including feeding, dressing, toileting; mobility, including transfers, indoor and outdoor locomotion, stairs with their speed, distance and safety; social function, including communication, comprehension and peer interaction. The child is compared to normally developing children and his functional limitations are assessed. A parent interview can be used and a child can be tested in his own environment. It evaluates the improvement in independence following therapy. Nichols and Case-Smith (1996) validated the PEDI.

The Wee Functional Inventory Measure for children (WeeFim) (Msall *et al.* 1994) from age six months to seven years and the Functional Inventory Measure (FIM) (Granger *et al.* 1986) from 7 years and older. These are measures of the degree of dependency of child or adult. This involves the 'burden of care' as it is scored to indicate how much assistance a person with a disability needs. There are 18 items in self-care, sphincter control, mobility, communication and social understanding.

The above Measures have been standardized with manuals of instruction and have been objectively tested for validity and reliability when used by the same assessor (intra-rater) or by another assessor (inter-rater). There are other functional Measures of activities of daily living or motor function which are less relevant to people with cerebral palsy and their programmes of treatment. These other Measures are designed for learning disabilities, strokes or developmental coordination disorder ('clumsy children').

The Measures above are detailed and graded to show that a skill is being achieved or learnt. It shows changes due to therapy interventions aimed at either increasing gross motor skills or increasing independence or decreasing assistance by carers as a child/adult becomes more independent.

Norm-referenced Measures of stages of child development compare a child with normally developing children. Examples are:

- *Alberta Infant Motor Scale* AIMS (Piper & Darrah 1994) is a measure of motor development from birth to 18 months and observes child in supine, prone, sitting and standing. It is devised for 'at risk' infants, detecting developmental delay. It is not useful for children with cerebral palsy as normal quality of movement is expected. Therapists cannot obtain details of what needs to be treated in cerebral palsy.
- *Bayley Scales of Infant Development* (Bayley 1993) is a measure of developmental levels of mental and motor skills from age 2 months to $2\frac{1}{2}$ years.
- *Peabody Development Motor Scales and Activity Cards* (Folio *et al.* 1983) measures gross-motor and fine-motor skills of children from birth to 6 years.
- *Griffiths Abilities of Babies* (Griffiths 1967) is an overall development norm-referenced test for infants and young children.
- *The Denver Developmental Screening Test* (Frankenburg *et al.* 1970) measures fine- and gross-motor skills, personal social intellectual skills and language in young children.

These Measures and many other developmental assessments detect developmental delay and give a broad picture of a child or older person's stages of development but not quality of movement for cerebral palsy. Therefore, these Measures cannot show the details of progress due to therapy.

- *Screening babies and children 'at risk'* and detecting cerebral palsy. As this book deals with established cerebral palsy, the reader is referred to the work of neonatal physiotherapists. Assessment and intervention are discussed by de Groot (1993), Morris (1996) and Campbell (1999). They also give many references in this field. Burns and MacDonald (1996) uses an assessment for screening and follow-up of any infant from 1 month to 6 years. It is called the *NeuroSensory and Motor Developmental Assessment for Infants and Young Children* and is for any children with neuromotor difficulties, including cerebral palsy. Prechtl *et al.* (1997) and other neuro-paediatricians are detecting cerebral palsy in infants but some of these abnormal motor patterns can resolve (Touwen 1978, 1987).

MEASUREMENTS OF IMPAIRMENTS

These are discussed under the headings of specific impairments.

OTHER METHODS OF OBSERVATION

These may or may not have measurements as well. Videos, films and photographs, either static or sequential (Holt *et al.* 1974), are useful for records and evaluation of progress. The viewing of a child needs to be the same each time a child is assessed to enable accurate comparison. Kraus de Camargo *et al.* (1998) use a video-based system.

Gait laboratories assist observations but are expensive and not always easily available. Some children are less natural in such assessments. Gait analyses have developed for the use of orthoses and pre- and post-orthopaedic surgery. Electromyography, recorded joint movements and force plates are some of the tools used.

A clinical gait analysis is given in Fig. 7.1 and is best used for a video, so that, if necessary, repeated viewing for all the details can take place. Footprints of a child have been used to assess gait for step length, base and amount of weight-bearing on each foot.

Notation methods such as that of Benesh and Laban have been used to observe movements. However, special training is needed for these notations.

SPECIFIC FUNCTIONAL ITEMS

The Assessment Test of Sitting (SACND) (Reid 1995; Knox 2002) and part of GMFM and

Chailey test (Pountney *et al.* 1999). See Long and Toscano (2002).

GRADING IN ASSESSMENTS

Observations of motor functions in assessments need to be graded as:

- 0 – No ability.
- 1 – Beginning, partially achieved, unreliable, insecure, momentary.
- 2 – Reliably achieved, efficient.

This grading is in tune with the way both normal and children with motor problems develop. There are other ways of grading in different centres. For example, The GMFM grades for scoring as 'cannot, initiates independently, partially completes and completes independently'. It is important not to have a 'yes' or 'no' grading which reveals no progress when a child has really achieved an active beginning of a new motor function or even a component. This also motivates parent and child and the older person with difficulties. The grading is used for individuals functioning without assistance to find out how a child copes on his own. However, manual assistance by parent, carer or therapist or by equipment reveal motor abilities in an individual. Haley *et al.* (1992) found assessment with handling less reliable than observation.

The assistance then needs to be recorded as clear descriptions of *how much*, *where given* and *for how long* within the duration of the motor act. Progress is then shown as the assistance decreases. The MOVE Europe programme (2001) is an example of how assistance called 'prompts' is recorded when given and decreased. It is a programme structured for teachers and carers. Therapists will have a greater variety of methods of manual assistance to offer in training carers, parents and others. Records of such advice given with training is needed. Videos or photographs are given to carers following assessments of the most effective methods for the carers involved.

Abnormal performance of motor functions are difficult to grade and record. Videos and sequential photographing and anecdotal descriptions are some methods used. In my experience of practical work with therapists, grading is only reliable if there is a broad category of a 'near normal pattern' as opposed to a 'very abnormal pattern' recorded on a chart or check-list. Fortunately, studies in this area continue in addition to gait laboratories offering more accurate information only on walking patterns. It still depends on a therapist's experience as to what abnormalities of motor performance are observed and which are given significance. Grading motor functions into *mild*, *moderate* or *severe* are usually very variable with different clinicians. Such 'labels' also change with time and the label of 'severe' may be unreasonably demotivating to those involved. (See Fig. 7.1 for gait analysis.)

ABNORMAL PERFORMANCE AND DEFORMITY

Observation of abnormal performance is the primary but not only observation of abnormal positions of the joints in posture and movement. These positions are the dynamic (unfixed) or the contractures (fixed) deformities. Specific examinations of the child's joints and muscles should also be made to check whether there is a fixed or unfixed deformity. Fixed deformity due to structural change, leg length or soft tissue contracture and muscle stiffness will explain abnormal performance on a mechanical level. Unfixed deformity is more complicated. It changes with position of the body, spastic muscle length and pattern of active movements, *and* with a child's mood and the time of day, temperature or any pain that may be present. Abnormal tone is particularly influenced by these factors. Retesting by the same examiner may reduce variability in assessments. (See Figs 7.2 and 7.3.)

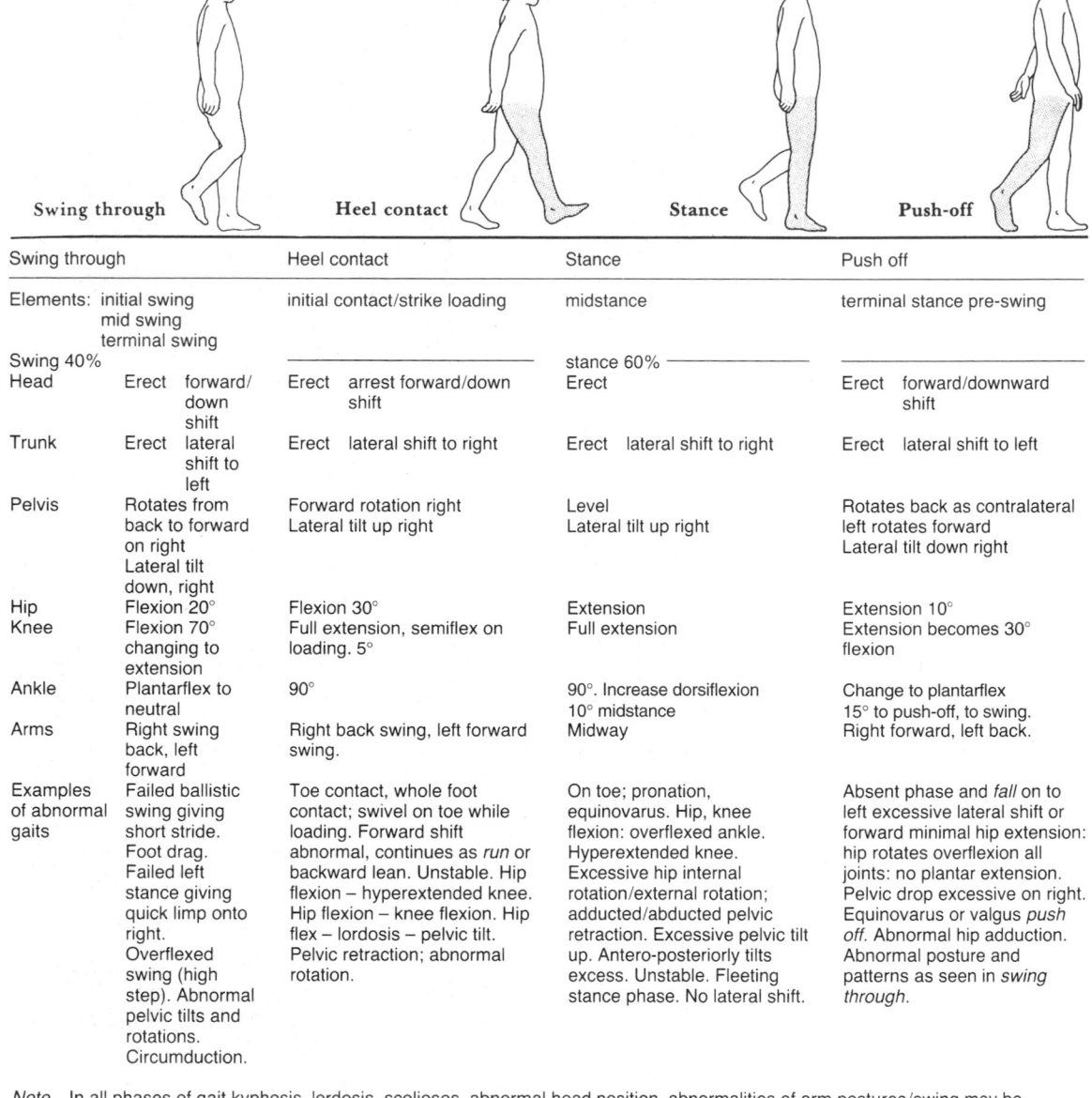

	Swing through	**Heel contact**	**Stance**	**Push off**
Elements:	initial swing mid swing terminal swing	initial contact/strike loading	midstance	terminal stance pre-swing
	Swing 40%		——— stance 60% ———	
Head	Erect forward/ down shift	Erect arrest forward/down shift	Erect	Erect forward/downward shift
Trunk	Erect lateral shift to left	Erect lateral shift to right	Erect lateral shift to right	Erect lateral shift to left
Pelvis	Rotates from back to forward on right Lateral tilt down, right	Forward rotation right Lateral tilt up right	Level Lateral tilt up right	Rotates back as contralateral left rotates forward Lateral tilt down right
Hip	Flexion 20°	Flexion 30°	Extension	Extension 10°
Knee	Flexion 70° changing to extension	Full extension, semiflex on loading. 5°	Full extension	Extension becomes 30° flexion
Ankle	Plantarflex to neutral	90°	90°. Increase dorsiflexion 10° midstance	Change to plantarflex 15° to push-off, to swing.
Arms	Right swing back, left forward	Right back swing, left forward swing.	Midway	Right forward, left back.
Examples of abnormal gaits	Failed ballistic swing giving short stride. Foot drag. Failed left stance giving quick limp onto right. Overflexed swing (high step). Abnormal pelvic tilts and rotations. Circumduction.	Toe contact, whole foot contact; swivel on toe while loading. Forward shift abnormal, continues as *run* or backward lean. Unstable. Hip flexion – hyperextended knee. Hip flexion – knee flexion. Hip flex – lordosis – pelvic tilt. Pelvic retraction; abnormal rotation.	On toe; pronation, equinovarus. Hip, knee flexion: overflexed ankle. Hyperextended knee. Excessive hip internal rotation/external rotation; adducted/abducted pelvic retraction. Excessive pelvic tilt up. Antero-posteriorly tilts excess. Unstable. Fleeting stance phase. No lateral shift.	Absent phase and *fall* on to left excessive lateral shift or forward minimal hip extension: hip rotates overflexion all joints: no plantar extension. Pelvic drop excessive on right. Equinovarus or valgus *push off*. Abnormal hip adduction. Abnormal posture and patterns as seen in *swing through*.

Note   In all phases of gait kyphosis, lordosis, scolioses, abnormal head position, abnormalities of arm postures/swing may be present.

Fig. 7.1   Right leg gait analysis (child over 2 years of age). Note also: speed, base, rhythm and step sizes, endurance (distance), EMG. (Source: Levitt S., 1984.)

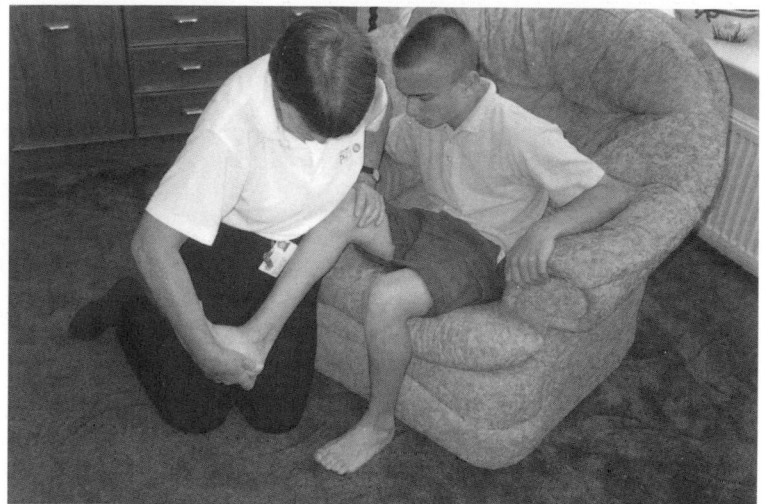

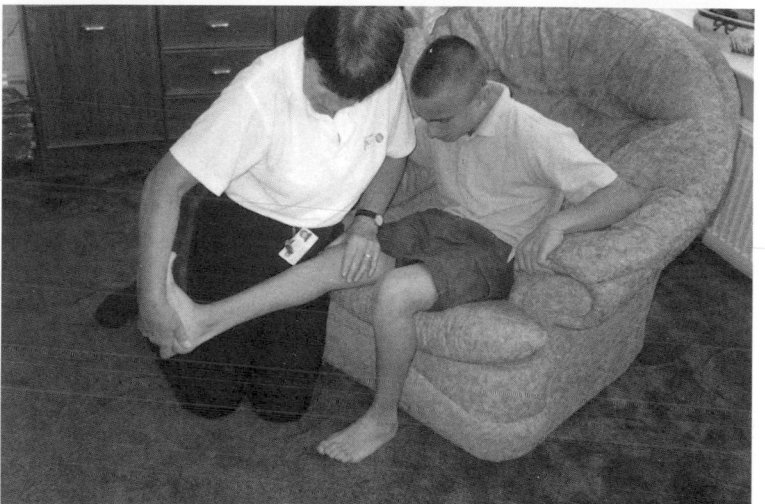

Fig. 7.2a,b Examining and explaining dorsiflexion with a person (see Table 7.1).

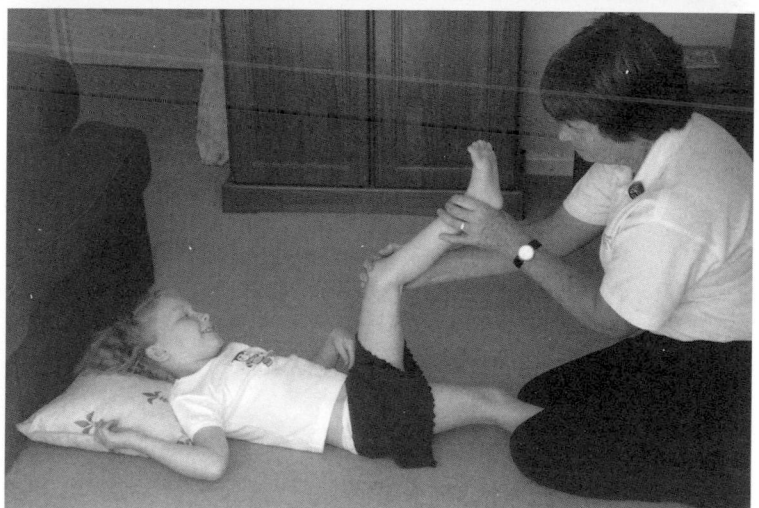

Fig. 7.3 Examining hamstrings and knee extension (popliteal angle) whilst relaxing a child (see Table 7.1).

Table 7.1   Assessment of joint range.

Assess:

Passive joint range: to demonstrate muscle length (extensibility, shortening), muscle tightness (spasticity, rigidity) and soft tissue tightness. Remember that muscle tightness (hypertonus) may or may not have full range of motion.
Degree of tightness or resistance to your passive motion, and where the greatest degree occurs in the range.
The difference between muscle and soft tissue tightness. Test *slowly*, use inhibitory techniques to inhibit muscle tightness and reveal true contracture (fixed deformity).
Active joint range for range and ability to move and *not* as equivalent to muscle strength. Quality of muscle action should be noted. Strength and the opposing degree of tightness affect active range.

Note: different positions may affect range of motion in some cases. Check in supine, prone, sitting, side-lying, standing as well. Lack of consensus on paediatric ranges exists.

Note any pain especially in the hip ranges.

Hip flexor tightness – extension range
Bend one knee to chest. The other may flex off bed. Overcome this hip flexion by downward pressure on the front of the thigh: Check how far this can be overcome, and how much pressure is required. Norm 0–20° age 2–5, 30° age 6–12.
or
Bend both knees to chest. Hold one bent and see how far the other can be stretched down to the bed.
Prone-hip extension is tested with other leg over edge of bed.

Hip extensor tightness – flexion range
Bend both hip and knee to chest. Note range and degree of extensor tightness. Hip extensor tightness also revealed in knee flexor test for hamstrings below.

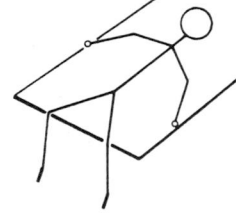

Hip adductor tightness – abduction range
Test in supine and in prone. Abduct hips with hips straight, knees bent. Abduct hips with hips and knees flexed. Abduct hips with hips and knees extended. These three procedures reveal tightness in different muscle groups and show which requires therapy and positioning; 45–60° is normal abduction with extended hips each tested separately in prone.
45° test together in flexion.

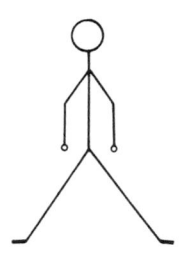

Hip abductor tightness – adduction range
Bring legs together and hips straight from *frog position* if present.
Note: keep pelvis level for abduction and adduction ranges.

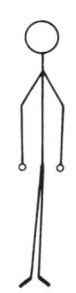

Table 7.1 Continued

Hip rotator tightness – internal or external rotation
Assess with hip and knee flexed and hip extended. Rotate thigh inwards and outwards.
Hip extended, knees over bed edge in supine or 90° in prone. Norm 45° between lower
leg and vertical supine; 45° prone; for rotation, internal or external.

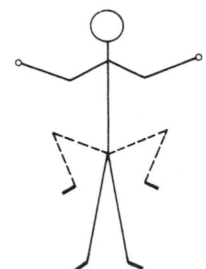

Knee flexor tightness – extension range
Bend one knee to eliminate hip flexion-lordosis and test the other. With hip at 90° fully
extend that flexed knee. Note popliteal angle only with other leg strainght.
Norm 30–40° between tibia and vertical femur.

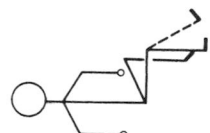

Straight leg lift also reveals tight hamstrings (flexor tightness at knees and extensor
tightness at hips). Norm 60°.

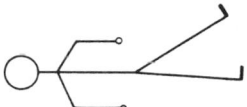

Press knees straight in lying supine or prone (limited range may be detected).

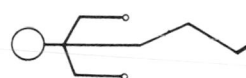

Knee extensor tightness – flexion range
Lying prone, flex the knee. If hip rises up into flexion, press hip down as far as possible to
detect tightness of rectus femoris (some ileo-psoas too).
Norm 130–140° from horizontal with hip straight
Note tibial torsion 10 15° norm between lines of thigh and midfoot. Age 2–19.

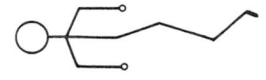

Sitting: flex knee for tightness of quadriceps.

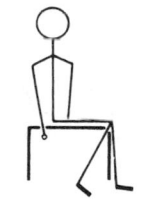

Lying knees flexed over edge of bed without lordosis. Bend one knee to counter lordosis
and also eliminate hip flexor tightness (if present) with test of quadriceps tightness.

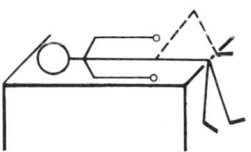

Foot plantar flexion tightness – dorsiflexion range
Bend hip and knee and dorsiflex foot by grasping heel and *avoiding* passive dorsiflexion in
mid-foot. Hold dorsiflexion with knee straight. Norm 10–20° with inversion.
Foot: inversion, eversion, plantarflexion tested with knee straight. Test forefoot and toes.

Note: keep pelvis level (stop antero-posterior tilt, lateral tilt) during assessments

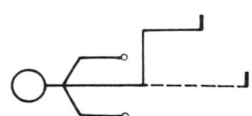

Table 7.1   Continued

Shoulder flexor tightness – extensor range
Bring arm straight back.

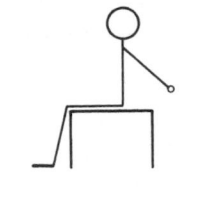

Shoulder flexor-adductor tightness – elevation range
Elevate arm forward and overhead.
Abduct and elevate arm.

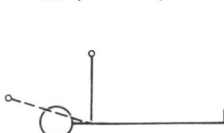

Shoulder rotations internal–external
Elbow flexor tightness – extension range
Slowly stretch *without* forcing elbow into extension with pronation and into extension with
supination.

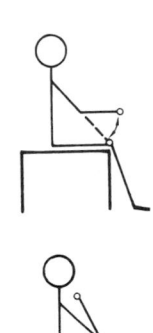

Elbow extensor tightness – flexion range
Bend elbow with pronation and test with supination.
Elbow pronation-supination
Carry out test with upper arm close to side of body.
Wrist flexion-extension
Wrist deviation radial and ulnar
Finger and thumb adduction and abduction
Finger and thumb flexion-extension
Remember to hold thumb at its base.
Head and trunk
Ranges assessed for torticollis or scoliosis.
Active ranges assessed as above but denotes action of antagonists overcoming tightness of agonists above. See also
assessment within functional examinations.
Check: speed – rhythm – endurance of active assessments here and in functional assessments.
Note: Goniometry is measurement used for degrees of joint ranges.
Grade strength can be accurate only as: present, weak, strong.

Examination of Deformity

The therapist should obtain information on:

- *Structure of joints* especially subdislocation or dislocation of the hips, varus or valgus neck of femur, spinal vertebrae.
- *Inequality in the length of legs* but not so much in the arms, as far as function is concerned.
- *Joint range* Passive range of motion carried out slowly may detect fixed or unfixed deformity as well as tightness of muscle groups.

Active range is also needed but has already been observed in the functional examination where it is of the greatest significance.

Passive range (figures and captions – Table 7.1). Passive range examines any limitations or excessive joint ranges. Goniometers measure ranges, provided a standard procedure is used, e.g. position and control of factors influencing tone. Stuberg *et al*. (1988) question the reliability of goniometer measures. Electro-goniometers are also used but not easily available. Ranges in paediatrics are not well documented (Long & Tocano 2002).

Active range (Table 7.1).

Active range is also observed in function as follows:

Head and trunk flexion, extension, rotation observed during head raise in prone, supine, sitting, standing developmental channels.

Shoulder elevation, abduction, rotation, flexion and extension movements are observed during the functional examination of, say, creeping, reaching and other arm movements.

Elbow flexion and extension observed during child's reach to parts of his body or toys. Forearm pronation or supination affects flexion and extension, and must also be seen in isolation.

Wrist and hand will be observed during hand function development.

Hip flexion and extension will be observed during all functions. Also ask the child to lie supine, bend his hip and knee to his chest and touch his feet and to sit and bend to touch the ground, to sit on very low stools and come up to standing and sit down again.

Knee flexion and extension seen with active hip flexion extension, as well as observing the child sitting using active extension to kick your hand or a dangling toy, and his knee extension in standing *tall*.

Foot movements need to be tested separately especially if there are abnormal feet.

If the child cannot achieve a full active range check:

(1) That it is not due to a decrease in the passive range of motion of the joint.
(2) That it is not due to weakness, primary or secondary.
(3) That it is not due to interference of abnormal reflex reactions occurring during any particular activity.

FUNCTION AND RANGES OF MOTION

Examination of ranges in supine necessary for muscle length and full joint mobility, may or may not transfer to a function. If possible this needs to be checked and suggestions are given under the heading of 'Active Motion'. For example, both active and passive ranges can be assessed in context of standing and preparation for stepping. A child or older person who can cooperate is placed in supported standing on one leg, on a block or on the ground. The other leg to be tested is not weight-bearing. Quick ranges of movement hip extension and flexion, knee extension and flexion and foot dorsiflexion needed for the walking pattern are tested. This will not be the full range usually needed as approximately a range of 25–35 degrees is usual. Muscle action of plantar flexion and hip extension for push off, hip and knee extension for stance, and hip flexion, knee extension and dorsiflexion for heel contact is also tested in this functional position. Training of these elements or components of standing and stepping can follow so that impairments of ranges are treated within a function. This approach is similarly used by Shumway-Cook and Woollacott (2001) for adults.

See Chapter 10 on deformity for details of the causes of limitation of ranges of motion and treatment. Equipment to improve ranges of motion are given in Chapter 8 in the context of positioning and developmental functional training.

Pre-operative and postoperative physiotherapy may require localized assessment to confirm that muscle groups which have been given the opportunity to act by the operation are in fact doing so. They and all other musculature need assessment and strengthening. Postural mechanisms need assessment in pre- and postoperative periods for function.

REACTIONS, RESPONSES AND REFLEXES

These should be known to the therapist so that she recognizes them during any motor functions on the developmental channels. These are summarized in Fig. 7.4 and Table 7.2 and linked with therapy suggestions. They

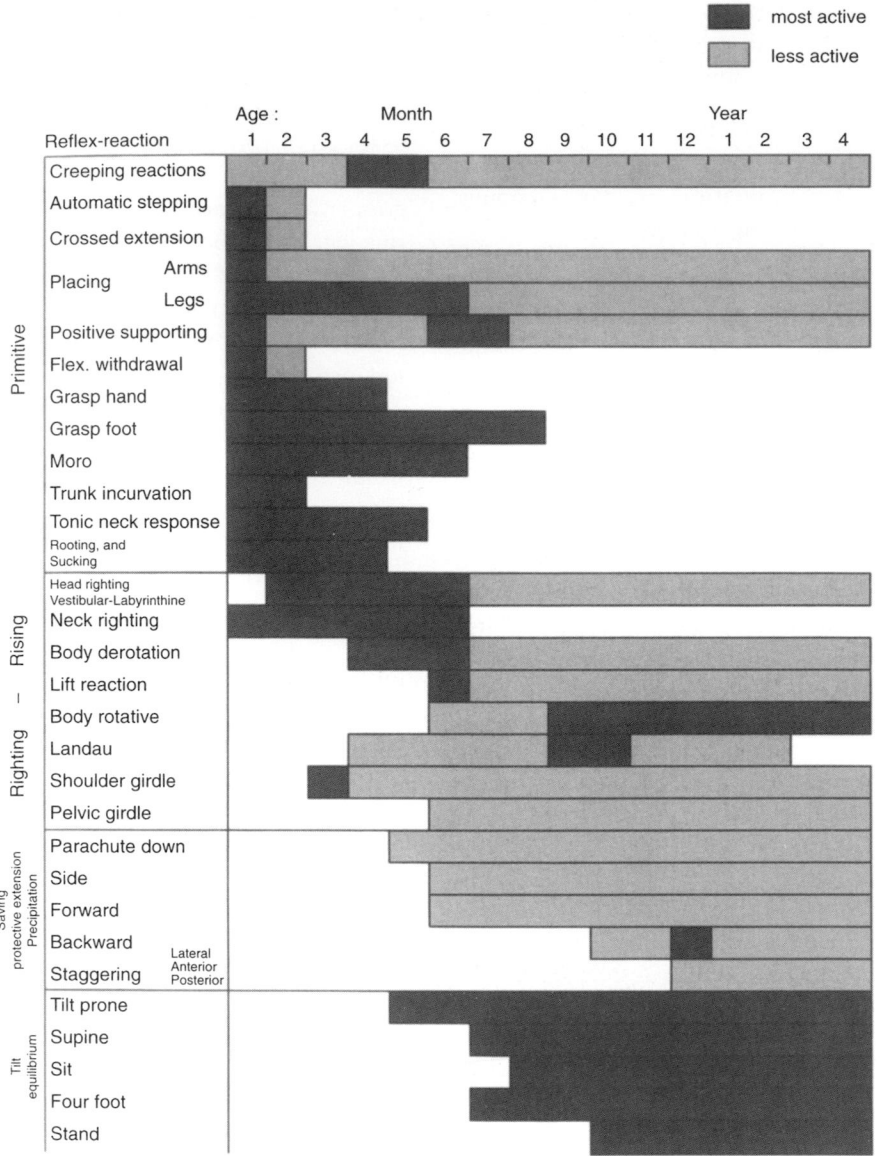

Fig. 7.4 Neurological reactions in development.
Note: This chart is not used as a test, but for background information. The content was selected by S. Levitt, based on Andre-Thomas *et al.* (1960), Paine & Oppé (1966), Milani-Comparetti & Gidoni (1967), Touwen (1976), Capute *et al.* (1978), Bobath (1980) and Illingworth (1983).

should *not* be examined by the therapist in isolation except as an academic exercise or with the doctor for diagnostic information. Normal postural mechanisms rather than infantile reflexes are all assessed within the channels of development of motor function on its own and within daily living activities. In this way the hierarchical reflex model becomes unnecessary as a list of tests (see Chapter 1, 'Abnormal Reflexes').

Table 7.2 Reflex reactions. A reflex conveys a stereotyped response to a stimulus. As responses vary in children the term reflex reaction is used.

Reflex reaction	Normal until	Stimulus	Response	Therapy
Sucking	3 months	Introduce a finger into mouth	Sucking action of lips and jaw	Train correct feeding
Rooting	3 months	Touch baby's cheek	Head turns toward stimulus	
Cardinal points	2 months	(1) Touch corner of mouth	(1) Bottom lip lowers on same side and tongue moves toward point of stimulation. When finger slides away, the head turns to follow	Desensitize face by child's own touch and other stimuli by therapist
		(2) Centre of upper lip is stimulated	(2) Lip elevates, tongue moves toward place stimulated. If finger slides along oronasal groove the head extends	
		(3) Centre of bottom lip is stroked	(3) Lip is lowered and tongue directed to site of stimulation. If finger moves toward chin, the mandible is lowered and head flexes	
Grasp	3 months	Press finger or other suitable object into palm from ulnar side	Fingers flex and grip object. (Head in mid-line during this test)	Weight bearing, stimuli over whole hand, hand opening in Development of hand function
Hand opening	1 month	Stroke ulnar border of palm and little finger	Automatic opening of hand	
Foot grasp	9 months	Press sole of foot behind the toes	Grasping response of feet	Weight bearing in Development of standing
Placing	Remains	Bring the anterior aspect of foot or hand against the edge of a table	Child lifts limb up to step onto table	Use in provoking early step
Primary walking (Automatic Walk: Reflex Stepping)	2 months	Hold baby upright and tip forward, sole of foot presses against table	Initiates reciprocal flexion and extension of legs	Weight bearing in Development of standing
Galant's trunk incurvation	2 months	Stroke back lateral to the spine	Flexion of trunk towards side of stimulus	Train trunk stability in Development of sitting and standing
Automatic sitting	2 months	Pressure is placed on the thighs and the head is held in flexion. Supine position.	Child pulls to sitting from supine	Train child's own rising in Development of sitting
Moro	0–6 months	Baby supine and back of head is supported above table. Drop head backwards, associated with loud noise	Abduction and extension of arms. Hands open. This phase is followed by adduction of the arms as if in an embrace	Train vertical head stability, use grasp, use prone position, use flexion position, shoulder fixation with grasp or hand support
Startle	Remains	Obtained by sudden loud noise or tapping the sternum	Elbow is flexed (not extended as in the Moro reflex) and the hand remains closed	Desensitize to noise by warning and experience

Table 7.2 Continued

Reflex reaction	Normal until	Stimulus	Response	Therapy
Landau	From 3 months to 2½ years, strong 10 months	Child held in ventral suspension, lift head	The head, spine and legs extend. Extend arms at shoulders	Use in therapy to activate extensor muscles
		When the head is depressed	The hip, knees and elbows flex	
Flexor withdrawal	2 months	Supine; head mid-position, legs extended – stimulate sole of foot	Uncontrolled flexion response of stimulated leg (do not confuse with response to tickling)	
Extensor thrust	2 months	Supine; head, mid-position, one leg extended opposite leg flexed – stimulate sole of flexed leg	Uncontrolled extension of stimulated leg (do not confuse with response to tickling)	Weight bearing, joint compression, knee splints and calipers in Development of standing
Crossed extension	2 months	Supine; head, mid-position; legs extended – stimulate medial surface of one leg by tapping	Opposite leg adducts, extends, internally rotates and foot plantarflexes (typical scissor position)	
Asymmetrical tonic neck (ATNR) reaction	6 months, usually pathological	Patient supine; head in mid-position; arms and legs extended – turn head to one side	Extension of arm and leg on face side, or increase in extensor tone; flexion of arm and leg on skull side or increase in flexor tone	Use both arms together and train head in midline, use prone position, only encourage in severe older child
Symmetrical tonic neck (STNR) reflex	Rare and usually pathological	(1) Patient in quadruped position or over tester's knees – ventroflex the head	Arms flex or flexor tone dominates; legs extended or extensor tone dominates	see Prone development Correct weight bearing on hands and knees. If correct abnormal posture in all development then usually ignore the STNR
		(2) Position as above, dorsiflex the head	Arms extend or extensor tone dominates; legs flex or flexor tone dominates	
Tonic labyrinthine supine	Pathological	Patient supine; head in mid-position; arms and legs extended. Test stimulus – is the position	Extensor tone dominates when arms and legs are passively flexed	See Development in supine; Development of sitting Overcomes excessive extension
Tonic labyrinthine prone *Reaction to prone*	3 months	Turn patient prone – head in mid-position. Test stimulus – prone position	Unable to dorsiflex head, retract shoulders, extend trunk, arms, legs	See Development in prone Overcomes excessive flexion
Positive supporting	3 months	Hold patient in standing position – press down on soles of feet	Increase of extension in legs. Plantarflexion, genu recurvatum may occur	See Development of standing Excessive anti-gravity response
Negative supporting	3–5 months	Hold in weightbearing position	Child 'sinks' astasia	See Development of standing
Neck righting	5 months	Supine, rotate head to one side, actively or passively	Body rotates as a whole in same direction as the head	See Development of rolling in supine Stimulate body rotative reactions
Associated reactions	Pathological	Have patient squeeze an object (with a hemiplegic, squeeze with uninvolved hand)	Clench of other hand or increase of tone in other parts of the body. Abnormal overflow	See Development of hand functions

Table 7.2 Continued

Reflex reaction	Emerges at	Stimulus	Response	Therapy
Rising Labyrinthine head righting Vestibular righting (decrease of head lag)	2–6 months	(1) Hold blindfolded patient in prone position, in space, as head drops	Head raises to normal position, face vertical, mouth horizontal	For all reactions, see all sections on Developmental training in Chapter 8
		(2) As above in supine position	Head raises to normal position, face vertical, mouth horizontal	
	6 months	(3) Hold blindfolded patient in space – hold around pelvis, tilt to the side	Head rights itself to normal position, face vertical, mouth horizontal	
Optical	6 months	As above, no blindfold	As above	
Amphibian	4–6 months	Patient prone, head in mid-position, legs extended, lift pelvis on one side	Automatic flexion outward of hip and knee on same side	
(a) Body righting, derotative	4–6 months	Supine – rotate head or one knee one side, passively	Active derotation at waist, i.e. segmental rotation of trunk between shoulders and pelvis	
(b) Rotative	6–10 months	Rotate hip and knee or arm or head actively	Active segmented rotation (hyperactive at 10 months, cannot lie supine)	
Lift reaction (*not* the pathological lift reaction (Tardieu)	5–6 months	Lift body through space	Head raises (lifts)	
Shoulder/pelvic girdle righting	3–6 months	Fix distal part(s) of limb	Rise up on to limb	

Postural fixation counterpoising (see the sections on developmental training in Chapter 8)

Tilt reactions (a) Supine and prone	6 months	Patient on tiltboard. Arms and legs extended, tilt board to one side	Lateral curving of head and thorax, protective reaction in limbs accompany trunk reaction	
(b) Four-point kneeling	7–12 months	Patient in quadruped position, tilt toward one side	Lateral curving of head and thorax. Abduction-extension of arm and leg on raised side and protective reactions on lowered side may accompany this	
(c)		Tilt forward and back (antero-posteriorly)	Forward – head and back, flex. Backward – head and back, extend	See Chapter 8
(d) Sitting	9–12 months	Patient seated on chair – tilt patient to one side. Tilt forward anteroposterior back	Head and thorax curve abduction-extension of arm and leg on raised side, other protective reactions may accompany this	
(e) Sitting		Tilt forward	Child extends head and back	
		Tilt back	Child flexes head and trunk	

Table 7.2   Continued

Reflex reaction	Emerges at	Stimulus	Response	Therapy
(f) Kneel-standing	18 months	Patient in kneel-standing position, pull or tilt patient to one side	As above	
(g) Standing	12–18 months	Patient in standing position. Tilt sideways. Tilt anteroposteriorly	Trunk as above	
Staggering reactions (see Saving from falling below)	12–18 months	(1) Move to left or to right side push or holding upper arm	Hopping, or step sideways to maintain equilibrium	See Chapter 8
		(2) Move forward	Hopping, or step forwards to maintain equilibrium	
		(3) Move backwards	Hopping, or step backwards to maintain equilibrium or dorsiflex feet going on to heels	
Saving from falling	5–10 months	Prone – sudden tip downward Sitting – sudden tip downward Standing – sudden tip downward	Immediate extension of arms with abduction and extension of fingers to save and then prop the child	
	6–9 months	Standing – sudden tip sideways – one arm		
	9–12 months	Standing – sudden tip backwards – both arms		

Note   Motor patterns of the responses may be abnormal. This is *not* a chart for testing a child, but as background information for observation in function.

SPEED OF PERFORMANCE

Independence of a child and older person with disabilities is not fully achieved if he cannot move fast enough for his particular needs in his particular environment. To help the children fit into regular (mainstream) schools or later normal work situations as well as live with people in society they need to be trained to function at reasonable speed. This could be slower than normal but not *very* slow. It is easy to assess when a child is very slow and therapy is adjusted accordingly. Other speeds have to be assessed if they are relevant to the child's life, and whether people are likely to wait for a person whose movements and walking are slow. In assessing speed there needs to be a simultaneous assessment of distances a child can walk. Assessment for electric wheelchair will also be associated with the problems of speed.

VOLUNTARY MOTION

This is part of the assessment of the motor developmental channels (Chapter 8, all sections) and is specially observed in the development of arm and hand function, and activities such as feeding and dressing. Arm or leg patterns in the postural reactions of saving from falling and rising reactions are *not* the assessment of limb patterns in voluntary or purposeful movement in play, feeding, dressing and other activities (see Chapter 9).

ABNORMAL TONE

This is really considered when assessment is made of the abnormal performance. It should not be assessed as such but rather as *tone* manifests itself in the functions and abnormal performance of the developmental abilities. The assessment of deformity also includes assessment of the manifestation of abnormal tone. Assessment of *degree and distribution of tone* is superfluous as the degree does not correlate with function, and distribution is obvious in the assessment of *motor delay and abnormal performance*. An Assessment Scale to measure spasticity is the Modified Ashworth Scale (Bohannon & Smith 1987) and tools used in gait laboratories.

MUSCLE STRENGTH

This is only assessed after the assessment of the functional examination as quite often it is no longer indicated then. The important observation is when muscles act *in function* and whether this action is a holding action for postural fixation or a moving action in voluntary motion or in rising, saving reactions or in stepping. The examination of deformity may have to include examinations of muscle strength. See active joint range (Table 7.1).

Measures of strength are used by Damiano *et al.* (2002) with children over 4 years. Hand-held dynamometers have been used as measures. However, measures are difficult with children so that there are general observations of 'present, trace/weak, strong or absent' muscle group action.

ADDITIONAL ASSESSMENT REQUIRED

Sensory examination. Loss of sensation in the cerebral palsies is rare having only been described in hemiplegia (Tizard *et al.* 1954). Also it is difficult to assess sensation in babies and young children with disabilities or older children with severe multiple impairments. Perceptual disorder or agnosias are much more common and various assessments are available and best done by neurologists, psychologists and specialized occupational therapists and teachers. Lack of body awareness and other perceptual problems may be lack of *sensory experience*. Poor sensory awareness is common in people with severe multiple disabilities.

Sensory unawareness can lead to pressure marks and pressure sores.

Assessment of daily activities. Assessment of feeding, dressing, washing, toileting, play and hand function must be made when planning therapy in collaboration with parents and child. However, this overlaps with the assessment of motor developmental channels, especially hand function (Chapters 8 and 9).

Assessment of equipment includes the selection, the measurements and the assessment of the child in or using the particular piece of equipment. Selection and provision of equipment should always be assessed and supervised by each child's therapists and medical specialists (see Appendix).

Select equipment according to the following considerations.

(1) *Assessment of the child's disabilities and abilities*, especially emerging 'unreliable' abilities. The correct amount of aid makes it possible for him to carry out tasks otherwise impossible, but too much aid prevents his own participation and development of emerging ability.

(2) *Assessment of the child's deformities* or threatening deformities. Good alignment in any apparatus and correction of abnormal postures must be maintained during the use of the equipment. For example, standing may be correct in a standing frame, but become abnormal on hand function in standing; sitting may be upright in a push-chair with special modifications but become abnormal when the chair is pushed!

(3) *Good design* of equipment takes account of adjustments for child's growth, removal of supports with increasing ability, a variety of modifications for different children in a clinic/school, is as portable as possible and looks as normal as possible. Simple designs

easily adjusted by busy parents and staff are desirable.

(4) Assess that special equipment provides a variety of additional motor experiences in different positions. Equipment needs to give individuals appropriate support so that they can participate in social and educational activities.

(5) Monitor different items of equipment for a variety of postures throughout the day as part of the prevention and correction of deformities. Check positioning at night and turn child. Equipment at night may interfere with sleeping patterns of a child and will need monitoring.

Ongoing supervision is important to check the following:

(1) *Measurements* of the child as he grows so that equipment is not too small.

(2) *Value of the equipment* in relation to achievements gained in therapy and daily care. Once again equipment must facilitate independence, not substitute for it.

(3) *Unexpected social problems* such as equipment being too cumbersome in a home or school; isolating the child from a family group too much; proving too fragile and requiring expense, time and worry on the part of people caring for the child, and other considerations of a similar kind. Home visits are a great help in discovering these problems as parents may not report these difficulties after 'all the efforts made' by staff to assess, provide and check the equipment in a clinic.

(4) *Provision of equipment, designs and new ideas* change with research and general progress in helping children with disabilities and this may help the particular child at the reassessments.

Assessment of Techniques Required

As the assessments are made the therapist collects her aims of therapy and daily care and selects techniques from any source to carry these out. In addition the selected techniques will be assessed during use. Assessment of techniques chosen *must* take place as one cannot always predict the individual child's response. There must be an *active* response or participation or whenever possible an active initiation on the part of the child with any technique. A change in a component/ability of function needs to be detected after using a method by the end of a session. If not it should be discarded within the first or first few sessions, and another method found. Passive correction of deformities is included as part of the therapy programme. Most passive procedures should in any event *not be totally passive*. They must be assessed to see whether the passive correction manually, with plasters, splintage, orthoses or equipment makes it possible for an *active* participation of other parts of the child's body or of the particular part of the body being corrected. Always assess how a child is positioned in special equipment and how he uses any walking and/or mobility aids to decide on their effectiveness. Parent's opinions are sought as these are significant (Chapter 5).

RECORDS

Considering the approach in this and the last chapters, the background information and therapy assessments are:

- *Background information* of medical history, drugs being used, comprehensive assessment of individual's other abilities and disabilities, and family background.
- *Developmental history.*
- *Priorities of child/older person, parents or carers.* These include social, financial and priorities other than motor function. Priority of an activity of daily living such as eating, drinking, washing, dressing, toileting and mobility of a child/older person on their own and that of parent/carer assisting the person with disability.

- A *daily living activity or task* is usually relevant to therapy programmes, but other daily activities in school and community may often be considered.
- *Current motor functions* of child/older person for the chosen task.
- *Current abilities/components* of motor function already achieved by individual.
- *Impairments constraining task* (observed within task and in isolation) such as deformities, joint range, strength, postural alignments, abnormal postural control, abnormal movement patterns.
- *Abilities a child still needs to achieve* includes *motor functions and components* at the next stages of development. (This simultaneously diminishes some impairments and enables him to control others.) Assessments of developmental delays and abnormal performance include both disabilities and impairments.
- *Outline of methods, equipment, orthoses* and other resources.
- *Outcomes of function and results of treatment of impairments*. This is observed in progress of motor developmental functions, components and less constraint by impairments. Assessment of motor delay and abnormal performance will show progress.

'Goals' need to be clarified as:

Ultimate aims. Child's goals; parents goals, even individual family members' goals.

Short-term aims. Therapists' aims are related to achieve these 'ultimate aims'. These are 'what a child needs to learn or achieve' and they include motor function, components of function and diminishing the impairments which interfere with that function.

Outcomes or results. This leads to modifications or changing of short-term and in time of long-term aims and of methods to implement them.

MEASURES

These may be of the child's current motor functional achievement, pattern of motor performance and measures of impairments. Progress or changes are recorded in available Measures.

SUMMARY

(1) Assessment is essential for a therapy plan which is relevant to each child.
(2) Assessment methods must be selected in *direct* relationship to techniques of treatment. Such a practical approach is outlined in this book.
(3) Objective, valid, reproducible assessments and records still need research, though many more are now available and increasing.
(4) The practical assessment includes a developmental functional assessment, examination of deformity (threatening or established), daily living activities and equipment and can be used for checking progress. Measures are outlined.
(5) Additional assessments of communication, perception and play and social behaviour are also needed.
(6) The way in which you approach a child in assessment affects the information obtained.

Note: see Appendix 1 for the Physical ability assessment guide and the Developmental levels illustrations.

8 Treatment Procedures and Management

MOTOR TRAINING

The therapist uses the assessment framework for motor training outlined in Chapter 7 for the management and selection of treatment procedures. The specific *motor developmental delays* and *abnormal motor performance* during an individual's attempted performance of his chosen daily activity are addressed in this chapter. Methods are suggested for the development of motor function with its components/specific abilities needed for the daily activity. Impairments are being simultaneously treated to a large extent in the therapy suggestions for abnormal performance. The active development of motor functions with their components also simultaneously minimizes impairments when this is possible. For example, achievement of postural control decreases the need to 'use' impairments as compensation. As discussed in this book, spasticity, abnormal reflexes or infantile reactions are used when a child tries to function as best he can manage without basic components of posture control and appropriate synergies (patterns).

The older child's use or observable overaction of reflex reactions normally seen in very early developmental stages are mentioned in each developmental channel. This alerts the therapist so that methods are selected which avoid these reflex patterns when they exist. Repetition of a limited repertoire of movement patterns whether reflex or for biomechanical compensations can lead to deformities into these synergies. A child is therefore being enabled to achieve motor function which modifies or controls his symptoms or impairments.

The treatment of deformities specifically includes impairments as well as the functional treatments (Chapter 10).

This chapter therefore offers techniques for *the assessment findings of* motor delay, abnormal performance and reflex reactions.

Motor function and component abilities are treated and managed in the context of feeding, dressing, washing, toileting and hygiene, playing or within other daily activities. However, learning motor function in these whole contexts can be too complex. Learning part of a whole function as well as the whole function is more helpful *provided* a child along with his parent is learning and understanding the connection. This maintains motivation.

Motor function needs to be isolated for specific concentration on the deficient motor apparatus. Similarly, perceptual problems, speech and language difficulties and special problems of hearing and severe visual impairment need to have structured separate sessions of specialized treatment and teaching. However, as Neistadt (1994) points out, the specialized training of perceptual problems does not transfer to other contexts. Like motor training they apparently need to be trained in context as well. Thus, therapy has two main related aspects:

(1) Techniques which integrate motor function with related areas of function of communication, vision, hearing, sensation, perception, and understanding in the contexts of whole daily life functions.
(2) Specialized techniques for specific motor abilities and disabilities to initiate dormant

motor activity, intensify correction of abnormalities and augment motor activity.

Although this chapter concentrates on the motor problems, they are not isolated from other aspects. Whenever possible, motor activities are interwoven with communication, vision, hearing, sensation and perception. Chapter 9 summarizes the motor functions trained in this chapter in the context of some daily activities, perception and communication and outlines developmental stages of these activities.

Developmental Levels and Techniques

The therapist will use the developmental channel most appropriate to the position in which a child might manage to carry out the chosen daily activity. This might be standing for transfers, sitting for eating and socializing or lying for getting out of bed. It is rare that only one channel is indicated as assumption of any posture crosses abilities in more than one channel. In addition, different positions for the chosen activity by a parent or carer which assists their management of an individual may not necessarily be the same as that of a child or older person. Both need to be considered. Sometimes, a therapist may well negotiate the use of an additional daily activity as well.

The assessment findings in an individual rarely suggest motor training at the same developmental level in each channel of development. Therapy plans involve *simultaneous* use of each developmental channel of prone, supine, sitting, standing and hand function. The developmental sequences in these positions provide a practical framework. However, the developmental sequences in each channel are used as guidelines and not as a dogmatic scheme. Variations within each channel need to be recognized once the therapist gets to know each child or older person. The functional severity and age of each person determines how much of a repertoire of motor items can be achieved in each channel. It is unlikely that all items will be pos-

sible due to the abnormal nervous system or abnormal musculo-skeletal system.

We cannot assume that obtaining a component *in one channel will transfer* to another channel, as muscle work, joint positions and gravity are not usually the same. However, activation and strengthening as well as lengthening or shortening muscle lengths can be more successful in one channel than another. Any preference shown by an individual for particular motor patterns of, say, flexion will need methods to emphasize motor functions with extension in a developmental sequence in any one channel. Such emphasis attempts to correct the preferred motor pattern in an individual so that he learns a variety of movements for all muscles.

Postural mechanisms and movements may be easier to achieve in one channel rather than in another. It seems to me that for this reason there are also cultural differences in the channels used for the normal acquisition of standing and walking in different environments.

Some suggestions for modifications of developmental sequences

(1) If head and shoulder control from 0–6 months levels cannot be activated in prone, then train them in well supported sitting or in a prone standing frame supporting the trunk, pelvis and feet. The child's head is forward and weight taken through forearms or hands on a table. Weight shift and counterpoising a head or one arm movement can also be trained in four-point standing which would be similar to prone. (See Fig. 8.33b.) Nevertheless prone development is often still needed for correction of abnormal postures with correct weight bearing and strengthening of extensor muscles which contribute to prevention and treatment of deformities.

(2) Programme for developing pelvic stability may be carried out simultaneously in prone and supine, on hands and knees, half-kneeling and in standing with hands supported on a low box. Vertical pelvic

stability can be trained with child in upright standing grasping a bar, in upright kneeling and in step standing with minimal support. Pelvic stability is activated in supine during 'bridging' of hips. Development of sitting develops head and trunk control which enables the pelvis to be positioned symmetrically, shift from side to side and tilt into the vertical or forward pelvic position.

(3) All techniques for arm and hand patterns ideally need to be trained in as many different positions as possible. The easier positions in lying, well supported sitting and supported standing are used initially so that movement patterns, perceptual-motor experiences especially with vision are developed as soon as possible.

(4) Supine development may be omitted if the developmental items of head raising are activated from side-lying to sitting. Bringing hands to midline, to touch body and grasp feet can be developed with a child in side-lying, sitting with forward lean or in supported and unsupported sitting and standing.

(5) Rising from prone or supine may be a choice needed for some individuals and rising sequences will be different. Ideally active rising in prone and supine developmental channels increases joint and muscle ranges and offers a person more strategies of getting out of bed or getting up from the floor. Rolling is part of these sequences as well as enabling a person to turn in bed.

(6) Development of standing and stepping seems to require training in the standing position. As in able-bodied babies at ages between 0–6 months, this can be activated early with appropriate trunk support and used in treatment for individuals of any age in the channel of standing and walking. The standing position provides the necessary visual and proprioceptive inputs. Vertical head stability may be stimulated but it is important that development of head and trunk control in the upright sitting as well as standing position is simultaneously being

trained. Pre-walking skills of rolling, crawling, creeping have not been shown to need establishment before training standing and walking in adult neurology (Shumway-Cook and Woollacott 2001). This is similarly so in the standing channel in this book. Nevertheless, rising from lying to standing, which is presented in the supine and prone developmental channels, needs training so that an individual does not remain dependent on others to be 'stood up' for walking with and without walkers. The disadvantage of focusing on standing and stepping is that a child with severe visual impairment or a lack of mobility along the floor through rolling, creeping, crawling or bottom shuffling will be deprived of spatial and other basic perceptual-motor experiences.

(7) Fears or strong dislike by a child when placed in any posture leads to initial use of one developmental channel rather than another. Prone can be disliked by children with breathing problems, gastrostomies, and severe visual impairment. Children whether able-bodied, or with cerebral palsy and severe visual impairment, who become bottom shufflers dislike prone sequences. Children with severe upper limb involvement or hemiplegia cannot use arm support and crawling in prone. Sitting, standing and walking can be achieved without prone development, but disadvantages have already been mentioned.

Therapy plans therefore need careful observation and clinical judgements which relate to each person's condition and lifestyle. With experience of an individual's needs, modifications become obvious. Therefore, start with all developmental channels until understanding of each individual is gained with experience.

Assessment and developmental function

Using the assessment findings of what a child can and cannot do, plan a programme to:

- Establish and practise motor functions achieved to give him confidence
- Attempt motor functions at the next developmental levels not just level. This is to check any flickers of response.
- Consider any omissions/gaps as possible contributions to abnormal performance or compensation. Omissions are not always important.

Age of Child and Techniques

Select techniques according to developmental level and *not* according to chronological age. Use similar ideas on the treatment of deformity. Commence *functional training* of feeding, dressing, washing for a baby and for severely and profoundly involved child, adolescent or adult. Developmental prerequisites for these activities will be treated (see Chapter 9).

It is unfortunate that some workers think treatment should be cut down in older children. Postural reactions and other motor controls may only mature much later and unless stimulated will remain dormant. Teachers and other personnel in the older child's life may be shown how to include motor development so that precious school time is not lost from the child's education. The physiotherapist at the child's school should work out ideas with the teacher to stimulate movement in the classroom, playground or in physical education. Extra effort also needs to be made to maintain contact with a school child or adolescent's parents.

Adjustment of techniques according to the size of child is obvious. However, the same methods may be used for any age. Instructions to babies and children have to be given according to the level of understanding in the baby or child and of an older person with cognitive impairments or learning disabilities. (See also the sections in Chapter 4 on The development of attention and Cues for learning.)

Onset and Techniques

Response to therapy sometimes seems much quicker if the onset is sudden on a previously normal nervous system. However, ultimately spontaneous recovery and motor development in acquired brain lesions may be as unpredictable as in babies born with apparent brain damage. Children with either congenital or acquired lesions warrant appropriate stimulation and therapeutic procedures given in this book so that the potential of any of their nervous systems is given every chance to reveal itself. There are more behavioural problems in many children following a traumatic brain injury which may interfere with therapy. Expectations of better results in children who have 'already known normal movements' may be more of a frustration than a help. It is not so much the memory and experience that matters but the amount of damage *and* the capacity of any particular damaged system to compensate for the abnormalities.

Diagnosis and Techniques

The techniques are not devised for particular diagnostic types but for motor problems of delay and abnormal performance. Different diagnostic types of cerebral palsy may have similar problems and even abnormal performances described may be seen. Other diagnostic types causing motor delay exhibit abnormal performance also seen in cerebral palsy, when mild or moderately involved, for example, rounded backs, hyperextended knees or pronated feet. This is especially so if abnormal performance is a compensation for delayed balance (postural mechanisms).

Application of Techniques

These should be carried out by qualified physiotherapists and occupational therapists and shown to anyone caring for the child with either motor delay or motor dysfunction. In this chapter, where techniques require a physiotherapist only, they have been labelled *physiotherapy suggestions*. Techniques which can be taught to others are labelled *treatment suggestions and daily care*.

Repertoire of techniques in this book cannot possibly include all those available. Firstly, not *all* individual problems could be included together with possible techniques. Secondly, it is difficult to describe techniques without demonstration and only those techniques which could be described have been included. Thirdly, those techniques which have been frequently used have been selected. There are many more. Techniques in this book are thus *suggestions* not *recipes*.

Lack of response to any technique given in this book indicates the need to try others in this book or in other publications or preferably from clinical colleagues. Check that if the child scarcely responds to any technique, it is not due to:

(1) Inaccurate assessment of the child's level of development.
(2) Inadequate knowledge of the child's non-motor areas of function, i.e. understanding, perception, or other problems which interfere with carrying out movement.
(3) Lack of skill of the therapist with the particular technique.
(4) A need to modify or change the initial aims of therapy.

MOTOR DEVELOPMENT AND THE CHILD WITH SEVERE VISUAL IMPAIRMENT

Motor delay will occur because of the visual impairment in otherwise normal children. When cerebral palsy is also present the delay will be augmented. Intellectual disability may be present or only appear to be present as the child is limited by the multiple disabilities. The therapist should learn what influence the visual problems have on motor development as they do not only delay but also create unusual patterns and sequences of motor milestones. Abnormal movements or *blindisms* such as hand flapping, waving over light sources, eye poking, rocking and other bizarre patterns are seen in children, especially in some of the

children referred late for training and parental advice. These will need special methods advised by psychologists.

The methods for motor developmental training in this book can be adapted for the visually impaired child provided that the following factors are kept in mind.

Hypotonia, Motor Development and the Postural Reactions

As discussed throughout the book the postural reactions are undeveloped in children who are hypotonic (see the section on Postural mechanisms in Chapter 1 and the Hypotonicity sections in Chapters 3 and 10). Blind or sighted immobile children, delayed in motor development, may also be hypotonic. Floppyness or hypotonia is thus associated in blind babies with lack of movement (Jan *et al.* 1977). Assessment and development of the postural reactions in the visually impaired baby and young child have been studied by the author. As vision is an important factor in detecting the vertical in the child's world and in appreciating any tilt of his world, it is not surprising that the blind baby's postural control is absent or poor. Blind babies prefer to lie safely on the ground and avoid the challenges of gravity. The development of the postural reactions is also the story of the development against gravity and changes in gravity. In effect it is the story of gross motor development. The visually impaired child, with or without cerebral palsy, will need careful assessment and training of the postural reactions using auditory, tactile and increased proprioceptive and vestibular stimuli. As fears are common, the techniques should be adapted to build confidence and provide fun and a sense of adventure. Large balls, rolls and swings should only be used *after* confidence has been established and in relation to the levels of development of the postural reactions present or just commencing in the individual child.

Thus, as for sighted babies with hypotonia, the development of the postural mechanisms will counteract the hypotonia and assist the development of motor abilities.

Poor posture such as rounded backs in sitting and standing, hyperextended knees and flat feet are common in sighted hypotonic children and particularly common in visually impaired babies and children (Fig. 8.1). The specific delays in postural stability, counterpoising, forward tilt and posterior saving reactions are often observed by the author to accompany the presence of round backs and shoulders. In addition, prone development which activates head and back extension is frequently poor. Vision provokes and monitors the postural mechanisms. Sugden (1992) reviews the studies on this aspect. It is the exciting object or person that a baby catches sight of that provokes him to look up. This then stimulates the head righting and postural stability of the head. It is also the effort to understand the visual stimuli that further activates exploratory movements and increasing postural control whilst exploring. Methods to develop the postural reactions or the motor abilities cannot be isolated from a child's total development (Zinkin 1979; Sykanda & Levitt 1982; Levitt 1984, Ch. 14; Sonksen *et al.* 1984).

Total Child Development and Motor Training

Mother-child relationships. The shock and stress in the mother who does not even receive the *primal gaze* from her blind baby (Goldschmied 1975), as well as his unusual reactions to her feeding and cooing, must be understood by any therapist attempting to help. All motor developmental training must be designed to build up mother's and father's confidence in parenting their child. Many of the gross motor activities in play help enormously in creating bonds with the child. The techniques in this book should all be adapted to take place on mother's lap, close to her body and face so that her kisses, touch and stroking and talking to the baby not only help motor development but also body image, movement enjoyment by the baby and demonstrate to the baby love and security which he needs so much. Clinging to mother in an unknown or puzzling world should be allowed for longer than in sighted babies and children. The weaning of the child with visual disability to a physiotherapist should be carefully done after mother-child bonding and confidence is established. Introducing more than one therapist or developmental worker may be disconcerting to the child and even the parents.

Figure 8.1
Hyperextended knees (a) being corrected (b) by training pelvic control (postural stability and counterpoising).

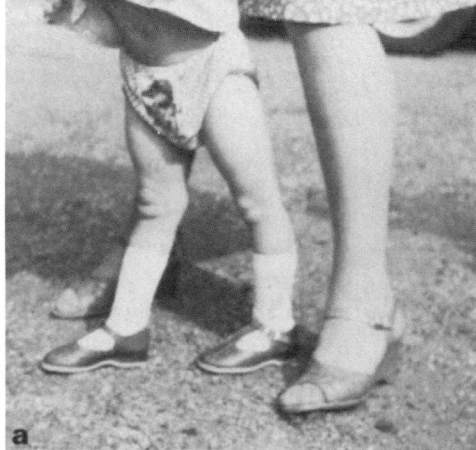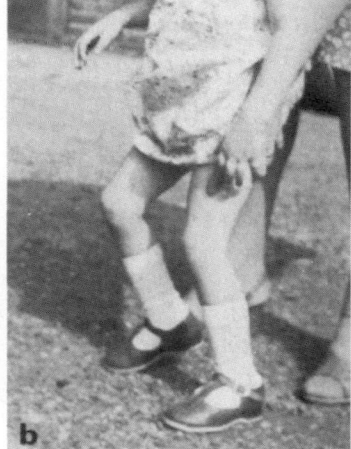

Other disciplines must advise one therapist rather than all handle the child themselves. Family participation in helping and in enjoying the motor programme with a child who is visually impaired is planned by therapists. If mother is under stress it is important not to overload her with exercises, but rather use corrective movements and postures within the daily living activities of the child. Social workers and other counsellors work closely with therapists to help the family (see Chapter 5).

Motor function and the child's daily life (Chapter 9 in this book) is usually the priority in the developmental motor training programme for the child with visual disability, not only from the parent's viewpoint, but also from the child's viewpoint. The purpose of motor function must be conveyed to each baby and child (Fig. 8.2). If not, he could be trained in basic motor patterns but never use them. He cannot *see* their purpose!

The assessments of the child's developmental stages in feeding and other self-care, play or sensory motor understanding and in exploration of his world must be obtained in order to introduce the corrective motor patterns appropriately. There are special stages and sequences for severe visual impairment (Reynell & Zinkin 1975; Kitzinger 1980).

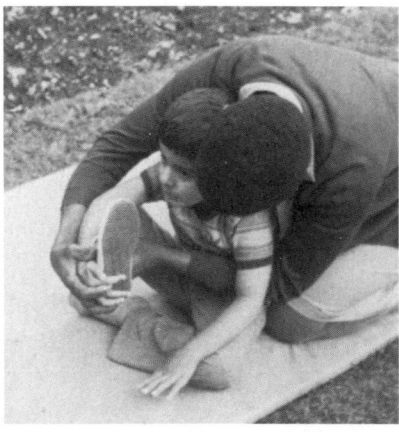

Figure 8.2 Movements for dressing.

Use of compensatory stimuli for motor development. As vision is not available, it seems obvious to use auditory and tactile stimuli to provoke motor development. However, it is vision which normally teaches the baby what makes sounds, where they come from in direction and in distance, how humans communicate and the association of sounds with situations such as meal times, bath times and so on. Therefore, first train the baby what sounds mean before they can really motivate him to move. Also use existing movements to confirm what sounds mean.

Auditory development is followed as observed in the normal child (Sheridan 1975) but with special adaptations for the visual impairment (Sonksen 1979). First, the baby is trained to listen, then to turn to sound and after that to reach for sound. He will first localize the source of sound near his ears horizontally and then above and below him. He must be helped kinaesthetically to search for the sound *kept stationary* near him. Developmentally this will be at ear level, horizontally, above, below and then behind the child. The child will *only* achieve reach for sound when his conceptual development includes *the permanence of objects* and their sounds. It is at about these stages that reach and move towards a sound will only be worth using to stimulate roll over, creeping, crawling or bottom shuffling. Until the permanence of objects is conceptualized, help the child locate sound and move towards it by providing tactile and kinaesthetic stimuli.

Similarly the appreciation of tactile stimuli, localizing and searching for them, has to be developed. Linking tactile with sound stimuli must be carried out. Encouraging the child to create sound himself should be included as he bangs a mobile, rattle, tambourine or a surface with hands or feet. The motor programme cannot be planned without these aspects which are devised by teachers, psychologists and developmental paediatricians together with the therapist.

Mother's voice and her touch rather than the therapist's will be more successful in the early stages. Vibration, smell, taste and air currents can be introduced. Link sound, touch, proprioception and vestibular stimuli. All these aspects are associated with the child's conceptual development (Sonksen *et al.* 1984).

Body image development. Poor body image is related to poor motor experiences and not seeing body parts static or moving. The tactile stimuli are used to develop the body image. However, it is the mother's and the baby's hands that should do the touching first. Hands of the baby are notoriously slow to move and explore because of many reasons, not least of which is the absence of *hand regard.* Help the baby bring his hands together in midline, *pat-a-cake* hand to hand, touch hand to mouth, hand to body and hand to feet (see Fig. 8.3). Later use as many other stimuli to his body such as rubbing with towels, soap, creams and powder at bath time. Use vibrating toys, bells, and playthings

placed for him to find on his tummy or legs, and similar ideas. The sections on Stages of hand function development in this chapter and motor function and perception in Chapter 9 offer ideas for the sighted child in this book. For the child without sight these stimuli offered in play activities should be emphasized and also *presented more slowly* and stage by stage. Do not bombard the baby with too many stimuli at once. Confusion or fear could be aroused if stimuli are not sensitively given. Thus, carefully introduce different surfaces for the child to roll on, creep, crawl, and walk on with bare feet.

Always give the child time to experience tactile and auditory stimuli and let him reach and find out about them himself whenever possible. He feels his own body movements and how he actively produced them. If he does not move himself, parents must move him, changing positions for him. He should feel his mother move about by being slung close to her body in a baby pack.

Proprioceptive and vestibular function. These aspects are also part of total child development. They are compensatory stimuli for visual impairment and also develop body image. All the postural reactions are dependent on these stimuli in a developmental context discussed in this book. Touch, pressure and resistance can be correctly given to stimulate movement giving clues as to direction and degree of muscle action. However, as with all therapy methods, observe whether the child understands and is not confused by what is expected of him. Do not use therapy techniques with handling, pressures, or other proprioceptive stimuli from behind him as he may well lean back or use his extensor thrusts to reach the stimuli or the familiar voice behind him! Body image training is also stimulation of proprioception and vestibular input for the visually impaired child.

Visual development. Not all blind babies are totally blind. Even reaction to light only, can be

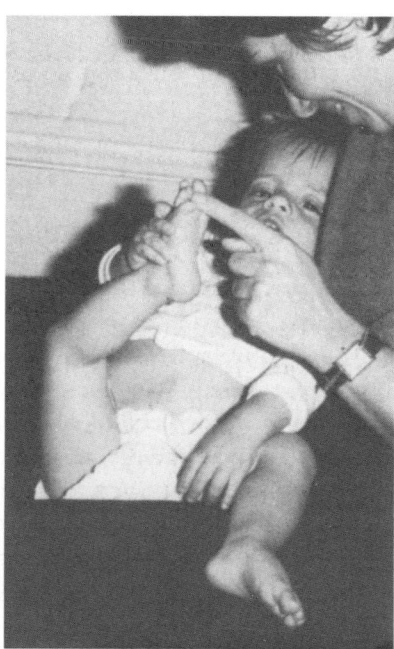

Figure 8.3 Body image development.

used and perhaps developed to the child's full if limited capacities. An assessment of the developmental *use* of residual vision is given by the development paediatrician and guides the therapist in her motor plan for the individual child. The physiotherapist should be told how large an object can be seen by the child, how far away, whether it can be seen if stationary or moving and which visual fields are present. Equality of vision in each eye and the acuity as well as any special visual defects which may affect handling the child and motor development should also be known. Vision for exploration and for learning is assessed by the developmental paediatrician. Development of visual potential is easily integrated with the methods for head control, hand function and all balance and locomotor activities discussed in this book. Once again, relate the appropriate level of visual ability with the child's motor programme. Also one may have to accept unusual head position and other patterns which make it possible for the child to use residual vision.

Language development. It is important to talk and clearly label the body parts used, the motor activity and generally encourage the child's language development. Delay is *normal* for a child who cannot yet understand the meaning of sounds, words and conversation as he cannot see what they mean, cannot see gestures and cannot link the stimuli from the external world. Psychologists and teachers work closely with the therapists to plan the language and speech programme.

Communication is also fostered through motor actions, touch and body language relevant to the sign system of a child. Psychologists and speech therapists will advise on these aspects.

Motor developmental sequences. The development of hand function is obviously the most important area for the child whose hands are his eyes on the world. The hand function chapter in this book should be adapted to use compensatory tactile, auditory and proprioceptive stimuli before motor actions can be expected to follow the normal rate of development. Do not force objects into the child's hand but train him to search for the nearby rattle, to orientate his hand to take it and to develop a variety of searching actions or finger moulding and feeling actions. Bilateral hand function will take more work than with the sighted child. Encourage both hands together in midline, holding and especially exploring both sides of a cup, bowl, ball or toy and transfer of toys. Train losing the toy and finding it and taking it apart, constructing it again. Also train crude and fine voluntary release. All these actions must link with the concept of object permanence and other intellectual development of the child. Remember that index finger pointing and associated index/first finger grasp is very much a visual skill and will be delayed. Offer toys and food to promote finger actions as mentioned in the chapters on hand function, motor function and play, feeding and other self-care activities.

Prone development is not popular with the baby with visual problems as there is no interest there, sounds cannot be heard as easily and he may be far removed from family and especially mother. There are no visual lures to provoke him to look up and progress to creeping and crawling. It is often noted that crawling is not used by blind children and that they prefer shuffling on their bottoms and then walking. It is possible to train prone development on mother's lap, on a soft cushion with attractive noises especially mother's voice and her stroking her child's back. The advantages are increased head and back muscle strength due to head and back extension and coming up on hands, hands and knees and development of an additional exploratory skill of crawling through space and of additional body image experiences for the child. The round backs and shoulders may be helped by stronger back extensors but additional postural training in sitting and counterpoising of the arms when reaching up for toys or mother's face helps more.

Crawling is not of course essential for the acquisition of walking, as bottom shufflers demonstrate. It is the crawling, rolling or movement across space and much learning experiences of space and especially that the floor is continuous that teaches the child to be less afraid and to walk alone. Walkers with wheels all around the child should be avoided as he will not develop his own postural and locomotive reactions. The child often sits or leans onto these walkers, stepping his legs but not learning to take weight through his legs and so learn to walk. Baby bouncers and rocking chairs are also of potential danger if unsupervised. Withdrawal into a rocking world can be engendered and bouncing may provoke abnormal leg patterns, excessive toe-walking (*blindism*) and spasticity and athetosis. Short supervised sessions in any equipment do often produce more desirable results, especially if mother–child interaction is included.

Blind babies develop postures slightly later or within the ranges of sighted developmental levels (Fraiberg 1977). However, there is more of a delay of moving into, or out of or forward from these postures. Thus, this book on developmental levels should be used as guidelines and not as rigid rules for developmental ages nor strict sequences for severe visual disability. The postural reactions of fixation, counterpoising, tilt and saving (protective) reactions and the methods given are in a logical sequence for therapy, but delays and modifications will be required according to the particular vision and hearing development, emotional and social situations and the amount of developmental intervention given. Rising reactions will require extra care as all workers in this field demonstrate how much visual lures promote posture changes. All other motor developmental training from 0 to 5 years presented in this book should be continued to avoid the frequently occurring clumsiness in the visually impaired. Co-ordination exercises, balance tasks, music and movement, dance, games and physical education are of great value to the children with visual disabilities. The older child will also be receiving mobility training from those employed for this work by the Royal National Institute of the Blind. Teachers for severe visual impairment will integrate their work on this and other aspects with the therapists, as there is a need to create a whole programme for each child and family.

PRONE DEVELOPMENT

The following main features should be developed:

Postural stability of the head (Fig. 8.4a–d) when lying prone (0–3 months), on forearms (3 months), on hands and on hands and knees (6 months), during crawling, half-kneeling hand support (9–11 months) or in the *bear-walk* (12 months) in normal developmental levels.

Postural stability of the shoulder girdle (Fig. 8.4b–d) when taking weight on forearms

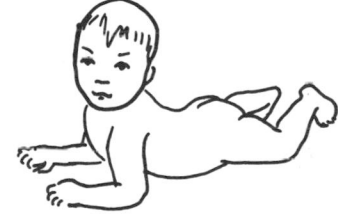

Fig. 8.4a Postural stability of head and shoulder girdle (on forearms).

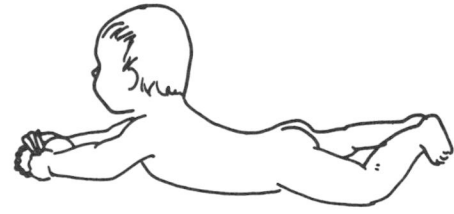

Fig. 8.4b Postural stability of head and shoulder girdle.

(3 months), on hands (6 months), on hands and knees and arms held stretched forward along the ground to hold a toy at 5–6 months also include postural stability. Pivot prone or the *Landau type* of posture with arms held extended and in the air also activates stabilization musculature (8–10 months). Maintenance of half-kneeling lean on hands or upright kneeling lean on hands or grasp a support are other normal developmental motor activities around 9–12 months which stimulate shoulder girdle stability.

Counterpoising of the head takes place in activities which include head turn and head movements whilst holding the head up against gravity.

Counterpoising the arm movements at about 5 months normal level when in prone lean on one forearm reach with the other or 7 months lean on hand reach with the other (Fig. 8.4c). Reach in all directions increases counterpoising ability

as well as other features of motor ability, such as weight bearing through pelvis.

Postural stability of the pelvis (Fig. 8.4d) on knees with hips at right angles (4 months), on elbows and knees and on hands and knees (4–6 months), on one knee with the other foot flat as in half-kneeling and upright kneeling with support (9–12 months) in normal motor levels.

Counterpoising movement of one leg takes place on knees with upper trunk and arms supported (5–6 months), on hands and knees (6–8 months) together with counterpoising of arm motion in crawling (9–11 months), in bear walk (12 months). Stand lean on hands on low table, carry out leg patterns in each leg also trains counterpoising in normal developmental levels (see Development of standing at 9–12 months normal developmental stages in this chapter).

Rising from prone (Fig. 8.5) head (0–3 months), on to forearms (3 months), on to knees (4 months), on to forearms and knees (5–6 months), on to hands and knees (6–7 months), to half-kneeling hand support (9–12 months), prone to standing without support (12–18 months). Change from and to prone, sitting, squatting, crawling positions (10 months) and other positions with further motor development.

Tilt reactions in prone (Fig. 8.6) Reactions seen on tilting the surface on which the child lies at

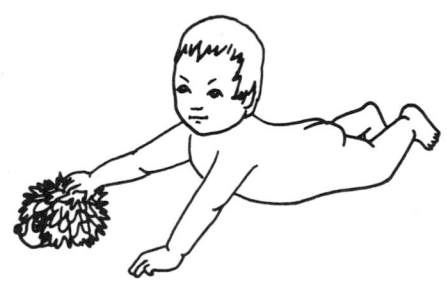

Fig. 8.4c Postural stability and counterpoising arm reach.

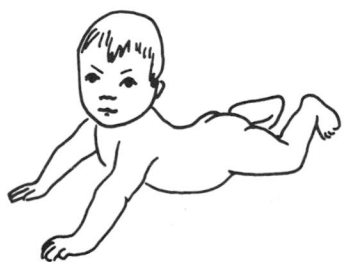
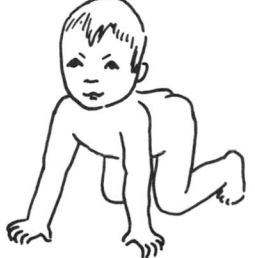

Fig. 8.4d Postural stability on hands and on hands and knees.

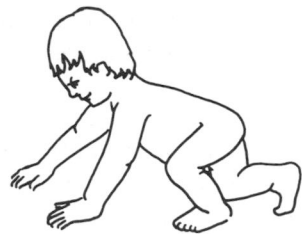

Fig. 8.5   Rising from prone.

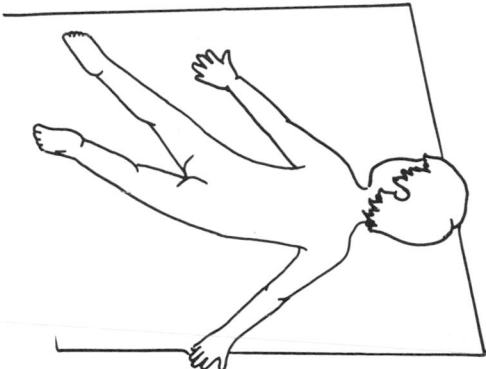

Fig. 8.6   Tilt reaction in prone.

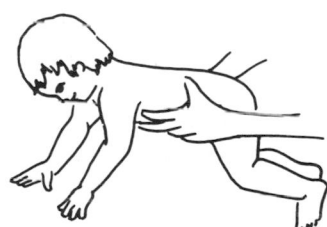

Fig. 8.7   Saving reactions in the arms.

about 6 months; on hands and knees at about 9–12 months.

Saving from falling reactions (Fig. 8.7) in the arms at 5–7 months downward-and-forward parachute, and propping. Arm and leg reactions accompany the tilt reactions in prone, especially if the trunk reaction is particularly poor. Other saving reactions are described in the sitting development. Arm saving sideways and forward can also be seen when a child is on hands and knees, if the child is suddenly pushed sideways or if pushed forward from a heel-sitting position, or when on hands and knees on a rocking board. Leg reactions also occur on pushing the child over sideways, forward, or backward when he is on hands and knees.

0–3 MONTHS NORMAL DEVELOPMENTAL LEVEL

Some Common Problems

Dislike of prone position. This may be due to early breathing difficulties, inability to turn the head and free the nose, inability to lift the head up, excessive flexion creating discomfort in prone, post-gastrostomy, severe visual impairment or even lack of opportunity given to lie on his stomach. Later a dislike of prone may be due to the child's inability to use his hands in prone.

Delayed development of head control, rising up on forearms, taking weight on forearms.

Delay in head turn without associated body turning.

Abnormal performance (Fig. 8.23) This includes asymmetrical head raise, rising on one forearm only, asymmetrical stabilization on elbows, excessive flexion of either of the arms (often caught under the child's body) or flexion of the trunk or legs, or all of them. The head may overextend when raised. Extensor thrusts persist. There may be more flexion-adduction in one leg than the other as the hips lift off the surface into flexion. One leg may flex and abduct into a forward creeping pattern with hips flexed off the surface or flat. This asymmetry of flexion is often greater in spastic diplegia than in tetraplegia.

Stages in prone development

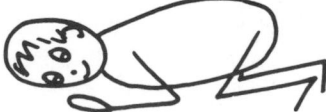

Fig. 8.8   Flexion posture decreases. Head turn (*0–3 months*).

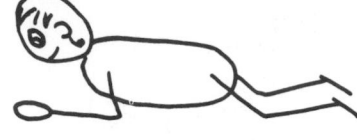

Fig. 8.9   Head raise and hold (*0–3 months*).

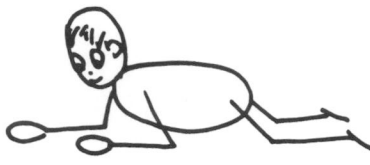

Fig. 8.10   Head raise, weight on forearms (*0–3 months*).

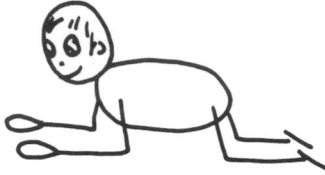

Fig. 8.11   On forearms and/or weight bearing on knees (*3–6 months*).

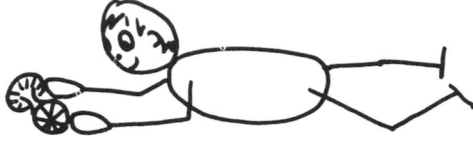

Fig. 8.12   Stretch forward to reach; stretch legs. Lean on one forearm and reach with the other arm (*3–6 months*).

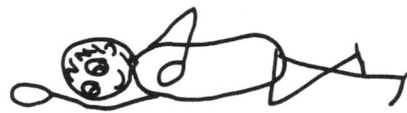

Fig. 8.13   Roll from prone to supine (*3–6 months*).

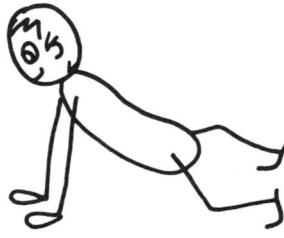

Fig. 8.14   Weight bearing on hands (*6–9 months*).

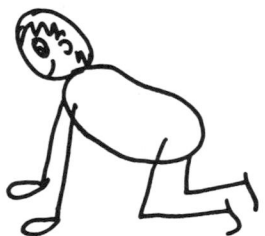

Fig. 8.15   Weight bearing on hands and knees (*6–9 months*).

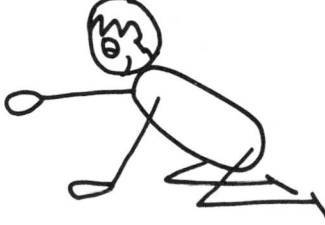

Fig. 8.16   Lean to one hand reach with the other (*7 months*).

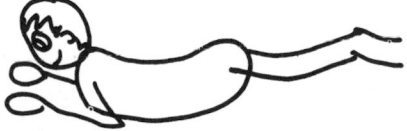

Fig. 8.17   Extend head, shoulders, hips pivot in prone position (*8 months*).

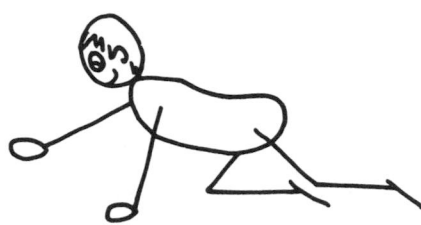

Fig. 8.18 Hands and knees, lift arm, leg or both (*8 months*).

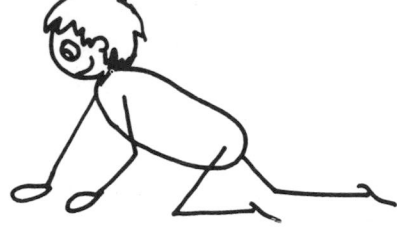

Fig. 8.19 Crawling. Rise into crawl position (*9 months*).

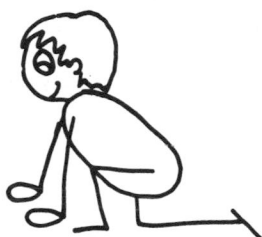

Fig. 8.20 Half-kneeling lean on hands (*11 months*).

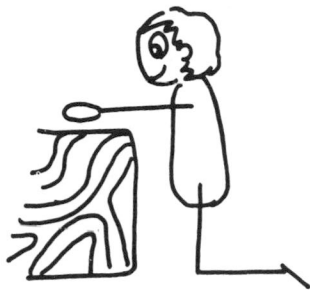

Fig. 8.21 Kneeling supported (*11 months*).

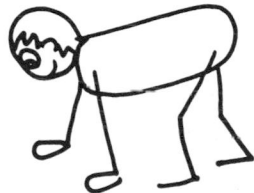

Fig. 8.22 Bear-walk (elephant walk) on hands and feet (*12 months*).

In tetraplegia and hypotonia very young children tend to show flexion-abduction of with flattened pelvis into the *frog position*. Hemiplegic children begin to creep and flex the good side whilst the hemiplegic side goes into extension-internal rotation. This is seen especially when the child raises his head and turns to the good side. Independent head raising in individual children is usually associated with flexion in the arms but extension of the back and especially of the legs into adduction-internal rotation. In normal babies the leg extension (especially at the next developmental level) is associated with abduction and external rotation.

Reflex reactions in prone. Flexor reaction to prone: arm flexor reaction: Galant's response, neck righting not beginning to diminish affecting head turn keeping body still. Appearance of head righting may be delayed.

Treatment Suggestions and Daily Care

Acceptance of prone position. Accustom the child to prone by placing him slowly on his stomach and on soft surfaces, such as sponge rubber, inflatable mattress, in warm water, over large soft beach ball, over your lap (adding a cushion if your knees are bony!). Gently bring his bent arms away from his chest and place them over an edge or curved surface, rock and sway a baby held in prone suspension. The child's face should be over the edge of the

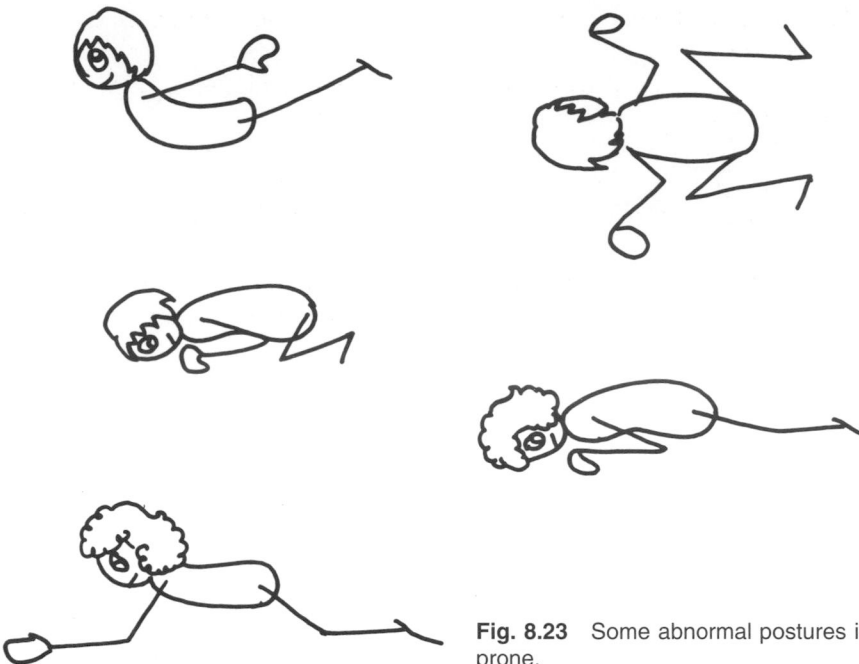

Fig. 8.23   Some abnormal postures in prone.

surface with the nose free. Training is given to help him turn his head to the side, if he cannot do this (see below).

The child may also be suspended in a blanket or hammock and gently rolled from side lying into prone lying and back until he accepts that last roll into prone lying. His nose should be over the edge of the blanket as he rolls over.

Note. Some children continue to strongly refuse to go prone and should not be forced to do so. Some of these are like able-bodied children who are *rollers* or *bottom shufflers* and a few others who do not use prone development in their motor development (Robson 1970). Cultural influences may affect use of prone.

Head control. Train these aspects of head control:

- Raising the head (righting).
- Holding the head steady (postural stability).

- Turning the head from side to side (counter-poising with movement).

(1) Place the child in prone across a sponge rubber roll, a beach ball, a wedge, pile of pillows or across your lap. Then elevate his arms and gently stretch them symmetrically across the surface or over the edge of the surface. Stiff arms may first have to be grasped near the shoulder joints and turned outwards as they are extended forwards over the edge of the apparatus or on the ball. If he reaches towards his object of interest, his head often raises as well. The child's legs may be abnormally bent or stiffly extended, turned in and held together, before or only during head raising. In such cases turn them out and keep his legs apart *while* he is initiating head control (Fig. 8.24). This allows anticipatory postural control without excessive use of adductor-extensor activity.

Rock the child forward and backwards over the edge of the roll/ball or inflatable mattress. Rhythmically tap under the child's chin to give momentum to lift the head. Tapping the child's forehead also helps, provided that he accepts having his face touched. Hold the child's shoulders on both sides symmetrically to keep his body stationary for head raise and turn.

(2) Bring his shoulders back and inwards towards his spine – this assists his active head raise. If the child persists in abnormal turning of his head to one side, then extend the shoulder girdle on the opposite side to activate head turn and raise to that side (Fig. 8.25). Place objects of interest on the opposite side as well.

(3) With the child's head over an edge continue to present him with interesting objects such

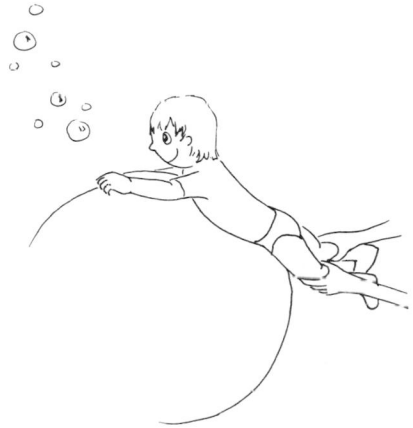

Fig. 8.24

as mobiles, Christmas decorations, mirrors, moving toys on springs or mechanically controlled, sounds from musical boxes, squeaky toys and mother's voice. At first use visual and auditory stimuli in the centre and progress to having them at each side of the child and move them slowly from centre to the side and from side to side. These stimuli obtain head control and eye fixation and tracking so that training of head control first associates with vision and also hearing. Later eye movements are learnt without head movement.

(4) Place wedge on a table or platform so that the child can see someone's face when he looks up. A friendly person obtains eye-to-eye contact by sitting in the centre and opposite the child, and sings or speaks to him and then gets him to move his eyes from side to side to follow her face.

(5) Keep wedge on the floor or in a sandpit or in front of a trough of water where other children are playing.

(6) Place child in prone on an inflatable mattress, large ball, water bed or trampoline and gently bounce him to stimulate and enjoy his active head raise.

(7) Swing a baby in prone over adult's arms or large child on a horizontal tyre suspended from a tree. Help a child to go down a slide while lying prone on a cushion. Place a child on a wedge on wheels or on a trolley with

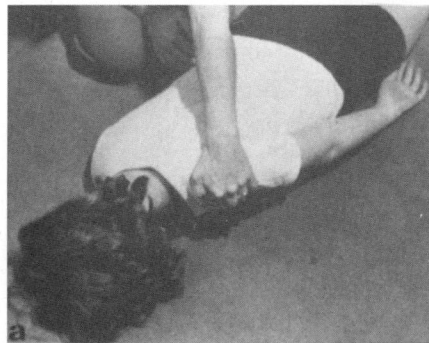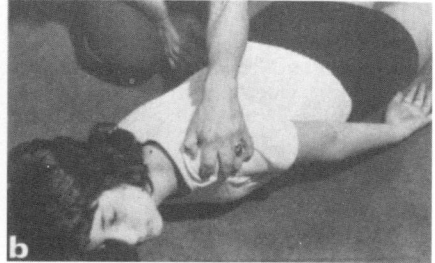

Fig. 8.25

a roll of towels between his body and upper arms.

(8) Weight bearing on forearms will also help the child's head control (Fig. 8.27). Give adequate support to a child's chest to prevent him hunching his shoulders. Check that the child's forearms are well away from the body, with elbows at right angles to body and, if possible, hands open. If the child's elbows still pull back against his

body, place a roll of towels between his body and his upper arms. Keep child's head and trunk centre, in alignment, legs apart, straight, turned out from hips.

Motivate a child to raise his head and look *down* and forward at a book or a toy in order to control hyperextension of head (Fig. 8.28). Help him with manual pressure down on his rounded back. Press his pelvis down for symmetrical weight bearing in lying. A small roll under his chest and between his shoulders overcomes hyperextension of head and body or retracted shoulder girdles. Reverse a child's position on the wedge so that he kneels over the

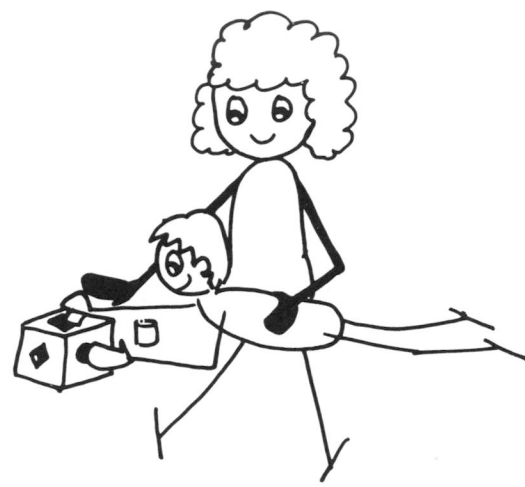

Fig. 8.26

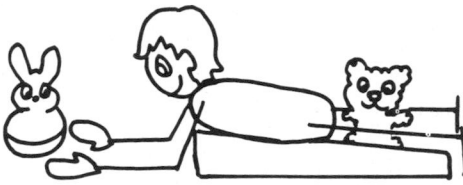

Fig. 8.27 Head control and weight bearing on forearms (on elbows). Prone, on forearms over low wedge, roll cushions. Keep legs apart and turned out in those cases where legs press together and/or twist inwards. Use a pommel, toy, small wedge or cushion for legs.

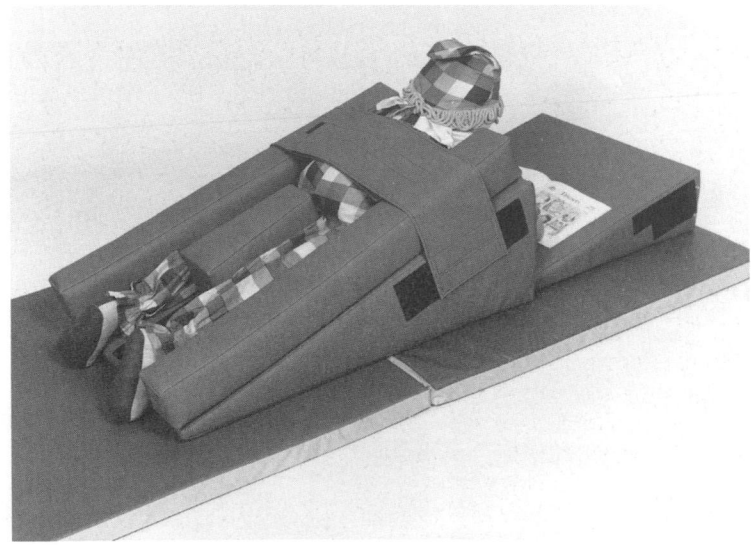

Fig. 8.28 Wedge with lateral supports, adjustable strap to prevent twisting of trunk, sliding or rolling off wedge. Abduction block to separate adducted legs. (With permission from Jenx, Sheffield, UK.)

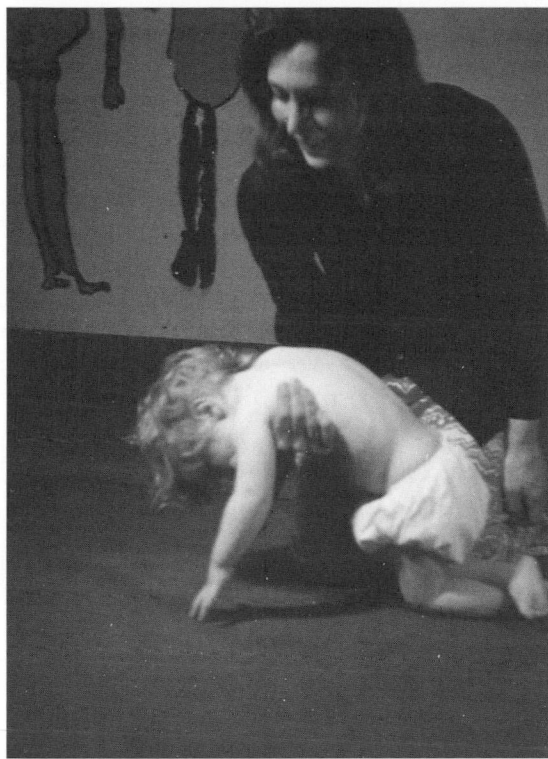

Fig. 8.29a Child needing head, shoulder and trunk control.

edge with his body fully supported in order to decrease lordosis and elongate a scoliotic spine (Fig. 8.29). Lying across your lap with his legs over the edge, feet flat on the ground, also overcomes lordosis and scolioses as he practises head control during play (Fig. 8.33, older child).

Equal weight on forearms. Weight bearing is often better on one side.

(1) Encourage the use of the more affected side by gently pushing the child's weight over it, whilst he is preoccupied with play. Also place toys in such a way that he leans on to the unstable side and uses his other arm to play. An older child should be informed, but not nagged, to do this as well. Give the child a toy to use with one arm while you gently

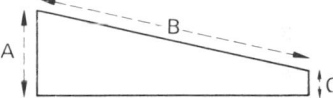

Fig. 8.29c Measurements for wedge for prone lying, arms over edge 'A'. A, Measurement from axilla to wrist. B, Measurement from axilla to 2 in (50 mm) above ankle. C. Length to top of foot.

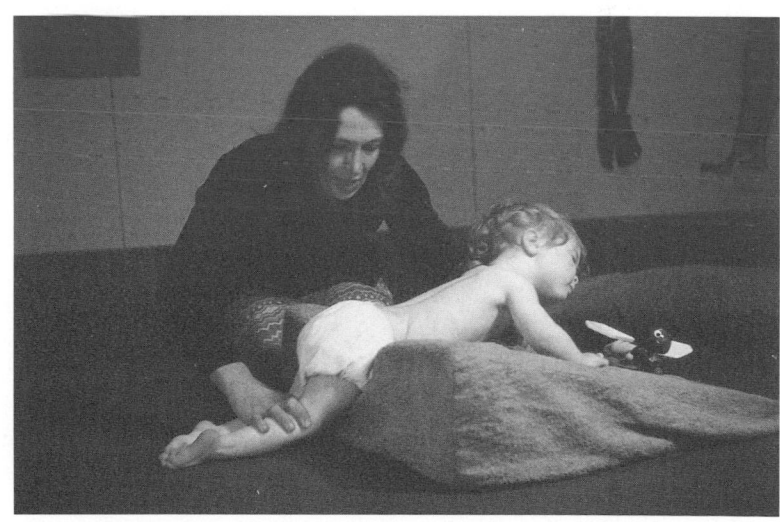

Fig. 8.29b Use wedge for weight bearing on knees. Straps may be needed to hold the child on the wedge. Also note child attempting head raise and a forearm support with pelvis support.

push his weight over and hold him on to the weaker weight-bearing side. As soon as possible remove your support and do not hold him during play. Reinforce this activity during feeding, washing and other functions in sitting and supported standing.

(2) When the child is in prone lying over a roll, pillows or wedge, press down on the top of his head in line with his neck (*chin in and long neck*) or down through the top of his shoulders increasing his weight bearing on to his elbows (see Figs 8.101, 8.102).

(3) Hold baby with his full weight through his elbows or on one elbow. Slightly shift his weight, first on to one elbow and then on to the other elbow. An older child can do this if you hold his legs up in the air while he takes weight on to his forearms. Hold his legs apart, turned outward and with straight hips and knees.

Note. Always try removing any supports given by your hands or equipment to check whether the child can lift the head or take weight on forearms on his own momentarily and with practice, reliably. Train a *long neck* with chin held in as well as head extension.

Physiotherapy Suggestions

Abnormal postures. Excessive flexion and other abnormal postures are corrected by the stimulation of head raise symmetrically, head turn to non-preferred side, weight bearing on forearms at right angles to chest, stretching child out symmetrically over rolls, wedges, mother's lap and by active extension movements and the active creeping patterns. General corrective positioning on special wedges with knee or elbow gaiters may be needed.

(1) *Activate symmetrical head raising* to look at therapist by either holding both the child's shoulders in extension or backward rotation. Try both arms elevated, abducted-external rotation behind the plane of his

head or by asking him to push his elevated arms back against your hands placed with pressure against his upper arms and straight elbows. Activate the chin in and long neck posture.

(2) *Facilitate head raise and turn* as in Fig. 8.25 or by lifting the child's elevated arm on one side back and behind the child's head to stimulate the creeping pattern (Fig. 8.30a). An older child can have arm on a cushion to actively practise the creeping action once the head turn is achieved.

Creeping patterns. It is difficult to describe these patterns without demonstration. Some aspects will be described as these techniques are particularly helpful to decrease flexion in prone, for muscle strengthening, lengthening and for activating early creeping on abdomen. Babies or severely involved older children are most responsive through automatic actions which can be used for learning the action later.

The *face arm* is elevated into shoulder abduction-external rotation (Fig. 8.30b). The *occiput arm* is brought down into shoulder extension-adduction internal rotation (Fig. 8.30c). The child may lie flat on the surface or over the edge of a roll, small pillow or wedge.

(1) Assisted active changing of the arms so that the opposite arm is elevated whilst the face arm moves down. These arm actions facilitate head raise and turn, back extension and, when on a surface, leg creeping movements.

(2) Use of stretch-rotation and appropriate manual resistance will activate the creeping movements of limbs with body-pelvic rotations.

(3) The child may continue active creeping on his own and so acquire one form of locomotion beginning at this level of development.

(4) Rising onto forearm can be stimulated by having the elevated *face arm* held stationary by your hand. You stretch the *occiput arm*

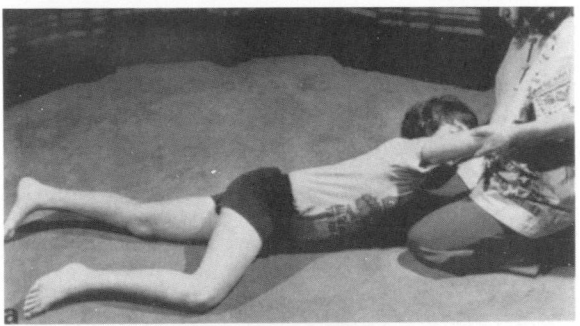

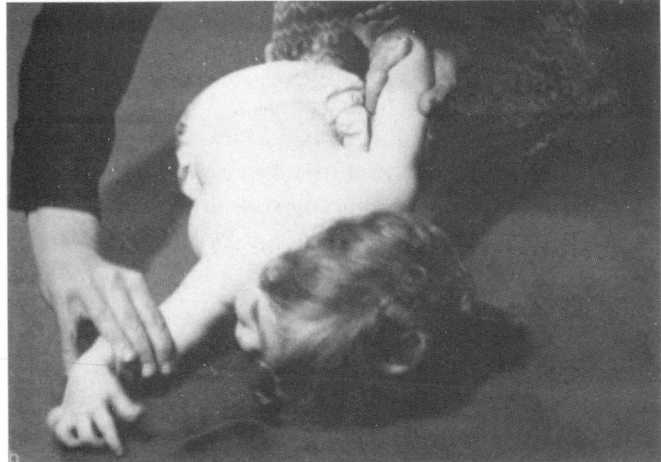
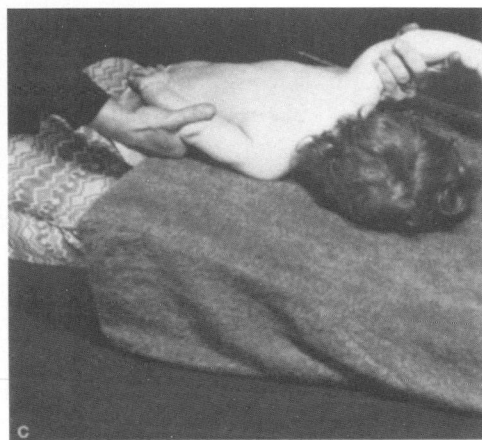

Fig. 8.30a–c

with manual resistance to the rebound creeping action response. If the child understands, ask him to pull his arm forward and above his head. An automatic rising reaction on to the forearm of the face arm occurs. As the child rises, he also raises and turns his head. Sensing the rising provides a strategy he can use later.

(5) Using action of leg for creeping involves single leg flexion-abduction-external rotation, preferably with pelvic rotation backward. The other leg is held in extension-adduction-*external* rotation. Legs should be held at the thigh and knee using stretch-rotation and resistance according to the young child's reaction. (See also Fig. 8.30a.)

(6) Active leg creeping may stimulate arm creeping actions. If the child understands, ask him to bend his hip and knee up and out against your hand on his thigh to have full pelvic rotation backwards. Offer him enough resistance to augment his movement so that an associated arm action to creep is gained.

This creeping technique is useful for activation of more affected arms or the hemiplegic arm of babies or severely affected children. Movement and/or rising is initiated.

There are many possibilities for automatic rising reactions and other stabilizing and movement reactions with Vojta's creeping techniques in addition to my own modifications. However, they are best demonstrated and supervision given by physiotherapists experienced in this approach.

Modified creeping over mother's lap or down a slippery wedge/incline is enjoyed by children. Once automatic creeping is experienced by a child, he needs to use it actively to reach an object or person he wishes to touch.

Train active rising on to both forearms or later hands at the same time. Hold the child's head by spanning his occiput between his ears. Ask him to raise his head up against your manual pressure. This pressure and sometimes manual resistance facilitates rising on to his forearms or hands, and teaches him to initiate rising with head action.

Augment head holding, and forearm support by asking child to maintain head posture as you push his head out of position. Encourage child to pull his chin inwards getting *a long neck*. Also give manual nudge or push to front, side, back of shoulders, as child is told to 'stay there' or 'don't let me push you down' or simply 'hold it'.

Note. Use of resistance is recommended for stabilizing and strengthening the athetoid (dyskinetic) ataxic and hypotonic types of cerebral palsy. In all types of cerebral palsy manual resistance needs to be controlled so that there is no abnormal overflow such as extensor spasms or flexor spasms.

4–6 MONTHS NORMAL DEVELOPMENTAL LEVEL

Common Problems

Delay in acquisition of rising on knees, rising on to hands with extended pelvis, weight bearing on knees, knees and forearms and on one forearm, reaching for objects, inability to lie prone with both or one of the arms stretched and reaching overhead, unable to roll over to supine, or unable to creep on abdomen, on elbows or using a variety of creeping movements of both arms and legs.

Abnormal performance. Asymmetric, abnormal positions of limbs, clenching hands during the activities, beginning *mermaid crawl* (see 6–9 months' level), asymmetric weight-bearing.

Abnormal rising patterns in prone include child pulling his knees up under his abdomen on his forearm support, then pushing up on to his hands; child rising on to his knees only with head and trunk flexed over bent arms; arms may not be used at all or he pushes up on semiflexed arms with clenched or open hands; child rising on to hands first and using his hands to push himself backwards into heel sitting (*W sitting*).

Although useful for a child, these patterns need modification to achieve weight bearing on hands, with elbows as straight as possible and avoiding excessive hip and pelvic flexion.

Reflex reactions may persist from the earlier level partly confirming diagnoses of cerebral palsy in young children. Back extension and head control activities counter any persisting reflexes.

Treatment Suggestions and Daily Care

Rising on to knees, forearms and knees. Encourage the child's rising on to knees instead of your lifting the child each time. Place one leg in creeping position and hold firmly or fix the foot against a heavy box, tip the child's *opposite* hip and pelvis up and back with a slight touch and wait for active rise on to knees, first on to the one that is fixed. The other leg creeps forward on to its knee. Carry this out without giving the child a *tip-up* at his hip, *if he can manage alone* as in Fig. 8.31. Use instruction 'Knee forward and get up!' Rising onto forearms, and later, hands are usually activated as well.

Weight bearing on knees, on forearms and knees (4–6 months), on hands and knees, on hands with abdomen on the ground, or on hands over a wedge (6–9 months) (Fig. 8.32).

Fig. 8.31 Rising onto knees and arms.

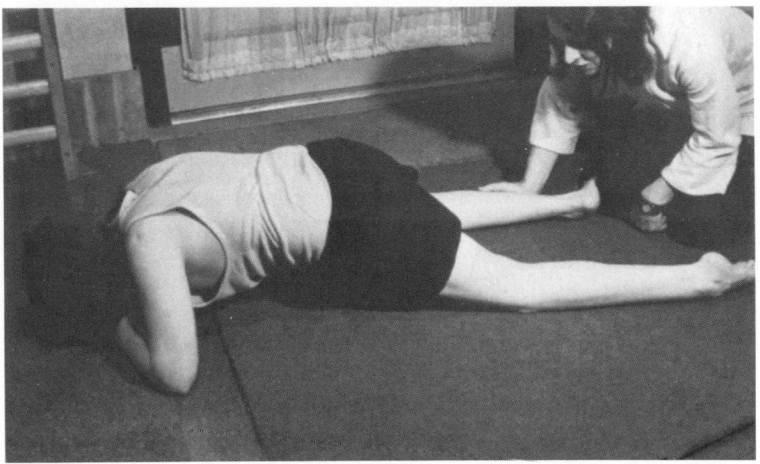

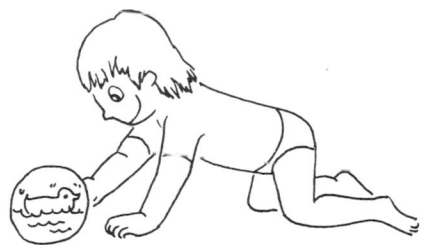

Fig. 8.32 On hands and knees unsupported (*6–9 months*).

Place the child on his knees, knees and forearms, hands and knees or on his hands with straight elbows with abdomen on the ground, according to what he can manage at his level of development.

(1) If there is tightness of hips and knee flexors, use *on hands* support with back, hips (buttocks) and legs straight. Press his pelvis down on both sides at the same time.

(2) Use your lap, wedges, rolls, pillows, suspension in blanket, sponge rubber shapes or big soft toys for support until the child can balance alone.

(3) Use interesting toys, balls, sand and water play in these positions.

(4) Have hips at right angles when he takes weight on his knees. Active use of the hands

also increases greater weight bearing on knees for stability.

(5) Press down on the child's lower back and buttocks to increase his weight bearing on his knees, and prevent sliding of his knees during his play with his hands, or *shoot out into extension*, or sideways into *frog position*.

(6) Use elbow splints to help weight bearing on hands with straight elbows, so that shoulders develop stability during these weight-bearing activities.

(7) Open the child's hands by pressing his weight through the heels of his hands; by gently bringing the thumbs out from their bases and not from their tips. Press palms flat with joint compression through the length of the arm. Keep elbows straight. Do this while a child watches television for interest so that he maintains the position for a period.

Unstable weight bearing through the arms (Fig. 8.33a–b) Joint compression through the arm to develop stability on hands in prone, in sitting or standing positions (Fig. 8.33a–b). A low table is used for child's arm-propping support. Press through the top of the child's shoulder and/or through the straight elbow. Arm must be in straight alignment with the line of pressure

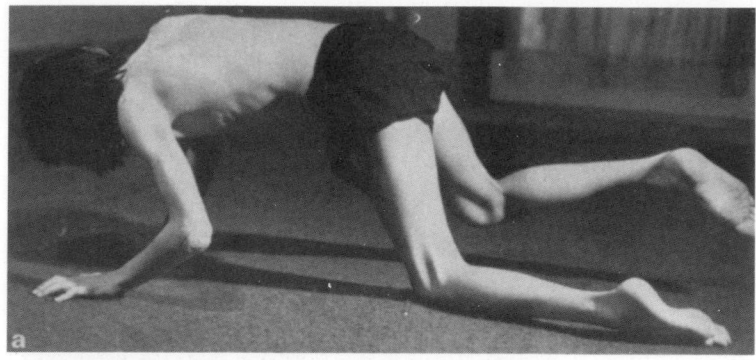

Fig. 8.33a Unstable shoulder and pelvic girdles with excessive action of elbow and knee flexors to maintain balance (postural control).

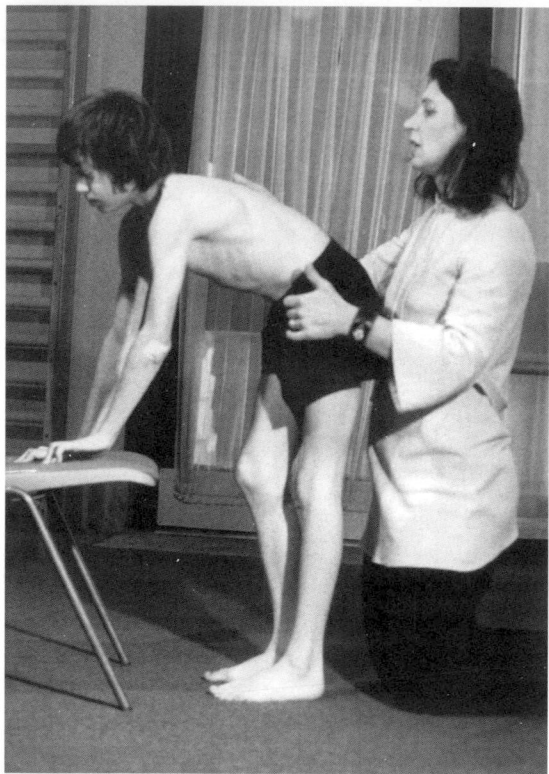

Fig. 8.33b Training stability with weight-shift of shoulder and pelvic girdles in four-point standing – a modification of developmental sequence.

through shoulder or elbow. Keep weight through heel of his hand to avoid finger flexion. Arms may also be placed on a surface below the child so that the weight of his body adds to the joint compression, e.g. on a stool below the plinth on which he lies. Child *walks on hands*

with his elbow splints, for similar effects. Use a variety of floor textures to increase tactile experience.

Motor control actions for daily activities. These can also be learnt in four-point standing and in prone-stander with table.

(1) Weight bearing on one forearm, reach with the other. Weight bear and shift from forearm to forearm. Encourage reach with one arm on floor, then above his head and in different positions to obtain objects.

(2) With the child bearing weight on both fore-arms give him toys in each hand to grasp and play with. Let him grasp the ends of a bicycle pump, concertina, plastic bottle, transparent cylinder with coloured water or marbles inside, grasp two balls or blocks to bang together or push a ball from hand to hand. Toys should move or make a noise if touched, patted, pressed or grasped. Remove any supporting wedge and hold the child on one of his forearms while he actively uses the other arm in play. Whenever possible remove adult support altogether (see the section on Development of hand function in this chapter).

(3) Child in prone lying on forearms on thick soft sponge, inflatable mattress, water bed, trampoline, press the surface down on each side so that the child tips on to his elbow. Do this to a song or rhythm to develop weight bearing and weight shift on forearms.

(4) Place a child on a low platform or low wedge on wheels with the legs held in abduction with abduction splint or a pommel. The child will move forwards and also *backwards*. If he is on a bed and wishes to get off he could then move himself backwards so that his legs come off the edge of the bed, his feet take the weight and he can stand up leaning on elbows and progress to supporting himself on his hands with his body against the bed (see Fig. 10.2).

Note. Do *not* use creeping on forearms on a prone-trolley or a 'forearm drag' along the floor in those cases where there is a tendency to tight elbow flexion and shoulder hunching, but rather practise weight bearing on one elbow whilst he tries stretching out for toys with the other arm and also stretching both arms well forward to toy or to push a big ball away. Use another form of locomotion as well.

Arms stretched overhead and forward: arm saving reactions in prone: propping reactions

(1) Encourage a child to reach forward and overhead for toys, to push away a ball, balloon or toy on wheels. Older children can walk their hands up a wall or wall bars as far as possible (Fig. 10.1). Use a small bolster or wedge to help him stretch his arms out *and* up towards toys on a box or suspended above him.
(2) Place a child over a beach ball or large roll with his arms over the top. Tip the ball forward and encourage him to reach for the ground to save himself from falling. Encourage him to prop himself on his hands by placing his hands on the ground, to *stand on his hands* whilst you hold his body safely on the ball. You can hold the body of a young child and tip him upside down near a surface, e.g. a table, and encourage him to put his arms out to save himself and then to take weight on them (Fig. 8.24). Provide different tactile surfaces for hand propping.

(3) Palce the child on his abdomen on a large cushion with his arms stretched forward, and help him to go safely down a slide head first.

Note. The therapist needs to check whether positions of arms and legs are correct during all the activities above, for example:

- Shoulders and hips at right angles in weight-bearing positions.
- Knees pointed outwards without a *frogging* position.
- Hips and knees straight, apart, and if possible turned outwards.
- Shoulders and arms turned out or in midline rather than in excessive internal rotation.
- Hands open and palms down if weight bearing.

It is important to recognize that *all the training* of weight bearing on elbows, one elbow, hands may be done in *sitting* or *standing* leaning forward down on to a low table or box. This reinforces the prone development *or* if prone is occasionally not indicated for a particular child, these activities can and need to be trained in these other positions (Fig. 8.33a,b).

Rolling from prone to supine. See physiotherapy suggestions for rolling and roll-and rise in the section on supine development. Weight shift from side to side with arm and shoulder, or leg and pelvic rotation to enable achievement of rolling from prone.

Physiotherapy Suggestions

Facilitate rising for assumption of four-point position which becomes more independent in the next developmental stage.

(1) Fix one of the child's legs in creeping position manually (Fig. 8.34). Press down through his buttocks. Alternatively, hold his other leg above or below the knee and stretch it into extension-adduction-

external rotation which stimulates leg forward creep and rise onto the other knee. If the child understands he should be instructed to *bend* a hip and knee. The child can then rise onto hands with or without chest support.

(2) When a child is actively able to commence or even complete rising up on to knees and forearms, but is weak, then manual resistance is used to reinforce his efforts. Apply manual resistance at the pelvis in a diagonal direction (Fig. 8.35) for better muscle activation and avoidance of stimulating spasticity.

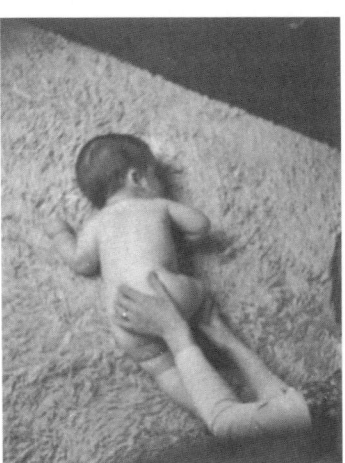

Fig. 8.34

Augment holding on hands and knees

(1) The child attempts to maintain this position as the therapist slowly pushes him:

- Laterally at each hip or each shoulder
- Anteroposteriorly at hip or shoulders
- At opposite shoulder and hip
- At shoulder and hip on the same side.

(2) Resistance to head movements and to shoulders *stay there* (see on forearms, above). Similarly use resistance for hips when child is on knees with chest and arms supported by roll or stool.

6–9 MONTHS NORMAL DEVELOPMETNAL LEVEL

Common Problems

Delay in weight bearing on hands and knees, in lifting one or two limbs, weight bearing on one hand and reaching for objects, crawling on hands or on knees, pivot position and absence of rising from prone to hands and knees.

Abnormal performance of motor abilities, over-flexed hips, knees or feet, internally rotated legs or arms, lack of reciprocation in crawling, *bunny hopping* both knees forward in heel sitting, asymmetrical weight bearing. Prone

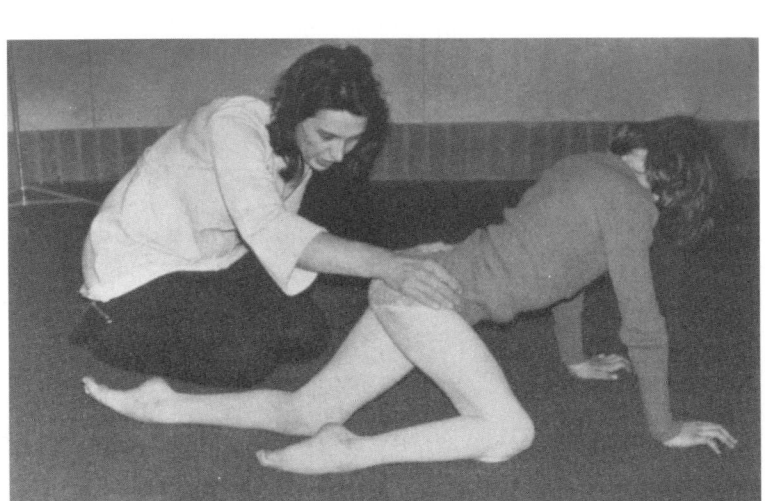

Fig. 8.35

mermaid crawl or *commando crawl* by pulling forward on his flexed arms with his legs stiffly extended, adducted and internally rotated. The hands may clench with each *pull* forward and often the legs adduct strongly with this pull.

Lack of postural fixation of the pelvis and hips creates creeping on the abdomen and masks the child's ability to take weight on hands at 6 months level of the development of crawling on all fours.

Absence of reactions expected at 6–9 months level in prone, absence of Landau, saving reactions in arms, tilting reactions in prone. Persistence of any early reactions, see 0–3 months level.

Treatment Suggestions and Daily Care

See Figs 8.32 and 8.33 and add the following.

Weight bearing on one hand, reach for a toy and on hands and knees lift one arm or leg or both. Place the child on hands or on hands and knees over rolls or your arm and when possible let him balance on his own:

(1) Lift individual limbs whilst he maintains balance to a song or counts.
(2) While child takes weight on his hands or hands and knees, encourage him to stroke different textures on the ground, e.g. carpets, linoleum, cool and warm surfaces, scratchy and smooth surfaces.
(3) While balancing on hands and knees he might scrub the floor, reach for a dangling toy, roll balls, move small toys on wheels, dig into the sandpit with one hand or a spade, on the grass he could pick flowers, handfuls of grass and so on. He can stretch a leg to kick tinkling toy bells, or touch a person in a game.

These activities develop counterpoising of limb movements. See 'counterpoising exercises' below, to augment ability.

Crawling. This can be trained with the child suspended in a blanket. Hold each end of the blanket and tip the child in it so that his weight is taken more on one side, releasing the other side for a 'step' forward. Guide the moving knee if necessary.

Note. It is important to avoid the use of crawlers and the training of crawling in children who have tight hip and knee flexors. In these cases use a wedge on wheels or prone-trolley with towels rolled under the child's chest so that his elbows are straight and his hands touch the floor. The child crawls on his hands whilst his legs are held extended on the platform. Play 'walking-on-hands' or 'wheelbarrow' with adult supporting child's legs in a straight hip-knee position. Weight-shift from hand to hand develops counterpoising of trunk muscles. In cases of severe knee and elbow flexion, splintage of these joints should be used as the child gets about on his platform on wheels.

Rolling. Encourage rolling on grass down a slight incline, on sponge rubber, on an inflatable mattress down a mound and on different surfaces.

Physiotherapy Suggestions

Flexion or lack of postural stability of head, shoulder girdle and hips in extension positions may be treated with techniques on wedges (small and large) already mentioned and with pivot prone. Pivot prone or Landau position is activated by a head raise to extend body and legs with legs held in abduction.

● This can be carried out on a large ball, roll.
● Also elevate-abduct-externally rotate arms behind plane of head to stretch spine and arms.

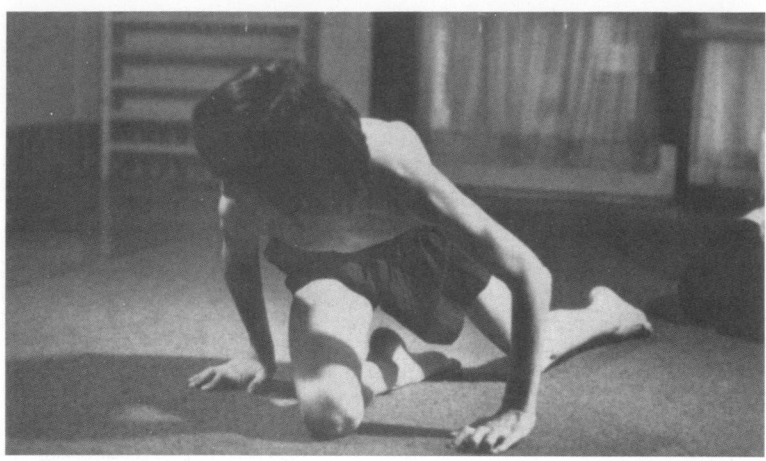

Fig. 8.36 Instability of pelvic and shoulder girdles and a poor counterpoising. Unstable crawling and stationary four-point posture.

- Older children using pivot prone and action of arms can strengthen shoulder girdle stabilizing muscles and trunk by pulling against weights over pulleys opposite them.
- Pivot to each side is taught to a child for some mobility on the floor. Weight-shift on the body and pelvis is developed and also overcomes abnormal weight bearing on only one side. Pivoting to each side is unlikely to transfer to standing owing to different gravity conditions.

Note. The extension in pivot prone is not enough for standing. Postural fixation of the head, trunk and hips in the vertical must be trained (see the section on Development of standing and walking).

Counterpoising exercises. Child maintains balance on hands and knees and carries out arm or leg patterns to achieve counterpoising. See Fig. 8.36 for person with instability needing the counterpoising (postural adjustment) exercises.

Leg pattern. Ask the child to bend one knee up to the ceiling; manually resist his knee flexion forward and outward. Then reverse to hip and knee extension with adduction and external rotation (Figs 8.37–8.38). Resistance given to leg pattern will also increase stabilization at the shoulder girdle and opposite hip at the same time.

Arm pattern. Use creeping pattern of child's arm from extension-adduction-internal rotation behind his back, facilitated to elevation-abduction-external rotation as described at the earlier levels (Fig. 8.30). Other arm patterns are arm flexion adduction across chest, change to abduction-extension-external rotation with trunk rotation backwards. As the child moves his one arm against resistance, he increases weight bearing or stabilization on the other three points. If he is on his hands only, abdomen on the floor, shoulder stabilization and counterpoising are stimulated, as follows: he balances on the one hand as single arm pattern of movement is carried out actively or against correctly given resistance.

(1) Continue pivoting in extension or other additional limb and trunk active extension for any continued flexion patterns.
(2) Continue rising on to hands *and* knees as above or roll-and-rise (see Fig. 8.65a and b in Supine development).
(3) Child crawls against resistance given to his knees. Grasp his knees and guide them outward as you resist each step forward (Fig. 8.39).

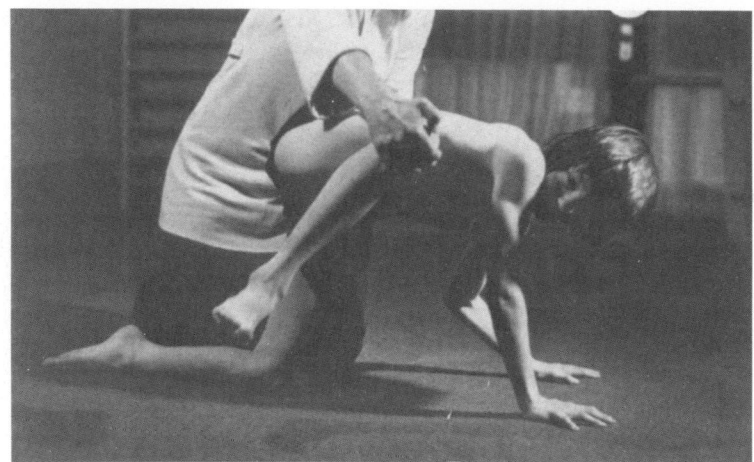

Fig. 8.37   Counterpoising exercises.

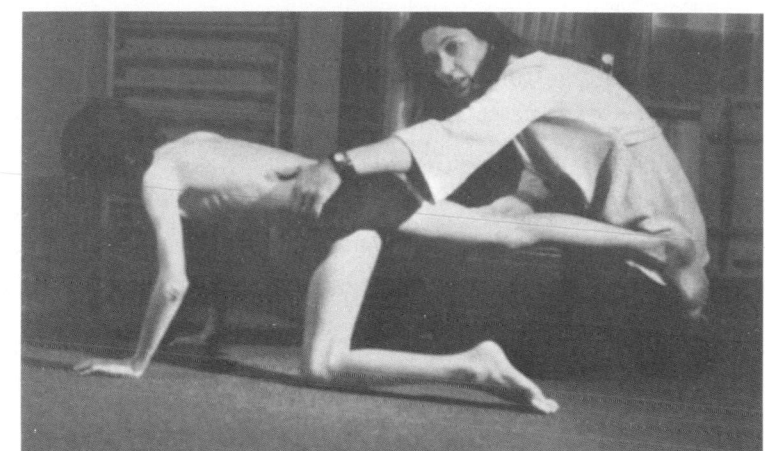

Fig. 8.38   Counterpoising exercises.
Positions of therapist's hands.
Child's leg flexion against hand on
thigh or pull against hand on tibia.
Leg extension against hand on tibia.

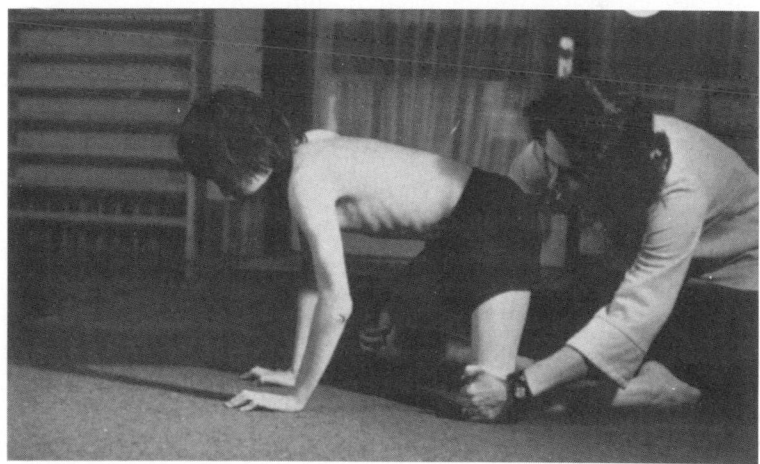

Fig. 8.39   Crawling against manual
resistance of therapist – guidance
or resistance of knee into external
rotation avoids adduction and offers
a wider base for balance.

(4) Augment holding the hands and knees posture against nudge or manual resistance. Concentrate on pelvic girdle stability for children who hop with both knees together in 'bunny-hopping' crawl. Suggestions to discourage bunny hopping are given below.

Items 3 and 4 overlap into the next stage of development.

9–12 MONTHS NORMAL DEVELOPMENTAL LEVEL

Common Problems

Delay in rhythmic independent reciprocal crawling, maintaining half-kneeling position hands on ground, on hands and feet and other more advanced postures. Absence of rising from hands and knees to standing holding a support, and inability to change from prone to sitting, prone to squatting, prone to supported half-kneeling while grasping support or hands on floor. Changes of posture are poor.

Abnormal performance. Excessive adduction-internal rotation of hips in crawling, in half-kneeling and weight bearing on hands and feet. If the child can *bear-walk* on hands and feet, he has his heels off the ground and/or excessive flexion of the knees with hips internally rotated and adducted. Pull up to standing uses an excessive leg extension with adduction and plantar flexion.

Absence of reflex reactions expected at 9–12 months in prone for example Landau, saving reaction in arms propping responses on tipping forward, sideways and backwards. Persistence of remnants of earlier reflex reactions, see previous levels.

Treatment Suggestions and Daily Care

Half-kneeling. Sit the child on the side of your lap when you sit on the ground. Bring his outside knee on to the floor, he is then kneeling on one knee, hold the other knee forward and outward. Remove your lap and place his hands on the floor for support. Encourage him to play in this position by moving a car or rolling a ball under the *bridge* of his knee, round his foot, or spend time in tying his boot laces, count his toes, paint his toe nails and so on. Later, he should grasp horizontal bars, at various levels, place his hands flat on the wall, low tables or your flat hands. Half-kneeling position should be maintained with the front knee pointing outward. Hold his knee out with his foot pointing out and placed out to the side. This is often difficult. Ask the child to press his front knee outwards against your hand and also maintain balance. Augment his balance by offering manual resistance to his hips at the side, shoulder girdle at the side and shoulder and hip girdles at the same time.

Whilst on hands in half-kneeling and also in upright half-kneeling, grasp a support. Manual resistance may also be used. In addition head lift against resistance applied between his ears across the lower occiput helps to augment the stabilization.

Rising from prone to standing. Once the half-kneeling position is assumed it should continue as a transitional position on the way to standing up. Assumption of half-kneeling takes place using the exercise in Figs 8.37–8.38. In Fig. 8.40 the therapist is helping the child place his foot flat on the ground. Figure 8.41 shows how to hold the knee and foot steady as the child rises. Another method is to hold the child's body under his chest whilst he controls his limbs, or for the child to grasp supports from the hands-and-knees position and pull himself up to standing via the half-kneeling position. You may also ask the child to rise against your hand, pressing his lower back and pelvis as in Fig. 8.41.

Note. The application of manual resistance must be done by physiotherapists as careful control of any abnormal overflow of undesir-

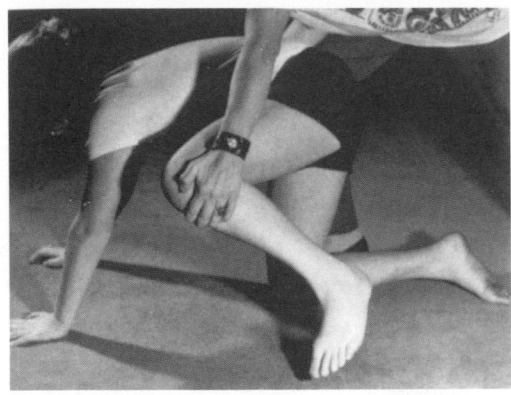

Fig. 8.40 Assumption of half-kneeling against the manual resistance or guidance of a therapist.

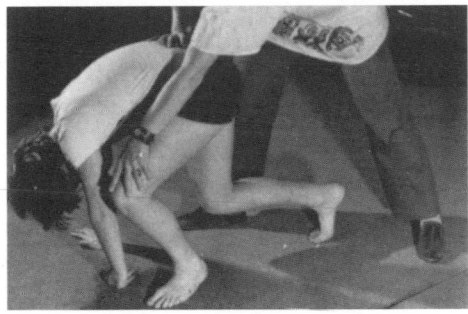

Fig. 8.41 Assumption of standing against manual resistance or guidance of a therapist.

able activity with appropriate degree of manual resistance is important.

See also other patterns of rising from prone in Fig. 8.179. Children have their own strategies which are acceptable provided that they do not aggravate deforming motor patterns.

Weight taken on hands and feet, and bear-walk. The child may place his hands on a low stool if he cannot easily reach the ground. Stabilization together with gentle passive stretching of tight hamstrings is carried out in this position. In addition the counterpoising exercises and activities of play, dressing, or other tasks can be done in this position and are illustrated in the development of standing at the 9–12 month developmental level (Figs 8.33b, 8.163, 8.164).

Stepping on hands and feet can be carried out using a stool on wheels, sliding a low chair, with a sledge or stable wooden toy on wheels. Hold the child's thighs and knees straight and turned outward if there is any abnormal flexion-adduction-internal rotation. Give manual resistance to the stepping leg whilst holding the standing knee straight, to stretch tight hamstrings or increase the action of the fixators of the hip. Wearing knee gaiters for the bear walk or for slow upright stepping prevents the overuse of knee flexion *and* activates the stabilizers of the pelvic girdle. Joint compression through hips or knees of the standing leg also helps this stability so that knee flexors do not need to overact.

Many normal children do not bear walk but this is desirable in cerebral palsy, or motor delay for stabilization of shoulder girdle (lean on hands) and pelvic girdle, stretching of tight hamstrings, stretching of tight heel cords (heels kept flat on the ground) as well as the counterpoising of each limb as a step is taken.

Hyperextended knees may be treated in the bear walk (see Fig. 8.170).

Increasing stability of the hips is associated with a decrease of hyperextension of the knees which may be a compensation for lack of postural stability of hips and pelvis.

Tilt reactions and saving reactions in limbs on hands and knees may be stimulated on a rocker board, inflatable mattress or thick soft sponge rubber (Fig. 8.42). However they are not as important in prone-kneeling as in the upright postures.

Changes of posture from prone kneeling (on hands and knees) to sitting and back again, to prone lying and back again, to half-kneeling and back again, and many other changes as in the righting reactions, should be trained at this level of development. See the development of sitting at this level. These activities overlap into all the other channels. They have been initiated at earlier levels in prone (see above).

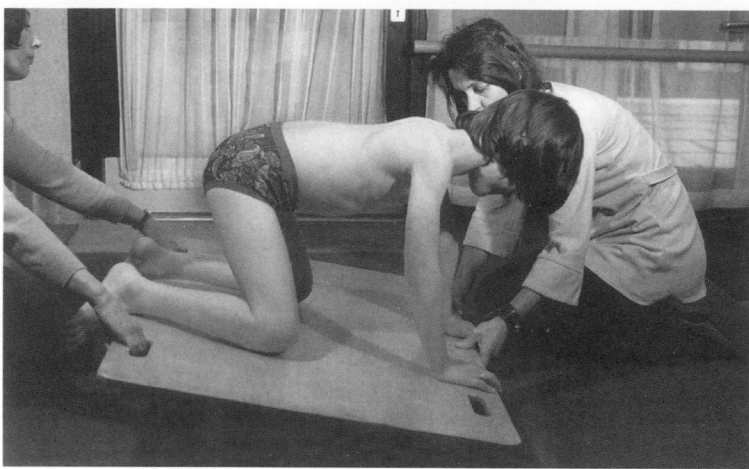

Fig. 8.42 Tilt responses activated on a rocker board.

Problem of bunny hopping. Reciprocal crawling rather than the continual bunny hopping of both knees forward is expected at this developmental level. Unstable pelvis, excessive tightness of hip and knee flexors and also habit, prolong bunny hopping and aggravate these problems, as well as adding deformities of the feet. Discourage bunny hopping by offering other means of locomotion such as the prone board on casters for prone lying with hips and knees straight, a tricycle, pedal car, and preferably walkers, with knees in gaiters, if necessary. Training children to bottom shuffle is also a good alternative and easily trained and learnt by many children. The child sits with feet in front on the ground. He leans on his hands at his sides, presses his feet flat on the ground and stretches out his knees and moves along the ground, backwards, or forwards. Avoid bottom-shuffling in side sitting to prevent any hip subluxation or asymmetry.

Encourage crawling on all surfaces, sand, grass, carpets, tiles, as well as using crawling on to a large step made with mattresses, wood or concrete, and climb in and out of boxes, cubby holes, through tunnels and under tables.

Discourage crawling in children with tight hip and knee flexors and equinus feet. Practise other forms of locomotion with extension of legs. Older people with cerebral palsy usually prefer not to learn crawling activities.

Training upright kneeling. This is discussed here as the child rises from prone positions to this position. Kneeling upright holding on to a support is expected at about 9–12 months whilst kneeling alone only at about 15 months in normal child development (Gesell 1971).

Do not use this position in children who persist with hip flexion, lordosis or hip-knee-dorsiflexion in this position and do not respond to control of these postures. Control this by pressure against the extended hip and keeping the knees at right angles. The back is held straight by the child leaning his trunk against a sofa or holding the arms forward with elbows straight for reach and grasp a support or for leaning on hands. However, all this may not really control every child's deformities.

Use upright kneeling if the abnormalities can be controlled (usually in athetoid and ataxic types of cerebral palsy and for motor delay) to develop vertical pelvic stability and postural stability of trunk on pelvis before standing supported is possible. Usually standing supported *is* possible if well controlled and is preferable.

However, in children with deformities of the feet, plantigrade feet are not available for the standing position. Upright kneeling achievement in such a child confirms the need for surgery or plasters for the feet which are then preventing standing. Naturally knee flexors must also be checked for deformity.

Upright kneeling balance in kneel standing, knee walking sideways and forwards and backwards and kneeling on a rocker board may be useful in some children, if, for any reason these activities cannot be carried out in standing.

SUPINE DEVELOPMENT

The following main features should be developed:

Postural stability of the shoulder girdle as the child holds the arm up in the air for reach, reach and grasp and other hand function and hand–eye coordination, beginning about 4 months normally when the hands are held in midline in, say, *hand regard*, at 5 months during reach for an object. (See the section on basic arm and hand patterns for all levels of development under Development of hand function and also Table 8.4.)

Postural stability of the pelvis as the child holds a leg up in the air, say, at 7 months in order to grasp his foot with his hand; at 5 months when a child *bridges* his hips off the surface *without* using back extensor spasm to do so.

Counterpoising the limbs in the air (Fig. 8.43). Children who cannot do this tip over when they are on their backs in water. Thus, holding a limb up in the air with absence of a hard surface increases a demand on the musculature needed for counterpoising, and reveals its inadequacy. Developmental level may be about 5–7 months when normal children hold their limbs steady in the air. Head, arm, leg raise and hold increases

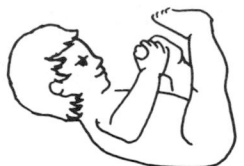

Fig. 8.43 Postural stability and counterpoising of the limbs.

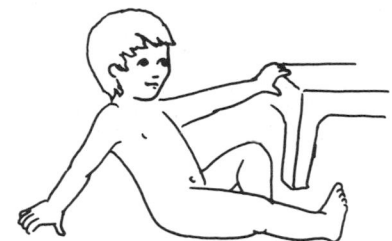

Fig. 8.44 Rising from supine.

weight bearing and weight shift on trunk and pelvis.

Rising reactions (Fig. 8.44). These are probably the most important reactions or activities to be trained in supine development. Many abnormal postures and abnormal reactions are particularly obvious in supine. Training the child to get out of supine involves counteracting most of these problems. This training seems to be preferable to spending time training the child's position in supine, except for severely immobile children who cannot manage this. Supine, *head rising* (righting) and the *overcoming of head lag* prepares and trains rising out of supine. Various *rolling-and-rising* sequences of motion, e.g. roll and rise on to hands and knees, roll to prone and rise; roll half-way to side-lying or side-sitting; roll half-way and grasp a support and pull to sitting or standing, should be trained. If these are impossible, other patterns must be found as, say, in the athetoid child in fig. 8.70. Rising is important as supine is a position of particular helplessness. Rising also contributes to a child's learning to get out of bed and turn at night.

Postural stabilization of the head (Fig. 8.45) is not head raising and requires special training. Head control is raising *and* holding of the head as well as head turning. Head holding is expected at 4–6 months normally, either in supine on surface with head held off the surface, or, if a baby is held suspended horizontally in supine and he holds his head alone in this position, in midline.

Note. Normal asymmetries, abnormal asymmetries and other aspects are discussed below. Pivoting on the back using weight-shift to each side and lateral arm and leg movements so that the child can move in circles may also be required in some children. *Tilt reactions* and *saving reactions* (Fig. 8.46) are less important in supine than in sitting and standing.

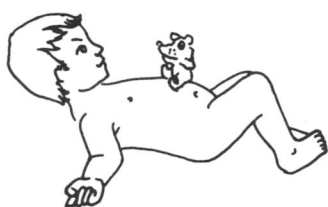

Fig. 8.45   Postural stability of the head.

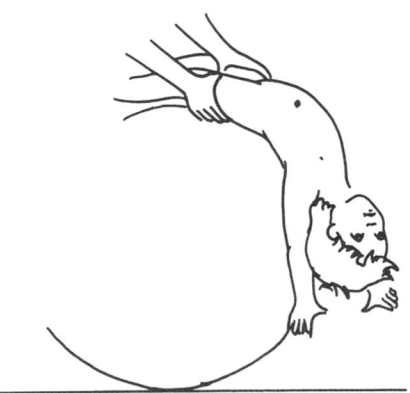

Fig. 8.46   Arms saving (parachute) reaction from supine.

TREATMENT SUGGESTIONS AND DAILY CARE FOR ALL LEVELS OF DEVELOPMENT

Supine Rise to Sitting and Development of Head Righting (Rising)

From 0–6 months normal development level. Help the child *to overcome head lag* using all or some of the following suggestions:

(1) First have the child lying half-way down against a back support or cushions, and encourage him to come up to sitting. Gradually lower the back support so that eventually he raises his head and trunk from supine to sitting.

(2) At first you will also have to hold his shoulders well forward, then later his upper arms and, as soon as possible, have him grasp your hands with his elbows straight. In these ways pull the child up to sitting, *waiting* for his own active head raise and later head and trunk (righting) raising. Some children bring their heads up first, their trunks follow. In others trunks may come up first and stimulate the head next (head-on-body righting; body-on-head righting).

Carry out (1) and (2) slowly from supine or half-lying to sitting and lower the child back from sitting to supine without his collapse.

(3) Many children manage to raise their heads if pulled to sitting in diagonal directions and, only later, can accomplish this coming straight up from supine to sitting. This diagonal direction is often preferable, as this is how the child will manage to pull himself to sitting. This is seen in normal motor development at about 9 months.

Stages in supine development

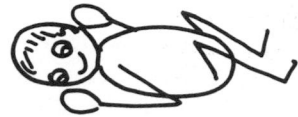

Fig. 8.47   Flexion: asymmetry of head (*0–3 months*).

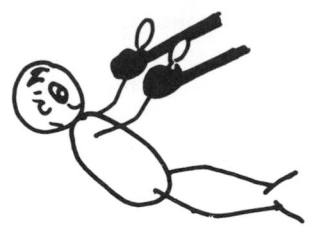

Fig. 8.48   Head lag (*0–3 months*).

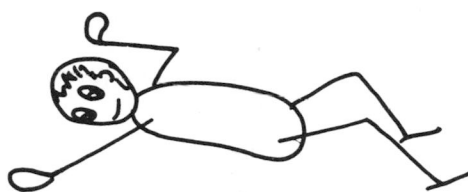

Fig. 8.49   Asymmetrical postures (*0–3 months*).

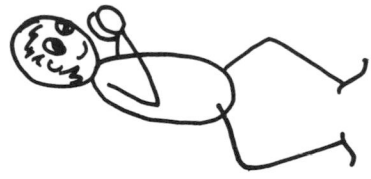

Fig. 8.50   Head, hands in midline (*4 months*). Symmetrical weight bearing on head and body.

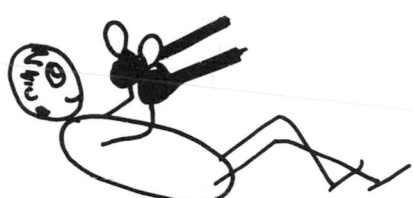

Fig. 8.51   Decrease head lag. Lifts head when about to be pulled up (*3–6 months*). Stabilizes pelvis.

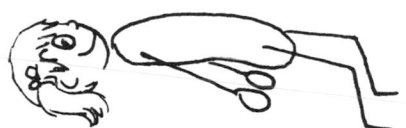

Fig. 8.52   Bridging hips (*3–6 months*).

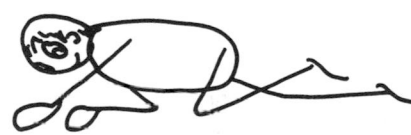

Fig. 8.53   Roll over (*6 months*).

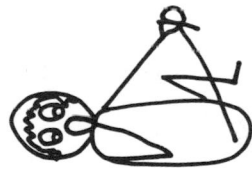

Fig. 8.54   Grasp feet (*7 months*).

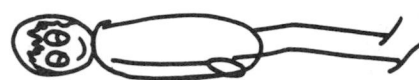

Fig. 8.55   Lying straight, symmetry (*8 months*). Head turn isolated from trunk.

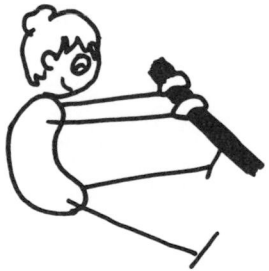

Fig. 8.56   Pull self to sitting. Dislikes supine (*9–12 months*).

(4) Pull the child's shoulder or arm diagonally across body to the opposite side (Fig. 8.57). Help him rotate his body and lift his head as he is brought up to sitting. As the child comes up to sitting he may automatically lean on a forearm and may require help to take weight on to this forearm. If he cannot use his forearm, for support, you may hold both his hands, arms or shoulders and pull them across and over to one side of his body as he comes up to sitting in this diagonal direction.

Note that in using methods (1) to (4) the child's legs should be observed as he rises to sitting. If his legs stretch, press together or twist inwards, then hold them apart, turn them outward on either side of a wedge, cushion or your lap or forearm (Fig. 8.58).

The child's arms need to be held straight at the elbows and turned outward if there is a strong tendency for his arms to twist inwards from the shoulders or bend tightly to his body.

Children who bend their knees excessively after the normal level of 3 months, and children who have tight hamstrings, may have them held straight by the therapist or by knee-pieces during these rising reactions.

(5) Rising to sitting may also be trained from the side-lying position, particularly in those children who are excessively extended in the supine position, have very poor head raising from supine, or require additional activity of the shoulder girdle muscles, back extensors, or arm elevation pattern (Fig. 8.59). Child in side-lying, hips and knees semiflexed, head forward and arm underneath the head with bent elbow. Lift the child's upper arm behind his occiput, turn the arm outward from the shoulder and gently pull this arm and thus the child up toward side-sitting, lean on elbow. Wait for his own active participation as he responds to gently pulling him up towards sitting. Later let him rise to

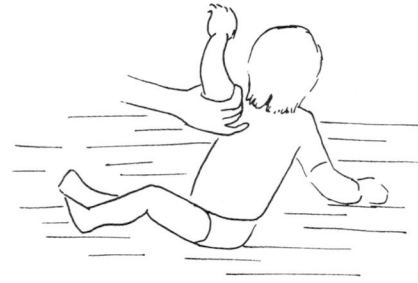

Fig. 8.57   Supine rise to sitting.

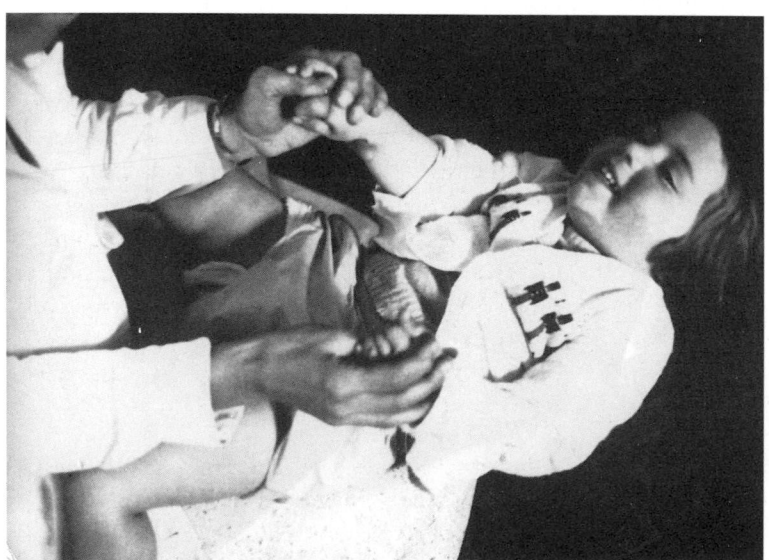

Fig. 8.58   Rising to sitting with the child's legs on either side of the therapist.

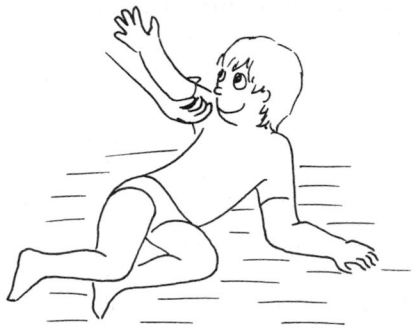

Fig. 8.59 Rising to sitting from side-lying.

side-sitting, lean on his hand instead of on his elbow. Check that his palm is down on the ground, his head is lifted up and sideways and his back is rotated and extended. Avoid side-lying with any sub-dislocated hips or when excessive hip flexion-adduction is present in the top leg.

From 6–10 months normal developmental level. Help the child *to rise* to sitting on his own in the following ways:

(1) Encourage his own head raise in supine by suspending him over the edge of a roll, your lap, a bed or a large ball. At first hold the child behind his shoulders, also place bells or toys on his tummy or feet so that the child is motivated to look up at them or at his toes (painted red if necessary!). Later, let him hang down over the edge of your lap, or down an inclined wedge with head supported and call to him to raise his head to look at you.

(2) Supine to sitting can be carried out by helping a child to grasp a rope, parallel bars or vertical bars with one hand across his body. He then pulls himself to sitting in a diagonal direction with half-rotation of his trunk.

(3) Supine to sitting can be accomplished by a child if he holds a short pole or stick, held by you as well, with help to sitting. Help him avoid hunching his shoulders and exces-

sively bending elbows and wrists to do this. You can press his wrists down during his grasp, so overcoming palmar-flexion.

Remember the normal child will first come up to sitting from supine in a diagonal direction with a half-roll to one side and lean on one elbow or hand. He will only come straight up to sitting from supine much later, as this is an advanced pattern seen in normal children over 4 years. Normally the child at the developmental level of 6–10 months may also roll over and rise to sitting. Rolling from supine is trained for this.

Physiotherapy Suggestions for Rolling and Roll-and-Rise

Rolling techniques will help the child to roll to side-lying where his hands might meet and he can see then. Well-chosen rolling methods correct the abnormal positions of the legs and arms and can also stimulate head righting, simultaneously decreasing infantile neck righting and activating various body derotative and rotative patterns. He is then, in effect, using his body to turn in order to rise from supine. Some children need rolling for locomotion and exploring space. Some of the many methods available are:

Reflex rolling or primitive reactions. Turn the baby or child's head to one side and hold his jaw firmly. Press down and across the fifth intercostal space towards the *opposite* site. A reflex rotation will begin at the pelvis causing both knees and then one knee to flex up and over to the side of the child's occiput. This technique initiates rolling in very young children and in the presence of severe impairments, also actively corrects leg adduction-extension, arm flexion, hand fisting and abnormal *roll-en-masse* (Fig. 8.60), and *frog position*.

Side-lying. Rotate the child's shoulder girdle forward while rotating his pelvis back. Change to rotation of the shoulder backward and pelvis forward, and vice versa (Fig. 8.61). If speed is

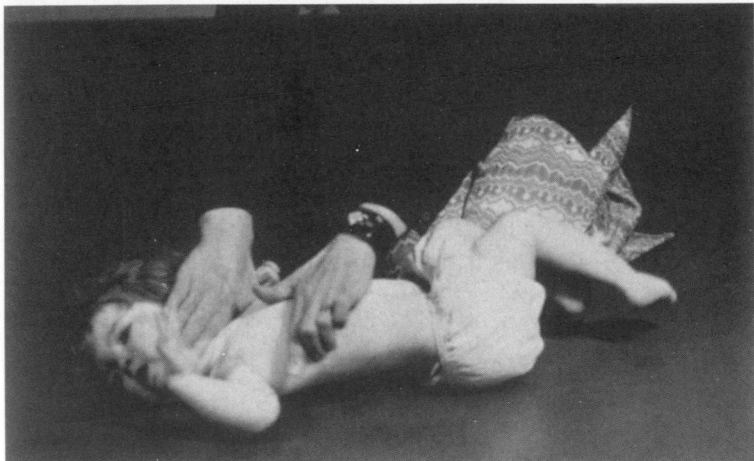

Fig. 8.60 Reflex rolling.

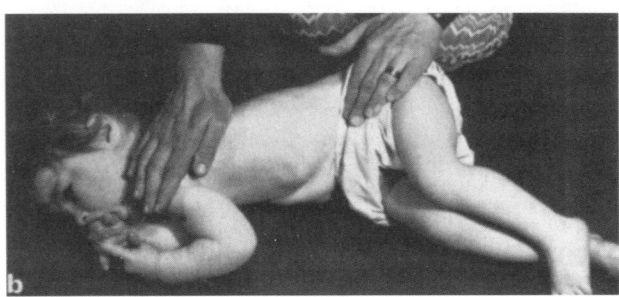

Fig. 8.61 Rotation of the shoulder girdles and pelvic girdles. Knees can be flexed and rotated to the opposite side.

correct and the rotary stretch on the trunk adequate, these *counter rotations* stimulate an active response in the child's shoulder or pelvis or in both areas. This also treats the rolling *in one piece* as seen, say, in the neck righting reaction. If rotation of the shoulder girdle is possible against some manual resistance, there is often an associated head raising with the rotation. Rotation of the girdles, pelvic/shoulder, not only facilitates rolling but also initiates arm movements and leg movements. Train shoulder rotation backwards as a preliminary to pulling the arm out from underneath the body in those children who get their arm caught in rolling over.

Supine. Leg patterns

(1) Bend both the child's knees across to the opposite side whilst rotating and holding his upper shoulder back. Release his shoulders and an active roll of the upper trunk follows.

This roll might be manually resisted at the shoulder as well, but check that correct amount of resistance is given so that a full flexion spasm does *not* occur (Fig. 8.61).

(2) Stretch one of the child's legs into extension-abduction as a stretch stimulates this leg to move to flexion-adduction to the opposite side. Wait for his upper trunk to roll over bringing the arm across (Fig. 8.62). A retraction of the shoulder often delays or even prevents the arm coming over within the child's roll from supine to prone. If possible augment leg flexion-adduction against manual resistance given at the knee and thigh. This shows him an active leg pattern, which he can learn to use later.

Arm patterns

(1) Bring the child's arm from his side in shoulder extension-abduction-internal rotation

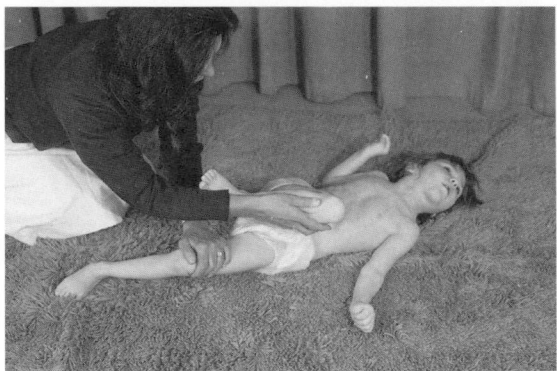

Fig. 8.62 Supine, leg patterns.

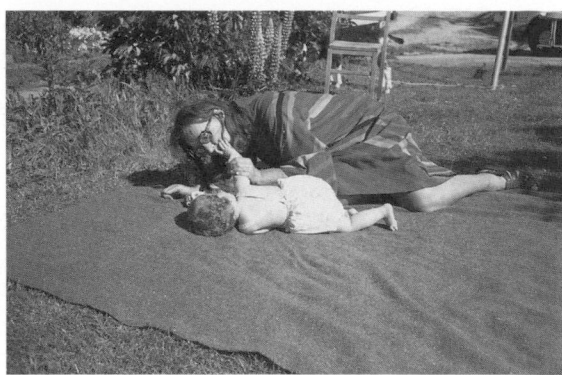

Fig. 8.63 Supine, arm patterns.

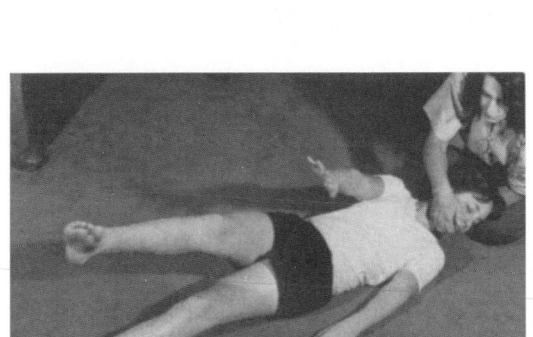

a

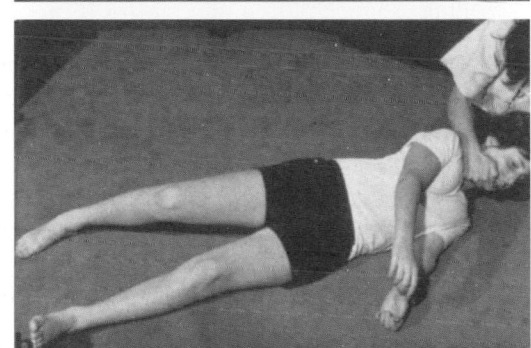

b

Fig. 8.64 Head pattern to stimulate rolling. *Note* limb action a, b.

and across his body to flexion-adduction-external rotation (child's palm must be towards his face) (Fig. 8.63). Wait for him to turn his head, trunk and legs. The therapist may guide the movement, activate it using stretch and resistance. A child actively reaches for a toy on the opposite side of the moving arm during this activity or as a result of this training procedure if he has no active reach.

(2) Bring one arm across to the other side to touch his mother's face as you give manual resistance to pelvic rotation forward which follows this action.

(3) If the underneath arm gets caught, initially hold it straight above his head.

Note

(1) Prone to supine rolling: use a pelvic rotation backward to turn.

(2) During rolling over, various leg patterns are themselves stimulated, i.e. leg flexes over with the roll from supine to prone in some children. In others the child may use the leg to *push-off* in an extended-abducted pattern (Fig. 8.64). During the roll from prone to supine, some children extend and abduct the upper leg. Other children flex the upper leg as they roll. Similarly arm patterns vary. The therapist must select the technique according to the action she wishes to obtain and which a child is most able to begin to do on his own.

(3) Combinations of head, arm and leg patterns also vary.

(4) All rolling patterns relax a stiff child and are enjoyed when repeated rhythmically supine to prone and reversed.

Head patterns. Gently raise the child's head into flexion-rotation and wait for him to follow with rolling towards the side to which his face is rotated. Hold his head lightly as he rolls. You may have to hold his chin up as he reaches prone. Resisted head flexion-rotation may be used as well in children who have good head control and respond with rolling in their waist and not in a total body action. Prone to supine rolling is carried out with head raise to extension-rotation. The arm patterns above may also activate associated head patterns. Some children may use an arm to push-off together with head patterns (Fig. 8.64).

Rolling to instructions. The facilitation patterns of either, head, or limbs need to be imitated as experienced for active learning by a child. Instructions used for say: *Prone lying* 'lift your head and one (right) arm up and back as far as possible', 'roll over'; 'lift your leg up and back, over to the other side', 'roll over'.

Supine lying. 'Bend one knee right across to the other side as far as it will go', 'roll over'; 'grasp your hands and stretch your elbows – bring both arms over to one side as far as possible', 'roll over'; 'lift your head and look over to one side as far as possible', 'roll over'.

A child selects the rolling pattern that he can actively manage. A carer works together with child and therapist in practising selected patterns that can be managed (see below).

Treatment Suggestions and Daily Care for Rolling and Rising

Rolling

(1) Place the child on his back, on his side or on his stomach (with face and neck over the edge) on a blanket. Hold each end of the blanket – two adults may be needed – and suspend the child in the blanket just off the ground. Tip the child gently from side to side, waiting for him to complete his roll over. If he cannot do this himself you can roll him in the blanket until he picks up the rolling motion himself. *Do not* do this with a child who arches his back or overextends when in prone position. However, training sideways rolling with a child suspended in a hammock or blanket prevents arching. This is because a child's head, shoulders and hips are bent in a hammock to counter extensor thrust or arching.

(2) Child lying on his back – bend one hip and knee well over to the opposite side and wait for him to complete the roll over (Fig. 8.62) during washing and dressing.

(3) Bring one of his arms over to the opposite side with the palm of his hand towards his face, or offer him a toy he likes on the opposite side, this may lead to a roll over (Fig. 8.63). Offer him a toy for rolling from side-lying or from prone.

(4) Child lying on his stomach – bring his hip and pelvis, or his shoulders, back and towards the opposite side and encourage rolling. Some children may push off on one hand to help roll from prone to supine, or rise on to their lower arms underneath their bodies.

(5) Child in prone or supine on a soft thick sponge rubber mattress or inflatable bed. Press down on one side of his body so that he tips over towards you and rolls. Rolling on such surfaces is often easier as he does not get *stuck* with his arm caught under his body. At first it is necessary to place the arm, which gets caught underneath, above his head.

(6) Encourage rolling on all surfaces, floors, carpets, grass and sand. Make an incline with a pile of mattresses or sponge rubber, or place the child on the top of a slight mound of grass or sand and let gravity help him roll downhill on his own.

(7) If a child can roll over *wait* for him to do so. In addition train him to roll over from

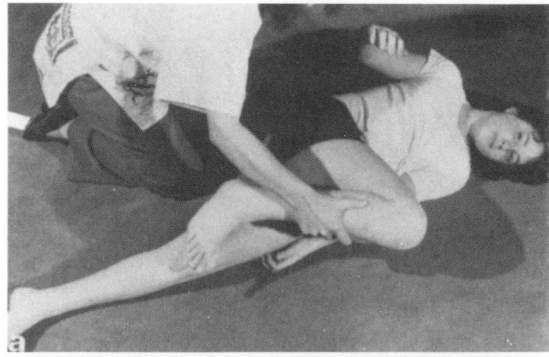

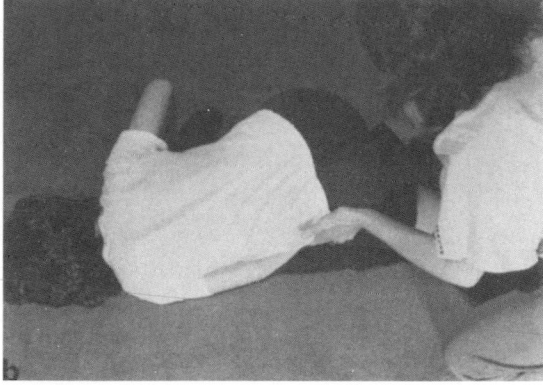

Fig. 8.65 Roll-to-rise onto hands and knees. *Note* many methods exist for this but must be demonstrated clinically.

his back to his stomach and then to get up on to his hands and knees (as described in prone development, 3–6 months level or Fig. 8.65a,b).

0–3 MONTHS NORMAL DEVELOPMENTAL LEVEL

Common Problems

Delay in gradual overcoming of head lag on pull to sitting. Inability to lift hand to mouth.

Abnormal performance (Fig. 8.66). Opisthotonus, or excessive extension of either head, shoulder girdle, back and legs or all of them.

Some arch into opisthotonus in infancy but become floppy later. Babies who are floppy (hypotonic) may have intermittent extensor spasms of head, spine and hips. They may also lie in 'frog' positions with the legs flexed-abducted-externally rotated, arms limp at their sides or in shoulder abduction, elbow flexion, hands open or closed. Apparently normal flexion positions may also be present in babies who later show spasticity. Kicking of legs begins and has abnormal patterns. There may be abnormal asymmetry in that one leg flexes, abducts and sometimes externally rotates, while the other flexes, adducts and sometimes internally rotates, or one may kick more vigorously than the other. This asymmetry may become so great that the legs look *windswept* to one side, especially when kicking stops. Later hip dislocation is threatening in the adducted-internal rotated leg. Persistent head turning to one side may occur. Pelvic obliquity and scoliosis may appear early or in later stages (Fig. 8.68).

Reflex reactions. Normally these include grasp reflex, Moro reaction, asymmetrical tonic neck reaction, leg crossed extensor reflex, withdrawal reflex, neck righting reaction. On passively pulling the child to sitting, his legs should flex-adduct and, by the next 3–6 months level, flex-abduct. A response of extension-adduction of the legs is abnormal. Some cerebral palsied children even extend the hips so much that their hips come well off the surface. Individual children cannot stabilize their pelvises against a surface and slide easily on it.

Physiotherapy Suggestions

See section on Physiotherapy suggestions for rolling and roll-and-rise as very young or very severely impaired children can only respond on an automatic level at this early stage. Continue into next stage of development, then add more advanced methods, which need active learning by individuals.

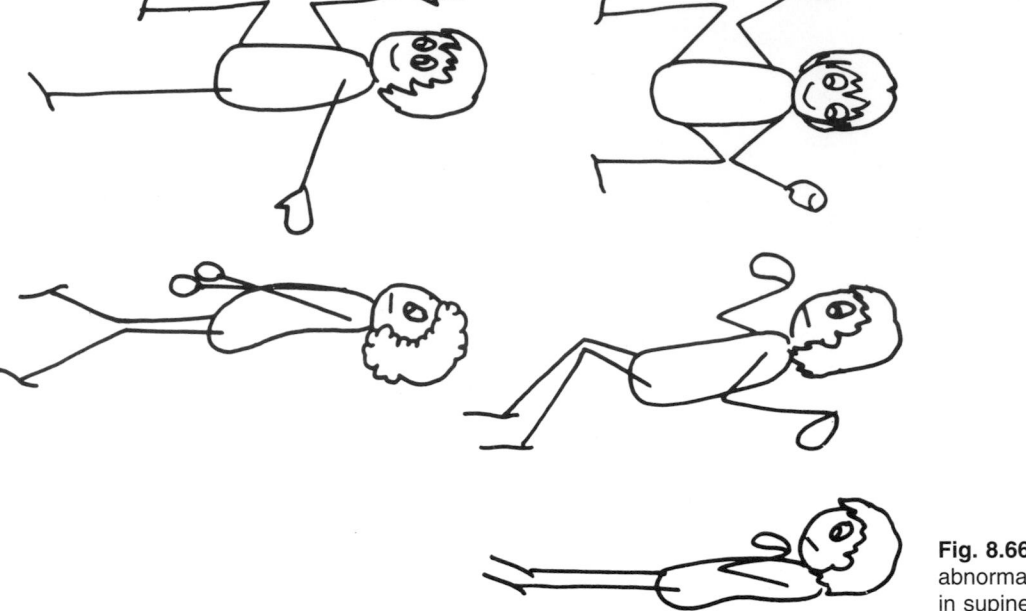

Fig. 8.66 Some abnormal postures in supine.

Treatment Suggestions and Daily Care

(1) See Supine rise to sitting and development of head righting (rising), from 0–6 months.

(2) Bring a child's arms well forward and turn them out from his shoulders, so that both hands touch your face, or make him touch his own hands, mouth, chest or abdomen naming these body parts. Stimulate visually and with noises in the centre to encourage his head holding in the centre and hands should make contact with bells or musical toys dangling in the midline.

(3) Eye-to-eye contact with your eyes parallel to his, at first in the centre. Keep your face close to the face of a child with severe visual impairment. Stimulate him to follow sounds, lights and mobiles from side-to-side (see development of hand function in Table 8.4).

(4) *Abnormal reflex reactions and abnormal performance* are modified as follows:

- *Discourage* supine if the child has marked ATNR (that is, asymmetrical tonic neck reaction) after 4 months, excessive Moro after 6 months or has extensor spasms. It is better that the child functions first in prone or sitting positions selected according to his level of development. Head needs to be controlled in midline and this may be too difficult in supine. If supine is inevitable during periods in the day, hold the child's head up into flexion in the hollow of a large cushion, use a hammock (Fig. 8.67) or special supine lying frames/equipment (Fig. 8.68) (see appendix). This overcomes the head falling or pressing back into extension. Head flexion often diminishes the ATNR, Moro or extensor thrusts. In this position have the shoulders well forward to counter retraction. Motivate symmetrical arm movements with toys, mobiles and so on.

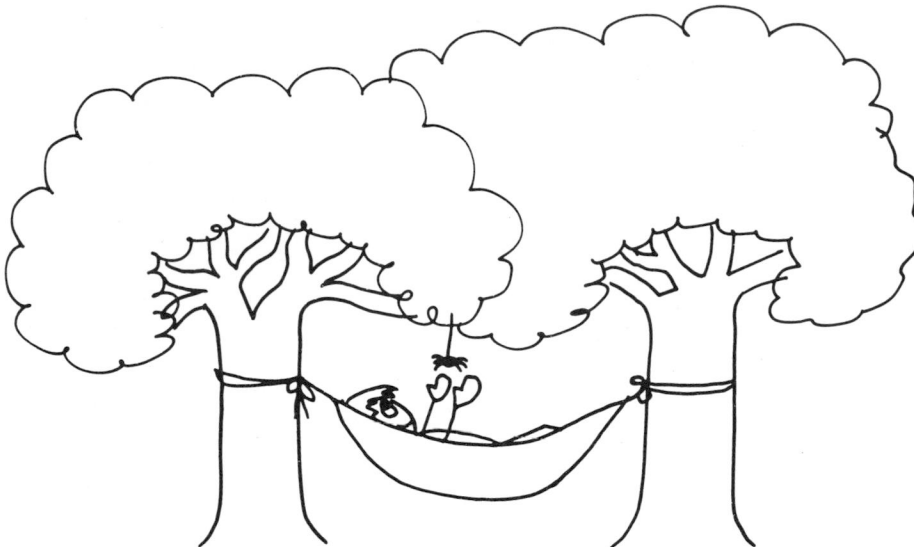

Fig. 8.67

- Excessively extended children should be flexed at head, shoulders and hips in side-lying or supine. The severely extended child, with arms in abduction, shoulders retracted and elbows bent, needs to be positioned in side lying with firm support from pillows or a *side-lying board* so that his hands will be able to meet and so that he can see them, so that they can touch his mouth and later reach for toys in front of him (5 months level). Place a toy between his hands that can easily be grasped (see Hand function), later train him to lie on his side alone. Show the child how to balance in side-lying with one leg on top of other, as well as one in front of the other.

- For a child with abnormally straight legs, pressed together and turned in, use abduction splints. For 'frog' position use sandbags to keep the legs together as you train rising to sitting or play with the child in supine. Pants that are well stitched down the centre can be used to bring the legs together when hypotonic legs can easily be positioned.

- Persistent head turning needs to be discouraged by motivating a child to look the other way. His bed should be on the opposite side of the room, offer toys, communication activities and even food from the side towards which the child rarely turns. Carry the child so that he can also look to the side which is not usually preferred. The physiotherapist must check that the child does not have a torticollis which requires stretching or even an operation. Plagiocephaly may accompany head turning. This strong head turning or preference has been observed in some babies who subsequently developed normally without therapy (Robson 1970).

- See therapy for grasp reflex in stages of hand function development, 0–3 months and 3–5 months levels. Methods to decrease a Moro or other startle reactions are mentioned in Development of sitting. Development of sitting simultaneously decreases any leg reflexes evident in supine. Rolling Techniques (Leg patterns, Arm patterns and Side-lying) simultaneously modifies neck righting or extensor thrusts seen in Supine.

- Abnormal synergies, i.e. leg extension-adduction-internal rotation are best corrected in the creeping patterns at this level in prone development. If prone development is not indicated in the particular child, train reciprocal leg movement in supine. Carry out active assisted full range of reciprocal motion. Hold the child's knees and bend one hip and knee up and out, holding the other leg straight and turned out. Change the motion by bringing the bent leg down as you move the straight leg up into flexion. This maintains joint ranges. Reciprocal leg motion is carried out to a slow song.

4–6 MONTHS NORMAL DEVELOPMENT LEVEL

Common Problems

Delay in acquisition of symmetry, in keeping head in the centre, in bringing the arms together and in hand regard. Delay in the disappearance of head lag and in acquiring ability to raise the head off the bed. The child is unable to *bridge* his hips off the floor, unable to reach for a toy (see Hand function, Table 8.4).

Abnormal performance. Flexed legs now abnormally extend-adduct and internally rotate in many children lying supine and when brought from supine to sitting position. Normally legs flex-abduct and externally rotate at this level. Presence of clenched hands (see section on arm function). Abnormal absence of isolated foot movements or knee movements, as these only occur as part of 'mass patterns'. Abnormal anterior pelvic tilt (see Fig. 8.68a).

Reflex reactions. May not be developing body derotation. Reflexes of 0–6 months level may not be disappearing.

Treatment Suggestions and Daily Care

(1) See Hand function (Table 8.4) and section on methods.
(2) See rise up to sitting and rolling techniques.

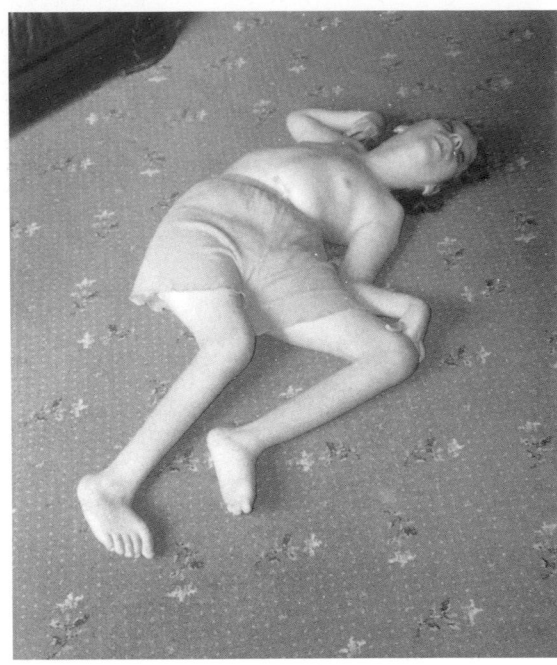

Fig. 8.68a Windswept posture, scoliosis and arms flexed.

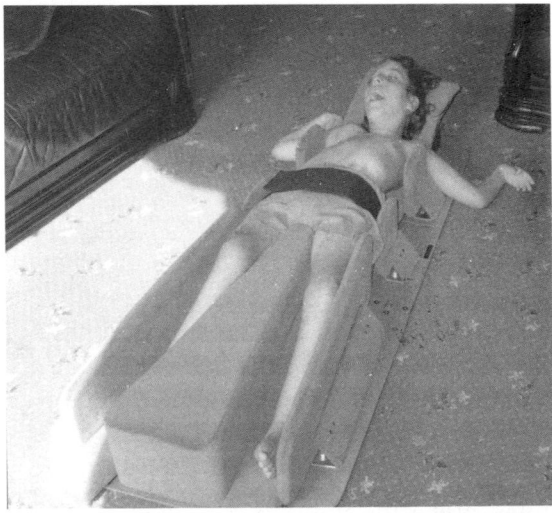

Fig. 8.68b Position to correct postures in supine.

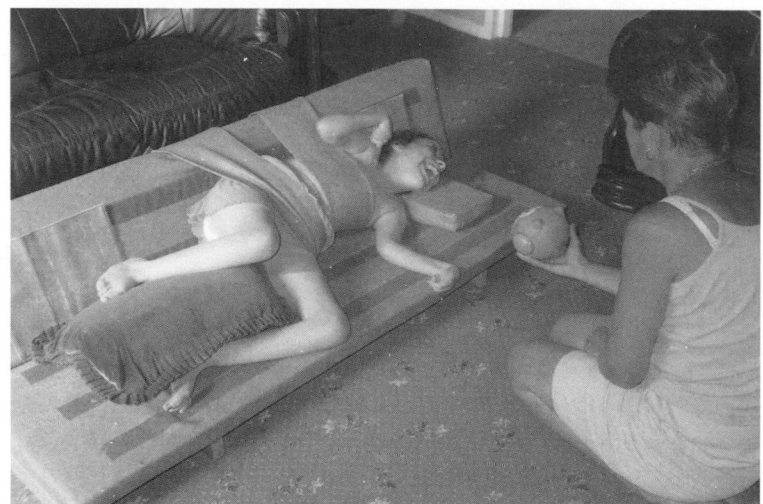

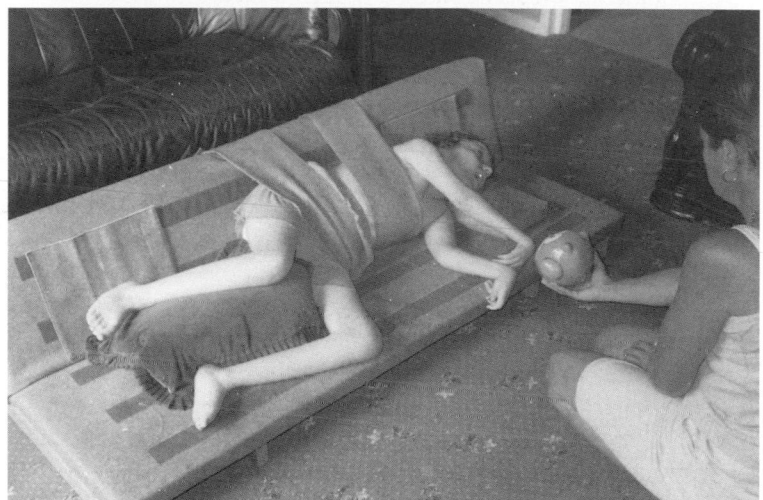

Fig. 8.68c,d Correcting posture in side-lying board. Her active arm reach for ball adds correction and communication.

Physiotherapy Suggestions

Arm reach. Child in side-lying and progress to supine. Train arm patterns such as flexion-adduction-external rotation with straight elbow and also with bent elbow, so that hands touch the child's mouth. Carry this out in side-lying and with both limbs in supine (see Hand function, Fig. 8.194). Place attractive objects in positions, near a child, which activate these and other arm patterns. A lack of shoulder girdle stability may cause compensatory shoulder

hunching and manual guidance is given to help control this (see Fig. 8.68d).

Bridging (Fig. 8.69). Hold the child's feet flat on the floor. He raises his hips to let a toy go *under the bridge*. Check that this is *not done* by using a lumbar lordosis. Check that arms do not flex up excessively and remain straight. Hold the 'bridge' steady while the wind tries to 'blow it over'. On this instruction the therapist gives manual resistance at the side of the child's pelvis, or on the anterior superior iliac spines,

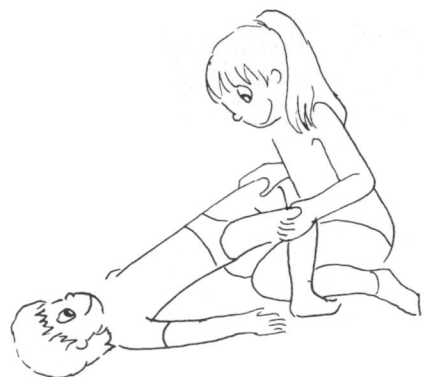

Fig. 8.69 Bridging.

or one hand in front and one behind to rotate his pelvis. The child tries to maintain the stability of the 'bridge' as far as possible. A pillow under his hips may help initially as he learns to maintain control against your manual pressure and resistance.

Note. Semi-bridging and moving backwards is a form of locomotion used by some children with dyskinesia (athetosis), athetoid children and more rarely by other children with cerebral palsy. However, this is often abnormal as it includes excessive hypertonic arching in the head and back and retraction of the shoulder. This should be discouraged and other forms of locomotion offered to the child.

6–9 MONTHS NORMAL MOTOR DEVELOPMENTAL LEVEL

Common Problems

Delay in grasping feet with legs in the air. The child is unable to roll over or pull himself towards sitting.

Abnormal performance. He cannot lie straight with arms and legs extended or with legs extended or with legs abducted-extended-externally rotated. A variety of abnormal postures may be seen including asymmetry of head,

trunk or limbs or all of these. Normally, the pull-to-sit should provoke extension-abduction of legs. Anterior pelvic tilt may persist abnormally.

Abnormal rolling patterns may be roll, leading with head and arms but with legs stiff and straight or passive; roll, using legs but upper arm bent and retracted at the shoulder; roll, using an action of *flexion into a ball*, or using an arching of the back and head to roll over. No rotation at the child's waist (body rotative pattern), i.e. either rolling in one piece or using the excessive total flexion or extension; roll to one side only, in say hemiplegia, towards the affected side only, using the unaffected side to carry out the roll over, or in tetraplegia or diplegia using the less affected side to carry out the roll. Others may be due to weakness.

Treatment Suggestions and Daily Care

(1) See, rising to sitting, 6–10 months level, Rolling Techniques (see particularly sections on Rolling to instructions and Treatment suggestions and daily care). Use arm and leg patterns against manual resistance to augment roll at this stage. See also Table 8.4 for a child's development of hand function. At this stage a child may show his own strategies of rising (see Figs 8.70 and 8.71). See also the section in Chapter 4 on 'A child's own goals and strategies'.

(2) Have the child in supine and help him to hold one or both of his feet. Turn his hips and knees outward and bend his leg so his foot is touching his hand. Gently stretch his knee and lift his leg so that he can reach for, look at and also grasp his feet and hold them. First bend his hips and lift his bottom off the bed if he is unable to reach his feet. The child needs to actively bend his hip and knee to his chest so that the full hip flexion is attained. Ask him to 'kiss his knee', 'to

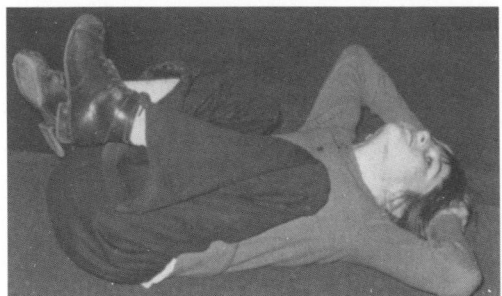

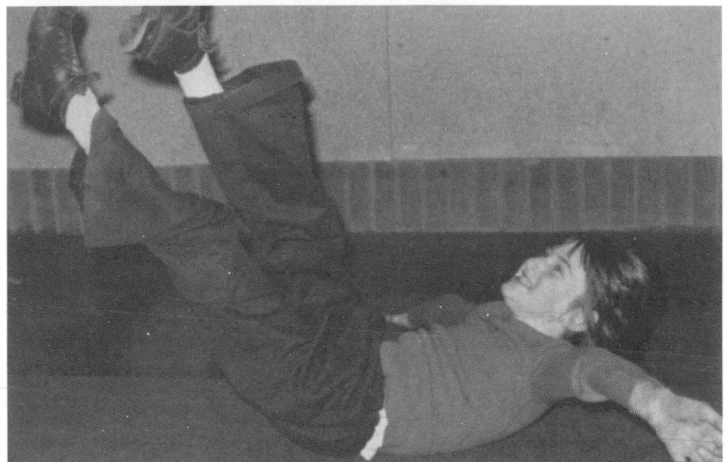

Fig. 8.70 Individual using her own method of rising (bend knees to chest and swing up to sitting, or grasp clothes and pull up to sitting).

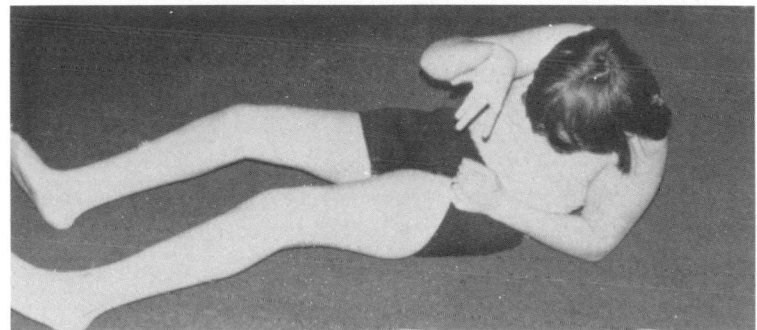

Fig. 8.71 Individual using his own method of rising to sitting. He grasps his clothes and pulls himself up alone.

pull his sock or shoe off his toes' or to 'hug his knees to his chest'. Holding his legs up above his face, play 'peek-a-boo' as he opens and closes his ankles and feet. All these actions help overcome abnormal pelvic tilts and activate abdominals.

Note that no further training is needed in supine as, from 10 months developmental

stages onward the child normally *dislikes* lying supine and persists in rolling out of this position or pulling up to sitting.

(3) Having trained the child to rise from supine to sitting *does not mean he can sit*. See Development of Sitting (Figs 8.77–8.90) which should be trained at the same time as Supine Development. Levels of development

of sitting stages may differ from rising to sitting stages. The postural mechanisms differ.

(4) Practise rising to sitting and rolling in order to get out of bed.

DEVELOPMENT OF SITTING

The following main aspects need to be developed:

Postural stability of the head or vertical head control. Normally developed by 3 months with trunk being supported.

Head righting or rising to the vertical position. Normally developed by 3 months with trunk being supported.

Postural stability of the head and the trunk (Fig. 8.72). Normally developed by 3–6 months and independent by 9 months. This stabilizes trunk on pelvis by 9 months.

Head and trunk righting or rising from sitting, leaning or slumped forward, backward or sideways, to upright sitting (Fig. 8.73). Normally developed between 3–12 months depending upon the positions and support given to the child to re-erect.

Note. Rising to sitting from supine, see Supine development, and from prone, see Prone devel-

opment. Rising from sitting to standing, see Development of standing and walking.

Postural stability of the shoulder girdle. Normally developed by 3–6 months. This is associated with the use of the arms for supports in sitting. Use of hands also activates shoulder girdle stabilization.

Sitting counterpoising head, arm, trunk and leg movements (Fig. 8.74). Normally developed by 6–12 months. Postural stability with counterpoising cannot be separated from hand function and daily life activities using limbs.

Tilt reactions (Fig. 8.75). When the child is tilted sideways, forwards or backwards (his

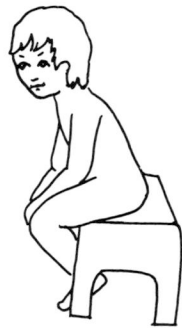

Fig. 8.73 Rising to upright sitting and reverse.

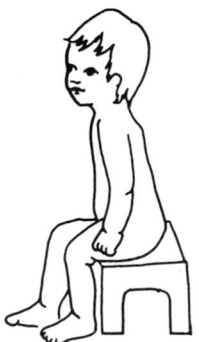

Fig. 8.72 Postural stability.

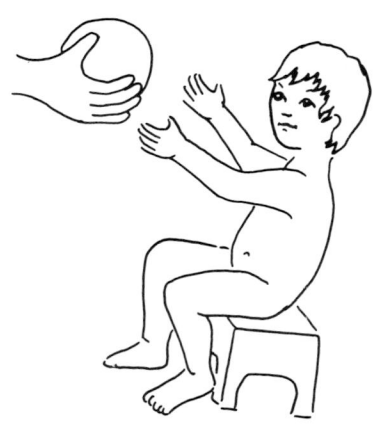

Fig. 8.74 Counterpoising.

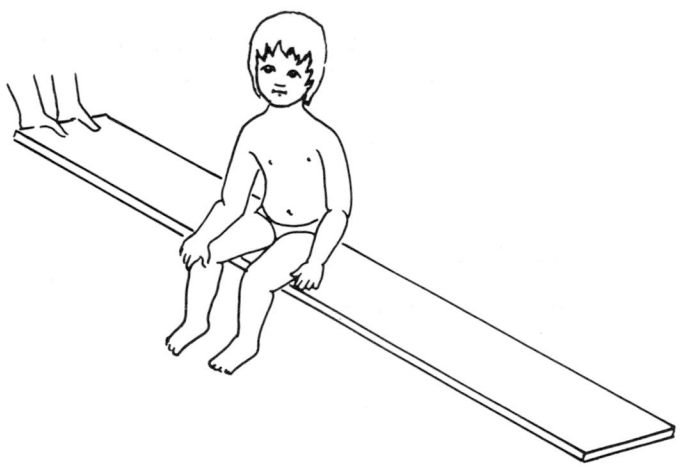

Fig. 8.75 Tilt reaction.

bottom is tilted off the horizontal). Normally developed by 9–12 months beginning with head followed by head and trunk adjustments.

Saving reactions (Fig. 8.76) and propping reactions if the child falls. Normally developed forward by about 5–7 months, sideways by about 9 months and backward by about 12 months.

ABNORMAL POSTURES IN SITTING AT ALL LEVELS OF DEVELOPMENT (Fig. 8.91)

These may be due to:

(1) Absence of the postural mechanisms and compensatory abnormal postures to obtain balance.
(2) Presence of hypertonus and short muscles.
(3) Attempts by an older child to control disrupting involuntary movements.
(4) Use of incorrect size and type of chairs, tables, pushchairs, wheelchairs and continual placement of child in only one or more poor sitting positions.
(5) Prolonged sitting in one special chair beyond two hours, even if positions are corrected.

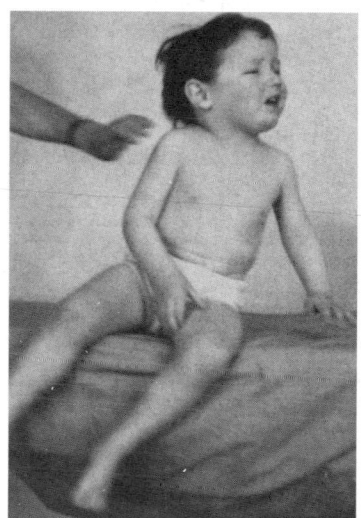

Fig. 8.76 Saving reactions in the arms and legs.

Absence of postural stabilization results in a child falling backwards or leaning back as he slides out of the seat of his chair. The normal postural stabilization holds the hips at right angles to the trunk as the pelvis and trunk are stabilized. In development the back is first rounded with pelvis tilted backwards and subsequently the back straightens with pelvis tilting upright and then towards the front. Delay in postural stabilization is compensated for by

Stages in development of sitting

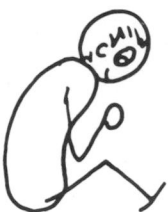

Fig. 8.77   Sitting head uncontrolled, flexion in total child (*0–3 months*).

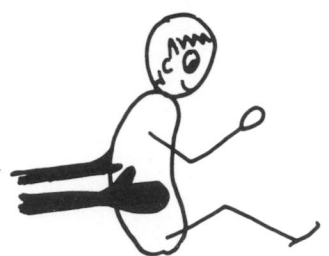

Fig. 8.78   Decrease of flexion, vertical head control develops (*0–3 months*).

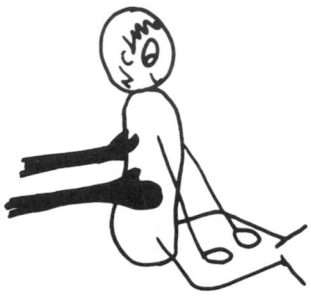

Fig. 8.79   Sitting lean on hands, flattening of upper back develops, lumbar kyphosis still present (*4–6 months*).

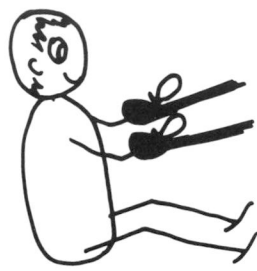

Fig. 8.80   Sitting with less support, back straighter, legs straighter, turning out and apart (*4–6 months*).

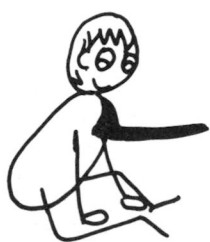

Fig. 8.81   Sitting lean on hands, hips flexed-abducted-externally rotated. Less support and without support (*4–6 months*).

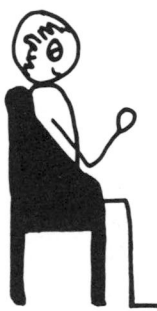

Fig. 8.82   Sitting in baby chair with back and sides supporting or propped on a pillow support (*4–6 months*).

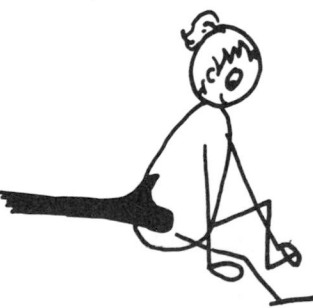

Fig. 8.83   Sitting lean on hands and lift one hand to play, with feet or a toy (*6–9 months*).

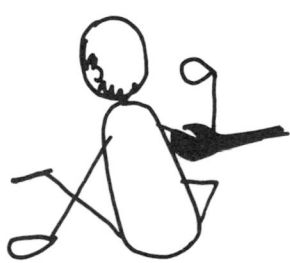

Fig. 8.84   Saving reactions and propping in arms (*6–9 months*). Tilt reactions begin.

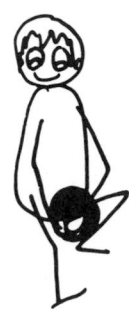

Fig. 8.85   Sitting alone on the ground (*6–9 months*).

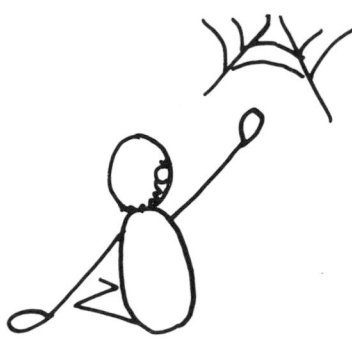

Fig. 8.86   Sitting reach in all directions, hand support (*6–9 months*).

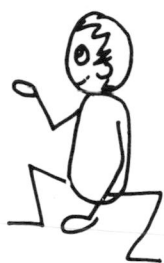

Fig. 8.87   Sitting turn reach, no hand support (*9–12 months*).

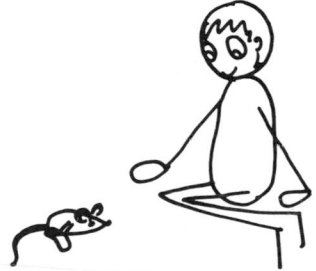

Fig. 8.88   Sitting in various positions (*9–12 months*). Pivot in sitting.

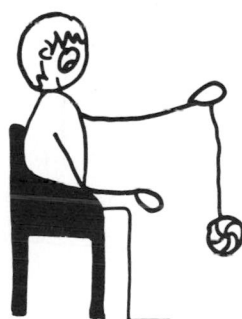

Fig. 8.89   Sitting in a chair for daily tasks, no hand support. Sit alone on stool (*9–12 months*).

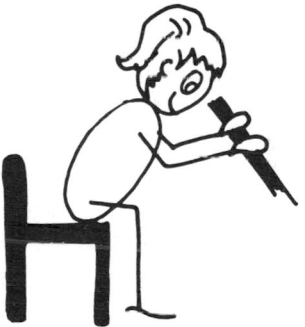

Fig. 8.90   Rising out of sitting and getting into all sitting positions. Tilt reactions complete (*9–12 months*).

various abnormal postures. These may lead to deformities. Abnormal postures may be:

(1) Head and trunk flex on semi-extended hips in *sacral sitting* (Fig. 8.91a and b). Arms

may flex and shoulders hunch tensely as a child avoids falling by grasping a support near his body. He may instead prop on his fists for support with his arms tensely internally rotated with straight elbows. He may

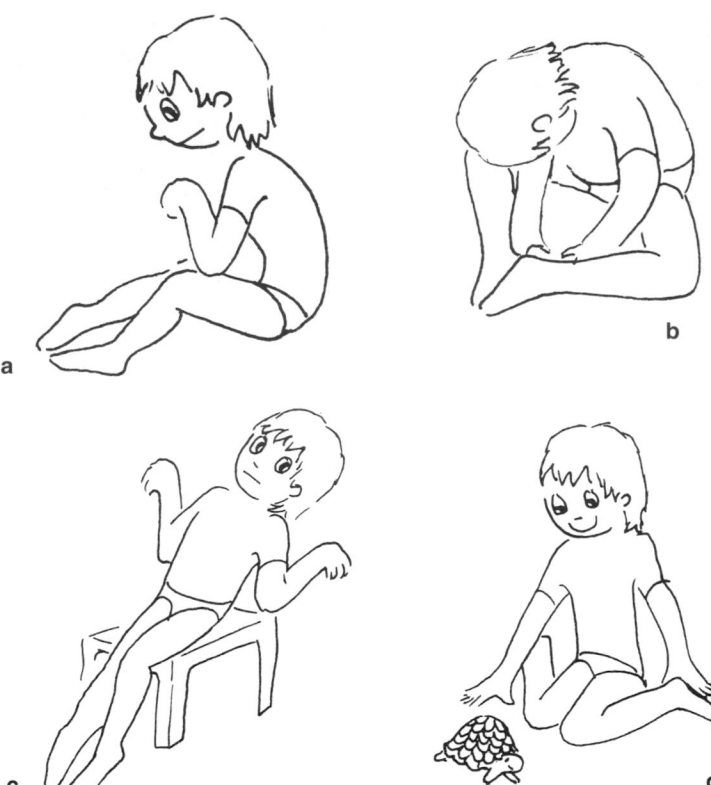

Fig. 8.91a,b,c and d   Some abnormal postures in sitting.

maintain his flexed position without hand support but has to hyperextend his neck to avoid falling forward and in order to look up.

(2) When a child leans back against a chair, his arms may be held up in abduction at his sides with shoulders hunched, protracted or retracted (Fig. 8.91c). He may instead elevate his arms forwards at 45–90° in the air with elbows straight, shoulders hunched in an effort to counterbalance his backward fall or extensor thrust. His feet may plantar flex to reach the ground for support or if the ground is near enough his toes flex to 'hold on' and his feet may press into valgus for support (Fig. 8.91c).

(3) A child sitting on a bed, the floor or on a chair which is too high may adduct and internally rotate his semi-extended hips with straight or bent knees. He may strongly bend his knees over the edge of the chair, twisting his legs around the front legs of the chair to avoid falling.

(4) Sitting on the floor with his bottom between his feet and his legs internally rotated and flexed is often seen in a child with cerebral palsy – W *sitting* (Fig. 8.91d). This is one way in which an unstable child can stabilize his pelvis and develop head and trunk control and hand function. Although this posture is seen in able-bodied children, it is not held for the many long periods which children with cerebral palsy persist in doing. Deformities of hip, knee and feet may develop unless there is more variety in floor sitting. Tailor sitting and long sitting with legs straight in front of a child also reveal very rounded backs and difficulty in using hands and reaching.

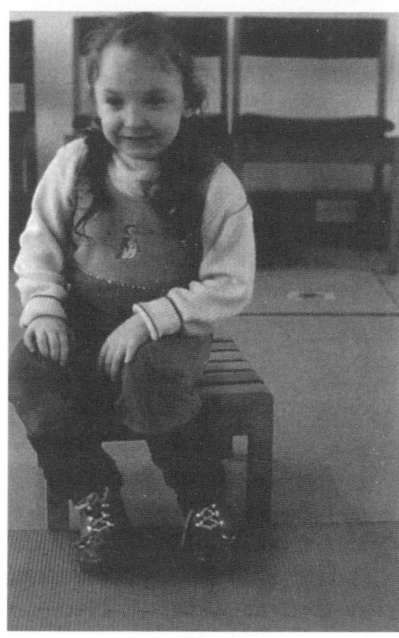

Fig. 8.92 Sitting with 'windswept' legs to one side. A mild example which may be much more severe in other children.

(5) Some children stabilize better on one side of their hips or trunk and prefer to sit sideways on to one buttock. This is obvious in children with hemiplegia but also in other types of cerebral palsy when there are *windswept* legs to one side (Fig. 8.92). Scolioses and pelvic obliquity may result from persistent asymmetrical weight bearing in sitting. If a child can only use one hand or one visual field this also increases asymmetry in postural stabilization and counterpoising.

Abnormal Sitting Postures in the Spastic Type of Cerebral Palsy

If the child is also hypertonic, he will assume the same postures already described, but the shortened or shortening spastic or rigid muscles maintain or augment these abnormal postures, as well as others. Thus prolonged sitting in any one position is particularly dangerous as it causes deformity and so disabling influences on the development of standing and walking and use of hands in situations other than sitting. Skin pressure points are likely when a child cannot ask, or is unable, to change his abnormal prolonged sitting posture.

The above postures associated with the tightness of spastic muscles will be seen as:

(1) Stiff extension so that the child cannot be flexed into the sitting position unless special methods are used. Some children can overcome their *extensor thrusts* or extensor hypertonus by using flexor hypertonus and sitting in excessive flexion.
(2) Some severely extended children may collapse into a flexion spasm or flexion and floppiness once the extensor hypertonus is overcome by the therapist. No sitting is possible in either position, showing absence of postural mechanisms.
(3) Most children achieve a position somewhere between full flexion or extension. The falling backward and extensor thrust seem to remain *in the hips* but trunk flexes with arms and head extends, legs assume various postures depending on the distribution of the short spastic muscles in each child. Trunk, head and arms also vary according to the child. Some children have hypertonus in the trunk, often on one side only. Scoliosis together with torticollis may be present.
(4) Tight hamstrings are often present with hypertonia. The pelvis is tilted back in sitting by the pull of the tight hamstrings. If the knees are extended as in long-sitting on the floor (Fig. 8.91a) the child may fall backward as his hamstrings do not allow this full extension. Many children can maintain long-sit with their pelvis tipped back in sacral sitting with a round back if they semi-flex at the knees. On a chair, the child's knees can bend fully and this often tips the pelvis back into position for upright sitting

with the child's weight on his tuberosities and not on his sacrum.

Knee flexion deformities are particularly threatening in these children, especially if they have prolonged sitting on chairs, where they find sitting so much easier.

TREATMENT AND DAILY CARE AT ALL LEVELS OF DEVELOPMENT

Practical Suggestions for Abnormal Postures and Balance

Abnormal postures are corrected as actively as possible. Special corrections may be given with special chairs (adaptive seating), for comfort, communication and hand function.

Kyphosis. Try active arm patterns involving elevation, as well as the general development of postural alignment and stabilization of head, trunk and pelvis in sitting and standing channels of development (see the section on Basic arm and hand patterns for all levels of development under Development of hand function).

Scoliosis. Make sure the child sits on both his buttocks. Reaching overhead is helpful on the side of the concavity. Sandbags or a roll of towels on his table under his forearm on the side of the concavity, or under the buttock on either the side of the concavity or convexity, should be tried to discover which props him into a more upright position. Corsets and special supports in chairs are needed for many children.

Abnormal postures of arms, trunk, head, legs are often corrected at the same time if the child sits on *both* his ischial tuberosities, leans forward from his hips, back straight to lean on his open hands with elbows held straight. Legs should be held apart and turned outward if they adduct. When knees are always in

flexion, sit on a inclined wedge with knee gaiters, in preference to chair sitting. Vary the angle of the incline according to the ability of child to keep his trunk straight. Feet should be flat on the ground if the child sits on a chair. Foot supports are essential if he is on a high chair (see Fig. 8.93). Correction of equinus feet, as discussed in Chapter 10, is important as this provides plantigrade feet as extra supports for sitting balance.

Some ideas to correct leg postures include sitting with any adducted legs apart and turned out on either side of large toys, a box of toys, bowl of sand or water, a small drum, straddling rolls, soft toys, the corner of the bed or chair, and across your hip or thigh. Avoid having a child straddle anything of too great a diameter as he then increases hip internal rotation with excessive abduction of his hips. Abduction splints may have to be worn during sitting for better hip posture. Tailor-sitting or side-sitting are preferable to sitting between his knees (Fig. 8.129), but should also be avoided if there is a threatening hip dislocation in one hip or there is too much flexion in the child's hips and knees as well as abnormal adduction and internal rotation. Feet need to be checked in case they deform in these sitting positions. Avoid

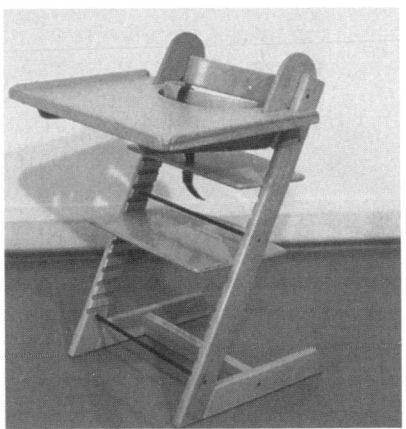

Fig. 8.93 Tripp-Trapp chair.

side-sitting which simulates a windswept preference, if present.

Avoid prolonged sitting especially if there is tightness of hip and knee flexors. Encourage standing up and standing positions or prone lying instead.

Excessive hip, trunk and head extension is corrected within the postures above, as well as having the child learn to sit on low chairs, sit in the corner of the sofa, or room, and use various special seating (see below). Carry the child in full flexion, to counteract severe extension and just before he is placed into his special chairs – see below and Figs 9.8–9.11.

Remember that when the child leans forward from his hips to reach his toys, feet or prop himself on his hands, he should lean from his hip joint. He avoids rounding his back if he does this. Help him by pressing your hand on the small of his back, if he cannot manage alone. Also make sure that the pull of tight hamstrings is not causing this and whether a small raise on to a platform for his floor seat is required. This is especially necessary if he is wearing knee extension splints. Sitting on a thick cushion, or sponge on the floor, may also improve posture of his back. If he sits on a forward-downward tilt on a wedge it may straighten his back (Fig. 8.110).

In all sitting postures a child develops postural control by first leaning forward then he re-erects to the upright posture where more control is needed. See Developmental stages in sitting.

Training Postural Control

The methods suggested below are used for each level of development provided that the *appropriate amount* of support is given to the child (Figs 8.94–8.108).

Support is at first given to the child's shoulders so that his total body is supported, and he should only achieve vertical head control (0–3 months level). Holding his upper arms and using shoulder girdle stabilization on forearms may act as a support to the whole child and

also facilitate head control at the first level of sitting development. With further training, support may be lowered to the child's body and waist (3–6 months level) and then to his

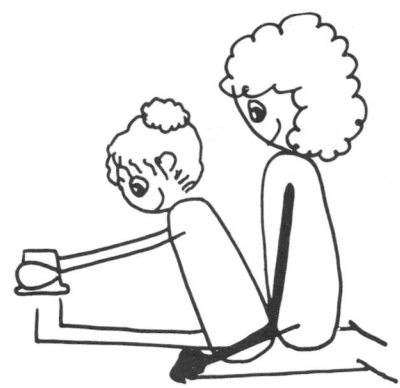

Fig. 8.94

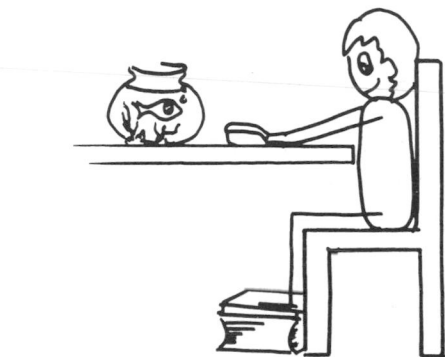

Fig. 8.95

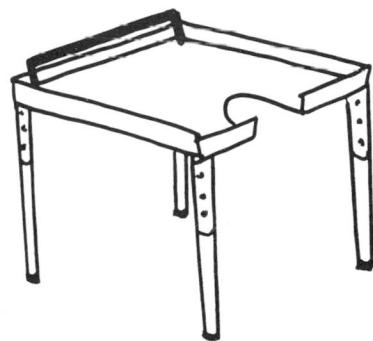

Fig. 8.96

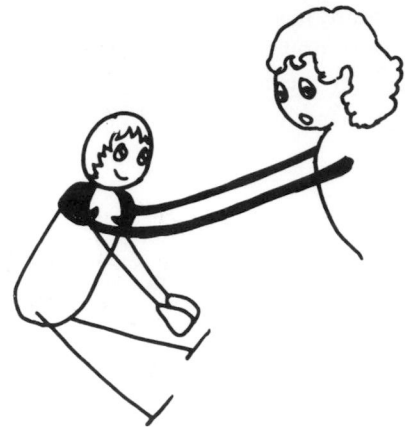

Fig. 8.97

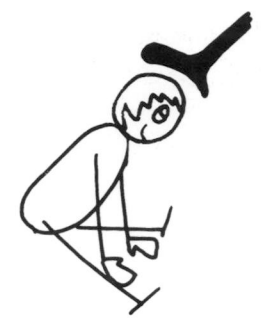

Fig. 8.98

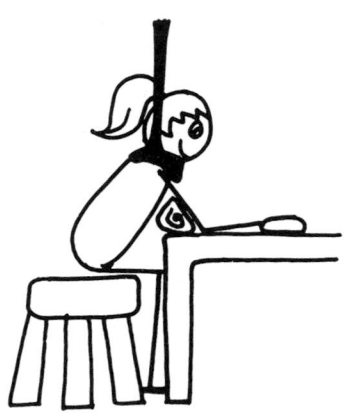

Fig. 8.99

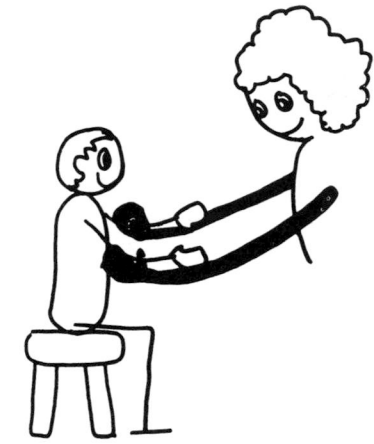

Fig. 8.100

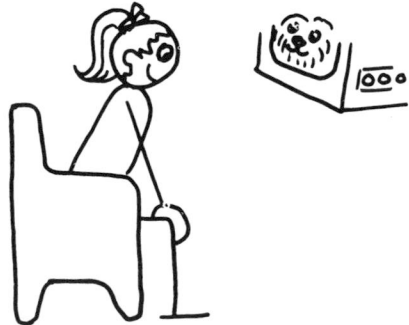

Fig. 8.101

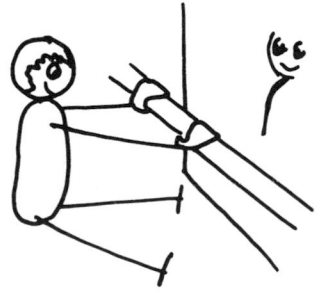

Fig. 8.102

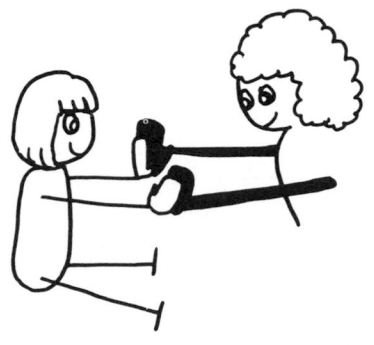

Fig. 8.103

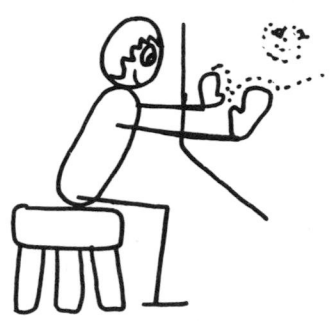

Fig. 8.104

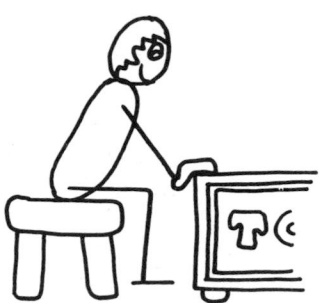

Fig. 8.105

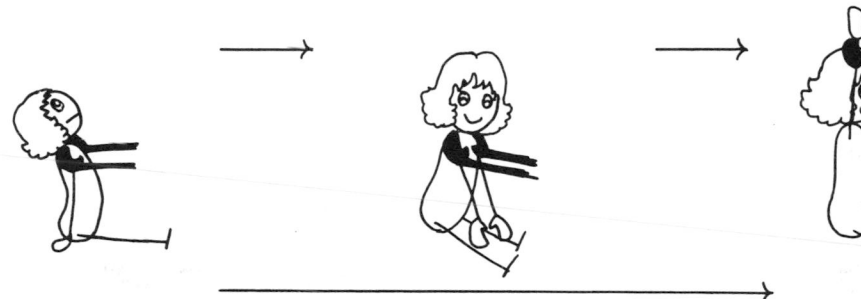

Fig. 8.106

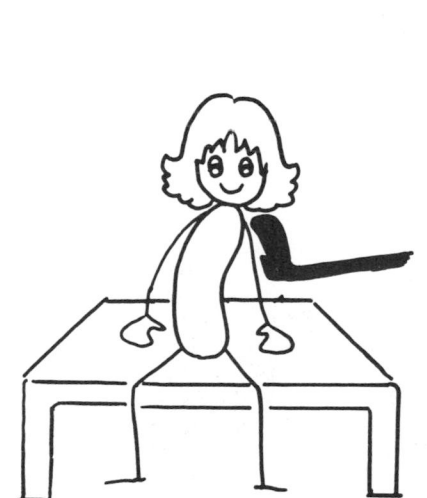

Fig. 8.107

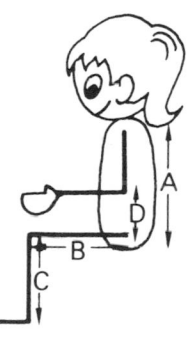
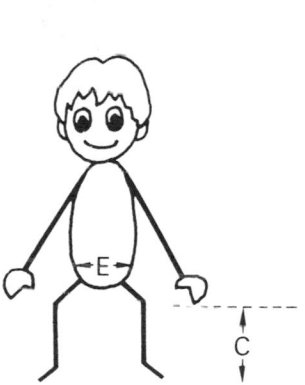

A   Height of backrest
B   Seat depth
C   Seat to floor
D   Armrest height
E   Seat width

Fig. 8.108

hips and thighs (6–9 months level), sometimes to his feet only, and finally removed at the 7–9 months level when sitting alone is normally expected.

Note

(1) All methods may be used for sitting on the floor and on the child's chair. Sitting on the floor is emphasized in babies and young children whilst in older children at the same early developmental level, chair sitting is emphasized.

(2) Sitting on the child's chair may be achieved before sitting on the floor in children with athetoid or spastic type of cerebral palsy especially if very tight hamstrings and poor sitting balance is present. Stable feet held flat on the ground are an additional aid to sitting in a chair, but is of course absent in sitting on the floor. If tight hamstrings still make him slide out of his chair, use a pelvic strap across his anterior hip level.

(3) *Involuntary movements* are decreased if a child pushed his own weight well on to his heels. Try tying ankles to chair or in foot pieces with straps, if this does not stimulate involuntary movements in the rest of the child. Grasping and leaning on forearms helps.

Various methods of giving and reducing support. Support may be given with the adult's body against the child's back as he is held on her lap or the child sits across a roll with the adult sitting close behind him. The adult then moves her body away from the child's back and support is only given at his waist level or at his hips and thighs (Fig. 8.94).

The child may be supported in front or lean against a table edge, preferably padded, at his shoulder level and this support is lowered to waist level and finally removed so that he sits at the table without leaning against it by 9 months normal developmental level. Feet should be supported on a firm surface (Fig. 8.95). Foot stools/boxes are not advisable when a child is able to get up to standing with help, or learning to step to chair and sit down.

The table may be used as a support together with the child grasping a horizontal pole attached to the table, the support of the table is removed and grasp alone can be used before total removal of table and grasp. The cut-out on the table offers more support at first, but should be removed as soon as possible (Fig. 8.96) to promote a child's postural adjustments.

Whilst training sitting, the support at the child's chest may be given by the adult instead of by a table. The child may hold the adult's shoulders or one of her hands, whilst her other hand supports his chest, subsequently his waist and finally his thighs, knees or just his feet flat on the ground.

Hold shoulders and child slightly forward for vertical head control. Train him to actively re-erect to the upright and maintain head control. Encourage head hold in the midline with eye-to-eye contact. Move support down child's trunk for next developmental levels (Fig. 8.97). Do this in forward position as well as in the upright posture. Sitting with a 20 degree forward lean is a functional posture for daily activities.

Joint compression through head in vertical alignment with trunk *or* hold baby/child and bounce him on his bottom on sponge rubber, trampoline, inflatable toy, beach ball or your lap (Fig. 8.98). Check that head with chin held in, trunk and bottom are in alignment. Use compression through head and/or shoulders during feeding, play, communication, and similar activities.

Child takes weight on forearms (Fig. 8.99). If child presses his arms to his chest use a roll of towels or sponge wedge to avoid this. Joint compression through shoulders or head may also be used.

Child is helped to lean on his forearms into adult's hands (Fig. 8.100). Adult reinforces this joint compression by pushing child's upper arm into his shoulder joint. Head and trunk control are thus activated within social interaction.

Visual and auditory stimuli at child's eye level for vertical head and trunk control in sitting (Fig. 8.101). Upright posture is encouraged.

Sitting grasping a pole, edge of a table or adult's hands (Fig. 8.102). Elbows should be straight and symmetrical. The support may be grasped with his arms at shoulder level, below shoulder level or above shoulder level. Child leans against table edge at lower levels of development (0–6 months).

Child pushes his open hands against adult's hands with wrists dorsiflexed (Fig. 8.103).

Child may also push against wall, make *hand prints* on powdered or soaped mirror or push firm toy to make a sound (Fig. 8.104). Trunk support may be given by leaning against a table edge or manually at 0–6 months level.

Child leans on hands on floor, child on a chair can lean on his hands (Fig. 8.105).

Stimulate head righting by bringing his shoulders forward and then take his upper arms, turn them out and elevate them to hold a toy in front of him or for dressing (Fig. 8.106). Make sure he tips his head forward when clothes are put over his head. *Active head righting is important* to prevent gagging or choking during feeding.

Stimulate head lifting from the chest by pulling shoulder girdle backwards or arms back against your hands to lean back on his hands with a straight back. Arms raise to extend rounded back and pelvic slumped posture.

Manual resistance may be given at the child's shoulder on its lateral aspect or anteroposterior aspect (Fig. 8.107). This reinforces head fixation, shoulder girdle fixation (stability). Do this also with the child leaning on forearms (Fig. 8.99), on hands (Fig. 8.98), or grasping a support.

Note: Give the correct amount of resistance so that abnormal reactions are not provoked in legs or body. Give him quick and slow

pushes expecting him to maintain balance ('Stay there').

Chairs and Tables

Special chairs (adaptive seating) are selected according to the child's developmental level to:

(1) Train sitting.
(2) Correct abnormal postures.
(3) Provide stimulation in the upright position to develop a child's social, visual and hearing abilities.
(4) Develop hand function in the *upright* position of *supported* sitting. Meanwhile training of sitting balance must continue and be associated with hand function as soon as possible. (See Basic arm and hand patterns for all levels of development under Development of hand function.)
(5) To enable better communication and oromotor function for feeding and speech.

Regular chairs are used:

(1) To increase development of sitting balance and independent good posture.
(2) To develop hand function together with sitting balance.
(3) To make standing up from sitting possible.

Measurements. If chairs are not of the correct measurements for the child they can obstruct the development of sitting, cause or increase abnormal postures and prevent hand function (Fig. 8.108). Only use an armrest if that support is needed. The back rest is 100° to seat. Slight forward lean to a table is active for daily activities carried out by a child. Table should be up to the height of child's waist or higher if he lacks trunk control. There should be a *large* area of work space.

If the chair is *too high* the child will find lack of foot support for his dangling feet disturbing to his poor sitting balance. Plantarflexed feet may become plantarflexion deformity. If the chair is *too wide* the child may take more weight on one side as he slumps to that side. The lateral lean or slumping decreases balance and may lead to scoliosis. Place rolls of towel, sponge-covered blocks, sandbags or magazines to decrease a chair which is too wide. The seat could be made to fit his buttocks. If the chair seat is *too short* the child may not be able to balance without support to his thighs. His feet may twist or curl around the chair legs in his efforts to balance. Deformity of his feet and of flexed, adducted internally rotated knees may be encouraged. If the chair seat is *too long* he may slump backwards to the back support and increase hip extension, adduction and internal rotation, knee extension and plantarflexion or hip extension adduction, semiflexion of the knees and plantarflexion of his feet. Rounding of the back is inevitable. In all the above situations the child's hand function is made impossible or difficult. Concentration on schoolwork, social situations and communication is usually disturbed.

Evaluating a Chair for a Child

Most therapists use trial and error to assess which chair and table is most suitable for an individual child. Research continues among therapists and bioengineers to clarify when particular designs are indicated for specific problems. Controversy still exists between different workers. The studies of the following are among many others which can guide clinical therapists: Trefler *et al.* 1978; Nwaobi *et al.* 1983, 1987; Mulcahy *et al.* 1988; Myhr & von der Wendt 1990; McCarthy 1992 (seating). Controversy about seating may arise when clinicians are really comparing children at different stages of development of quiet sitting versus sitting for hand function, vision and communication or for balance training. An *assessment chair* with different elements which can be removed according to each child helps to make decisions as to which chair is suitable. Try this with a child in quiet sitting and during functions

and where relevant during transport. Bardsley (1993) describes an assessment chair which affects details of design which can be custom made if this is financially feasible. Zacharkow (1988) has written a book with useful suggestions for seating.

Potential Seat Elements (Fig. 8.109a–d)

There is an increasing range of seating systems for children produced by different manufacturers as well as custom-made individual seating and the use of orthotics for desirable sitting positions. For most mild and moderately involved children with physical disabilities, for babies and for children with motor delay, mass-produced regular chairs and tables are suitable. A few modifications with foot rests and foam pieces or firm cushions can be used to obtain the desirable posture in each child.

General considerations in selecting a chair/wheelchair

(1) Parents and child find the chair aesthetically acceptable.
(2) The chair should be comfortable not only during quiet sitting but also when a child moves his head, body and arms. It should be comfortable and safe when the chair is moved from place to place.
(3) The chair needs to be portable from room to room or transportable for outings. It should not be too cumbersome for homes, classrooms or doorways.
(4) A chair should enable a child to join his family, friends or classmates around a table, on the floor, in a sandpit or at picnics and camps.
(5) A chair does not substitute for therapy and periods of a child's own development of locomotion and postural control.
(6) A child may need more than one chair: one for practising his emerging postural adjustments during looking, listening, reaching out and hand use in all directions; another

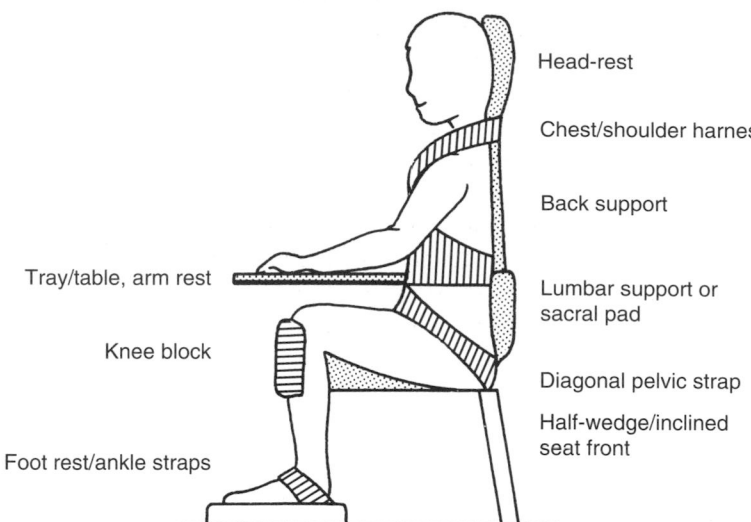

Head-rest

Chest/shoulder harness

Back support

Tray/table, arm rest

Lumbar support or
sacral pad

Knee block

Diagonal pelvic strap

Half-wedge/inclined
seat front

Foot rest/ankle straps

Fig. 8.109a First stages.

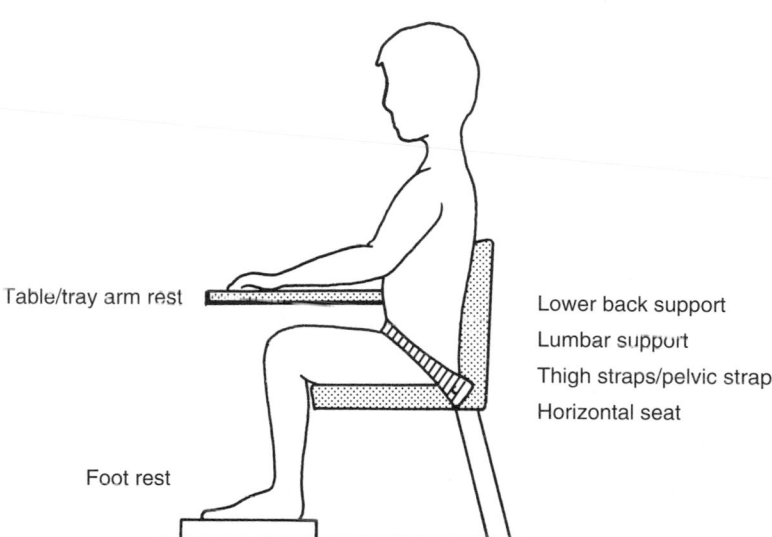

Table/tray arm rest

Lower back support

Lumbar support

Thigh straps/pelvic strap

Horizontal seat

Foot rest

Fig. 8.109b Second stages.

for safely supporting him during transport
and when he is unsupervised and may fall.
The additional support maintains postural
alignment and stability at times when a
child concentrates on difficult communication, visual, hearing and self-care activities.
He may have a floor seat and one for a
regular table, or, the floor seat can be
strapped to a frame at table level with prox-
imity to others at home or at school. An

armchair for relaxation is also appreciated
by many individuals. There are supports
and abduction wedges included in those
available on the market.

Specific considerations. See Figs 8.95, 8.109,
8.110.

Pelvis, hips and thighs. The position of a child's
pelvis is the keystone for better alignment of his

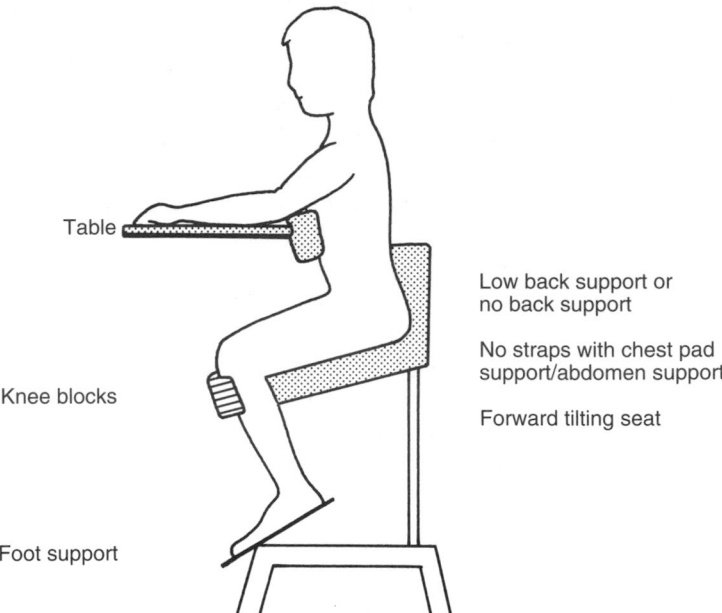

Table

Knee blocks

Foot support

Low back support or
no back support

No straps with chest pad
support/abdomen support

Forward tilting seat

Fig. 8.109c   Third stages.

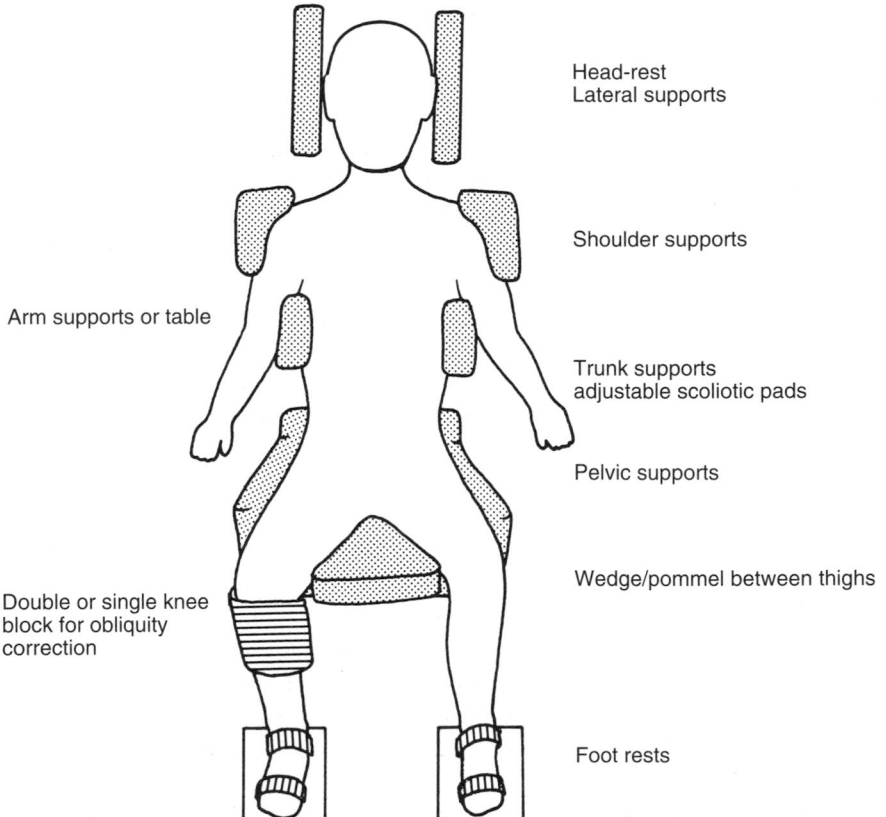

Arm supports or table

Double or single knee
block for obliquity
correction

Head-rest
Lateral supports

Shoulder supports

Trunk supports
adjustable scoliotic pads

Pelvic supports

Wedge/pommel between thighs

Foot rests

Fig. 8.109d   First
stages.

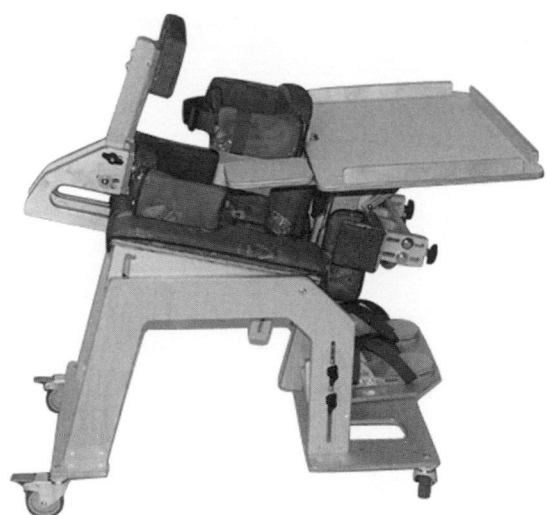

Fig. 8.110 Tilted seat with chest support. Tilt is adjustable and back of child can be observed for symmetry and weight bearing on buttocks. A table can be attached. Image supplied courtesy of Jenx, Sheffield.

head and trunk. It is positioned in association with hips, knees and foot rests. As in postural control training, a child is taught to sit well back in his chair and take weight equally on hips, thighs and feet. When his pelvis is smaller in girth than his trunk, then a sacral pad supports his pelvis as his trunk is supported by the back of his chair. When his body and buttocks change in size then the sacral pad is removed so that protruding buttocks can be accommodated and a lumbar support used. At the same time assessment is made of the developmental stage of a child's pelvic tilt forwards and lumbar mobility. A lumbar support promotes the normal minimal lordosis with vertical pelvic alignment, when a child is at that stage. If not, discomfort and pressure marks are caused.

In order to hold a child's pelvic alignment when he cannot yet do so himself use the following suggestions according to each child.

- A diagonal strap across the front of his hips which ties below the level of his seat to keep

hips back against the sacral pad or back of chair.
- A thigh strap for each leg nailed well back between a child's thighs and tying behind and below seat level. Use padding or rubber tubing on the straps to prevent chafing.
- Incline the front of the child's seat (half-wedge) so that his hips flex and his thighs receive support while his buttocks rest on a flat contoured seat. This prevents a child sliding forward, sacral sitting or hip extensor spasticity. When extensor thrust or tension is severe, then a roll of towel under the knees may help to overcome it by the increased hip flexion. The head and back may also flex as a result and a firm back support with lumbar padding may correct this. If not, try flexing the child's hips with his chest supported in a forward leaning chair with table (Figs 8.109c, 8.110) or against a padded table edge as he stretches his arms forward to grasp bars or lean on forearms.
- Some therapists prevent extensor positions of the hips and sliding out of chairs by tilting the whole chair backwards with the hips flexed between 95° and 110°, as 90° creates forward sliding. This backward tilt has advantages in that it can be a relaxed position for those children who do not have a Moro response, head and trunk thrust in semi-lying or increased athetosis. Backward leaning also fixes the vertebrae in alignment in some cases of scoliosis and in severely involved children with excessive flexion which cannot be straightened otherwise. Most therapists prefer to avoid backward leaning chairs as a child can only see the top of a room, cannot explore visually or locate sounds below him or make face-to-face contact with children on the floor. Reaching and hand function is more difficult and feeding development needs either a slight forward lean (about 20–25°) or an upright and slightly flexed head posture. This head posture prevents swallowing problems, and gagging. Backward leaning gives a sensation

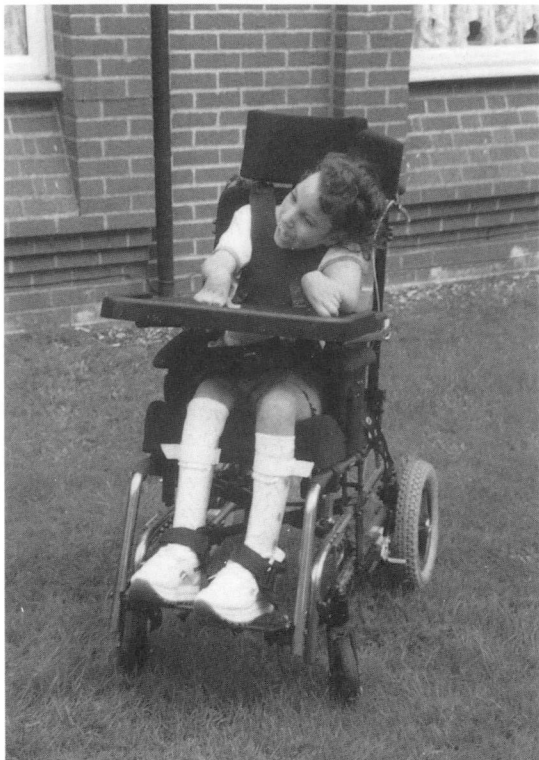

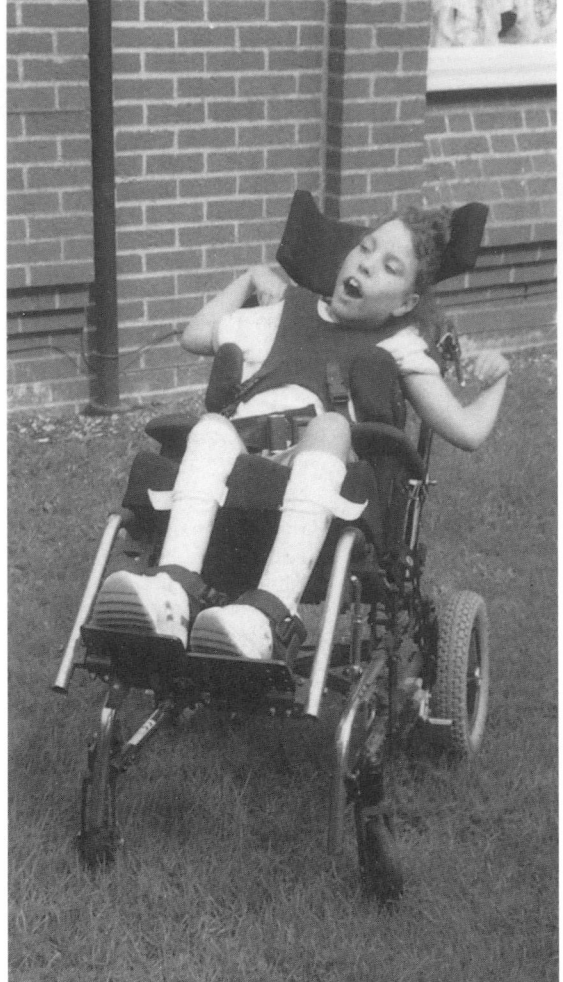

Fig. 8.111a,b Effect of backward tilt and upright position of a chair. Upright position with tray assists head control and arm function for daily activities, use of vision and communication.

of falling without the proprioception of the vertical posture essential for the development of postural stabilization (Figs 8.111a and b).

- Knee blocks hold the child's pelvis in position against a sacral pad or back support. They are also used in the forward leaning chair or forward tilted seat for back extension.
- Thigh supports with foot rests may have to be adjusted in relation to the hip flexion used. Take care to avoid pressure behind the knees. Thigh length discrepancies may require shortening of one side of the seat. Observe the position of the knees and check whether pelvic obliquity is the cause of the apparent shortening when knees are not level with each other. Thighs may also straddle a bolster seat (Stewart & McQuilton 1987) in this special design which provides a wider base for head and trunk control (Fig. 8.112).

- Knee block to correct for pelvic obliquity is needed when this is part of *windswept hips*. A wedge-shaped pommel, thigh or diagonal straps suffice in mild cases. For more severe windsweeping the abducted thigh is pushed back to position the pelvis backwards if it is rotated forwards on that side. The other thigh is abducted as far as possible (Scrutton,

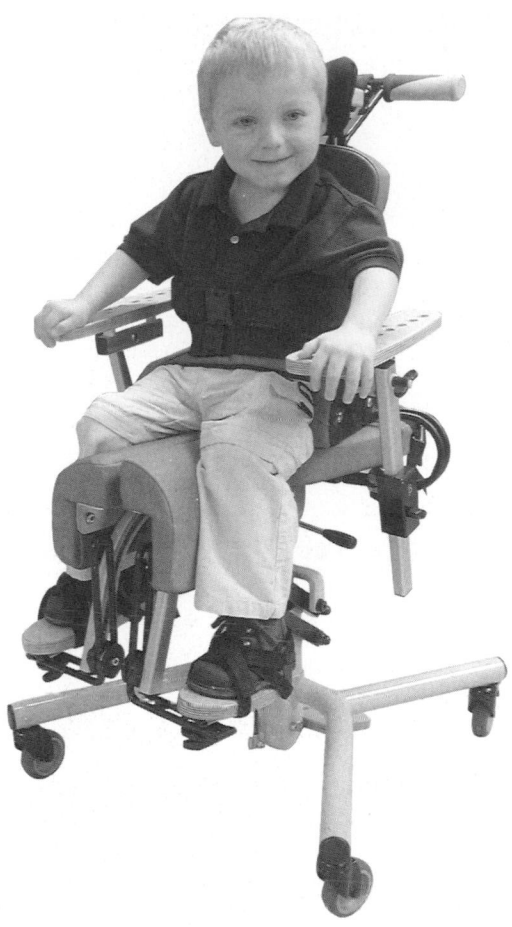

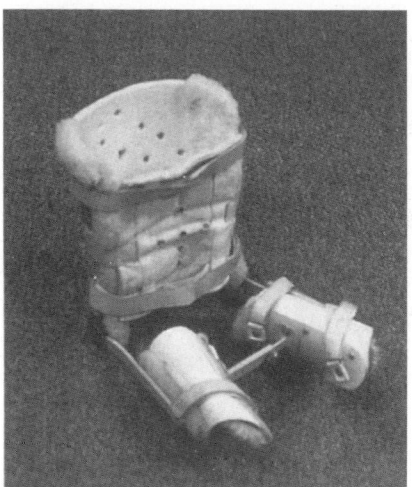

Fig. 8.113a

Fig. 8.112   Image supplied courtesy of Jenx, Sheffield.

personal communication). If the pelvis is rotated and tipped down on one side then the thigh on that side is flexed on to a small wedge to position the pelvis up and level with the other side. Some severe children benefit from thigh abduction splint alone or when attached to a trunk corset (support) (Fig. 8.113a,b). Trunk posture is then supported and checked for correction of scolioses.

- Lateral pelvis supports and pommels for a wider base also stabilize the pelvis (Fig. 8.109d).

Head and trunk. Once pelvis and hips are aligned then head and trunk are examined further. Add the following if necessary:

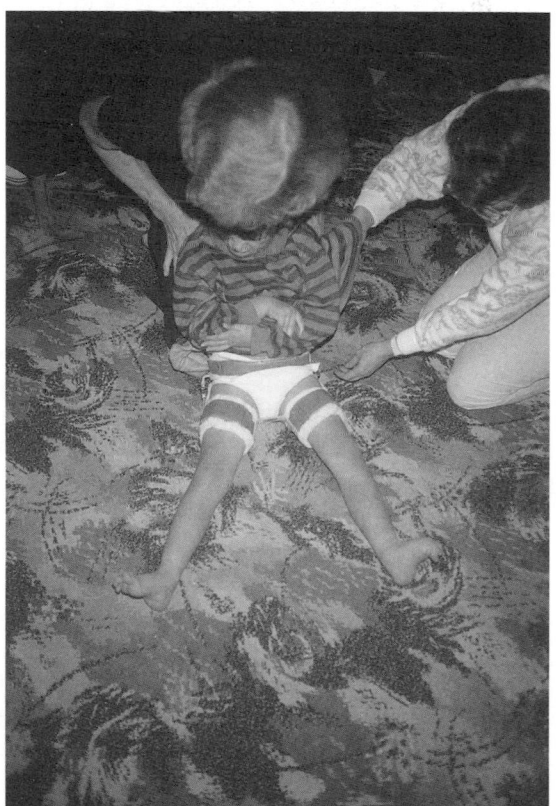

Fig. 8.113b

- An H harness or shoulder straps to maintain the upright position. A V or crossed harness may be dangerous if a child often drops his head and catches his neck in the harness. Harnesses may be tied behind a child if he enjoys playing and opening the harness buckles.
- Lateral chest supports with lateral pelvic supports hold some children in midline if they frequently tip to the side.
- Shoulder supports together with pelvic supports or with trunk supports or even all three supports can hold a child more upright.
- Shoulder supports may be used to bring retracted shoulders forwards so that a severely involved child can reach the table or touch his hands and body.
- The table needs to be adjusted so that kyphoses are corrected and both a child's arms can be lifted to correct lateral tipping or other asymmetries.
- Hand grasps on correct tray/table heights also assist head and trunk alignment.
- Scoliosis pads are attached to some chairs. The pads need to be moulded to the child's ribs first on the convexity and also on the concavity side at the axilla and at the pelvis.
- Scolioses cannot be corrected by seating on its own and trunk orthoses are necessary. When wearing a corset or other orthosis the child can be upright and the backward tilt of the chair may then be avoided. Sacral pads or other lateral padding need to be removed to give space for a spinal orthosis. Check that the orthosis does not rub against the child needing chair adjustments.
- Head control is often activated with adequate trunk and pelvic support with or without a trunk orthosis (see trunk-and-thigh orthosis in Fig. 8.113a,b). Stimulation to hold a child's head up in a chair is usually necessary. However, severely involved children may still benefit from a collar or chest and chin support.
- Usually severely involved children are placed in moulded seats custom made to the shape

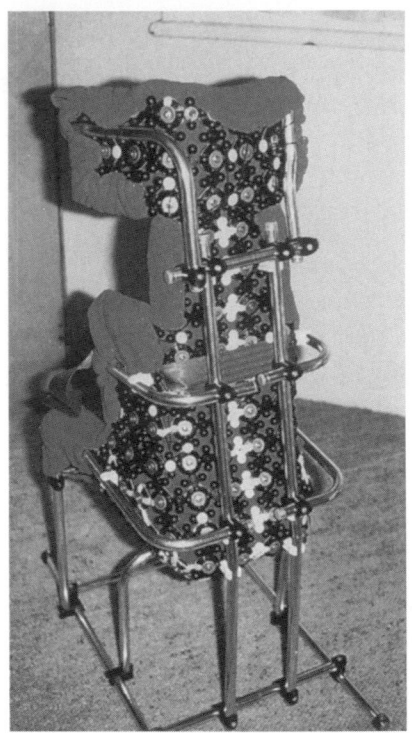

Fig. 8.114 Matrix seat.

of their own heads and bodies or to their bodies only (Bardsley, in Eckersley 1993) (Fig. 8.114).

- Lateral head supports remind children to keep their heads centred, but are unfortunately ineffective in many cases. A child often drops his head outside these head blocks.

Floor seats Select the correct floor seat so that the young child can play with toys on the floor or join other children playing on the ground in playgroups, playgrounds or sandpits (Figs 8.115–8.117).

(1) A well-padded pommel for adducted legs. Two small pommels may be used close together and gradually moved apart as the child develops more abduction of legs for a wide base.

(2) Height of the back should be at shoulder level of the child if he tends to fall back or

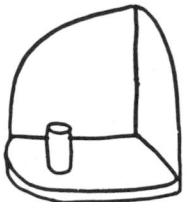

Fig. 8.115

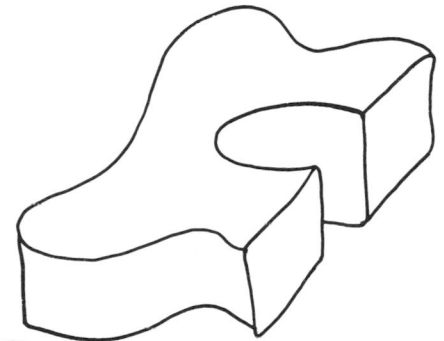

Fig. 8.116

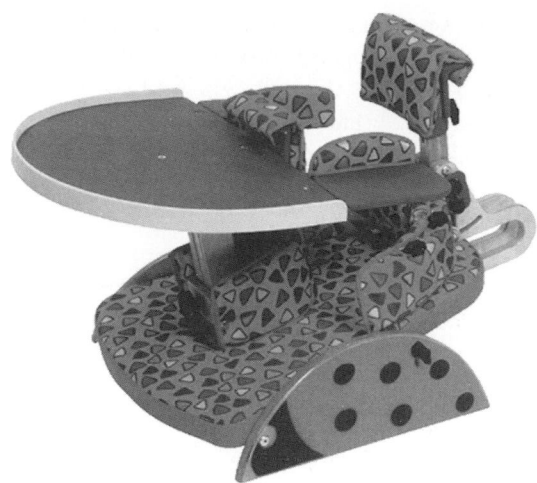

Fig. 8.117 Floor seat with tilt down and forward. Image supplied courtesy of Jenx, Sheffield.

arch back when sitting. Occasionally the head may require a padded back support. Curve the chairback to prevent shoulders and back of the child arching into extension. See cylindrical chair (Fig. 8.116).

(3) Height of the back and sides of the floor seat should be cut down to the child's waist level as he acquires more head and trunk control. A square back may be used, as well as triangular and cylindrical ones.

(4) The width of the chair should be such that the child does not slide from side to side. Pad up the sides with sponge or newspapers so that this does not occur. A canvas or inflatable seat allows the child to sink into his own area of support. His thighs become supported by the front of the seat.

(5) Seat of chair is measured from child's hips to his knees.

(6) The floor seat may be placed on wheels for locomotion if the child requires this; it may be used in a toilet seat; it may be tied on to a sturdy adult chair next to the family table. A table can be fitted to it.

(7) The floor seat may have to be raised off the floor for those children who have a very rounded back. The height of the floor seat off the floor should be tested to see whether the child's back straightens. If this does not occur, it is important to give him a table which is high enough for his arms to be elevated to that point where his back straightens. A small firm pillow or back support may help to hold the back straight. Adjusting the position of the pommel or abduction wedge may help. If none of these methods corrects a severely rounded back then a *floor seat should be used* with a tilted seat (Fig. 8.117).

(8) The seat is inclined down and forward to augment back straightening (Fig. 8.117).

Other Equipment for Sitting

(1) Chair swings, back and sides on toy trucks, rocking horse or pedal cars. Inflatable chairs, car seats, various special bath seats and also toilet seats practises supported

sitting. There is more independence if a child can grasp a horizontal bar to sit.

(2) Toilet seats (Figs 8.120–8.124). See also Chapter 9, Figs 9.1, 9.2.

(3) Pushchairs and wheelchairs (Figs 8.109a–d, 8.111a).

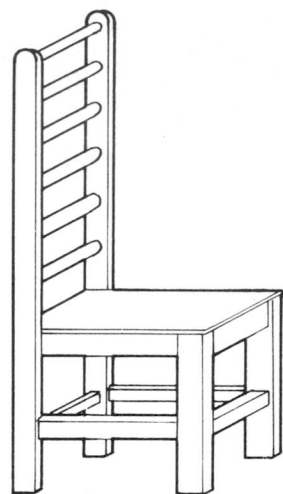

Fig. 8.118 Slatted back based on a design by Petö Institute. Child can sit sideways and hook his arm through slats for balance; use slats to push chair for walking aid. Stabilize base by using a box as base or skis attached. A box base also prevents legs twisting under the seat.

0–3 MONTHS NORMAL DEVELOPMENTAL LEVEL

Common Problems

Delay in lifting the head up from flexed or extended posture when the body is fully supported in a sitting position. Unsteady head holding in supported sitting. (Head lag in pull-to-sit, see Supine development.)

Abnormal performance of vertical head control. The head is held in an asymmetrical posture either laterally flexed, rotated or both. Arms, trunk and legs may be in infantile or other abnormal postures (see above).

Treatment Suggestions and Daily Care

Carry out any relevant methods suggested in Figs 8.94–8.105, but *giving support* to the child's shoulders and trunk and emphasizing vertical head control. Correct and train active head raise for a backward drop to avoid gagging, and correct forward drop to avoid breathing and swallowing problems.

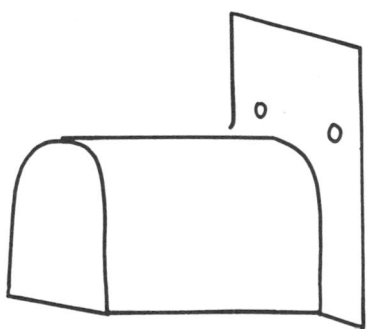
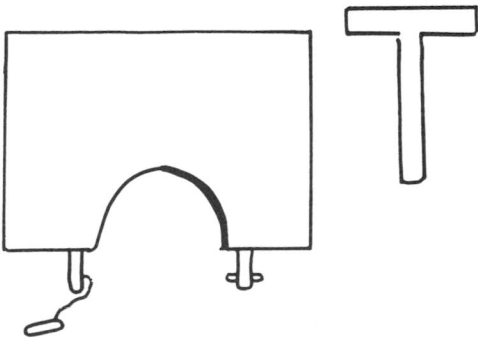

Fig. 8.119 Legs are abducted over this roll chair (based on a design by Finnie). Knees must be just beneath the top of the roll, and the roll not too wide for the child. Check that the child does not slide down one side of the roll. Ordinary low table or fitted cut-out table is used. Leave 50 mm (2 inches) between the child's body and the cut-out edge for postural adjustments.

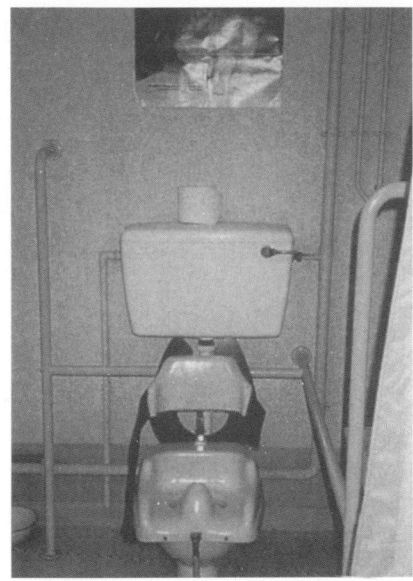

Fig. 8.120 Toilet seat.

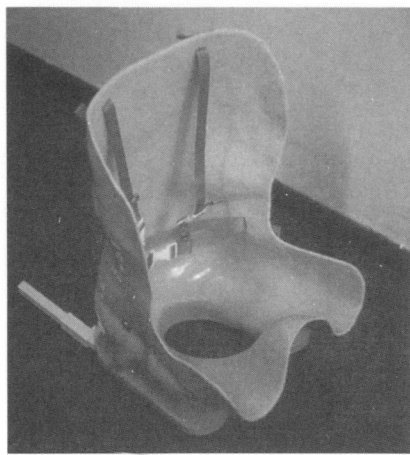

Fig. 8.121 Toilet seat.

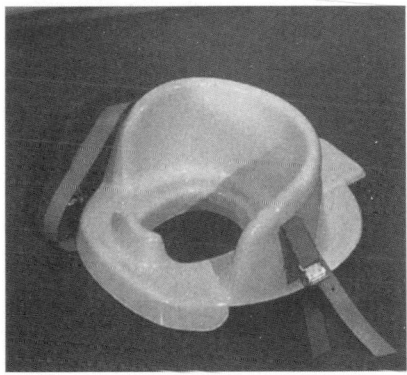

Fig. 8.122 Toilet seat.

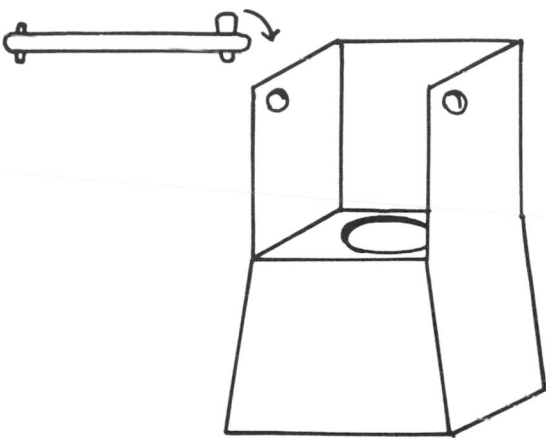

Fig. 8.123 Watford potty chair. The bar is made from 1 inch (25 mm) dowelling. For a tall child the back height needs increasing and the 10 inch × 10 inch (250 mm) seat needs enlarging. Feet must be flat on the floor. Use foot stool or box for increase of flexion of hips and knees for a very extended child.

3–6 MONTHS NORMAL DEVELOPMENTAL LEVEL

Common Problems

Delay in sitting propped up in a chair with back and sides or similar support, in the straightening of the back from the dorsal area and subsequently of the whole back, sitting leaning on his hands for support. Delay in re-erecting from lean to upright position (5–6 months level). (Delay in overcoming head lag in pull-to-sit, see Supine development.)

Abnormal performance. Therapist can anticipate abnormal postures in sitting (see above), which *may* be seen when support is given to a child at either shoulders, upper trunk, waist or hips during training and use of special chairs.

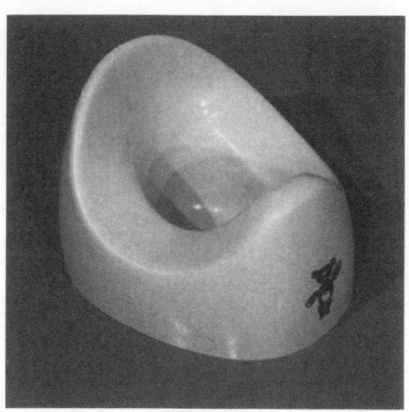

Fig. 8.124   Potty.

Reflex reactions

(1) Abnormal presence of extensor thrusts, flexion spasms, Moro or asymmetrical tonic neck reaction from 0–3 months.
(2) Arm saving reactions forward, if tipped in sitting is expected.

Treatment Suggestions and Daily Care

(1) Carry out any relevant methods in Figs 8.94–8.107, but decrease the amount of support so that head on upper trunk then on lower trunk can now develop.
(2) Tip young child whilst carrying him on your hip. Encourage him to come up to the vertical position again.
(3) Holding a young child in upright suspension and testing tilt reaction will be positive and playful for a child. However, tilt and righting in sitting is only expected at the next level.

6–9 MONTHS NORMAL DEVELOPMENTAL LEVEL

Common Problems

Delay in acquiring independent momentary sitting, sitting lean on one hand and use the other, inability to use a variety of sitting positions, once sitting has been acquired.

Special chairs still needed to support a child's body due to delay in achievement of sitting with hips supported, or child still needs to use both or one hand support for sitting. Delay re-erecting to the upright from backward forward or side leaning positions. Poor counterpoising of limb actions near the surface, shoulder level and later above shoulder level.

Abnormal performance

(1) See Abnormal postures in sitting above, only *without* support to the child.
(2) See Abnormalities of arm reach in Hand function, Figs 8.187–8.189.
(3) Turn head in all directions with abnormal trunk alignment.

Reflex reactions

(1) Reactions 0–6 months developmental level may persist abnormally in the absence of sitting control.
(2) Expect saving reactions in the arms when falling sideways and forwards.
(3) Expect head and trunk adjustment toward the vertical if the child is tipped *slowly* sideways, forward or backward.

Treatment Suggestions and Daily Care

(1) Carry out any relevant methods in Figs 8.94–8.107 *without support* at this level of development.
(2) Use methods for sitting whilst encouraging a child to *use one arm* movement whilst the other arm is grasping a support, leaning on a support or propping as a support. One arm is used for movements in feeding, dressing and playing (Chapter 9). Reaching down and in front with maintenance of sitting is first achieved followed by reach to shoulder level and later above shoulder level during activities. Decrease other arm support later to estab-

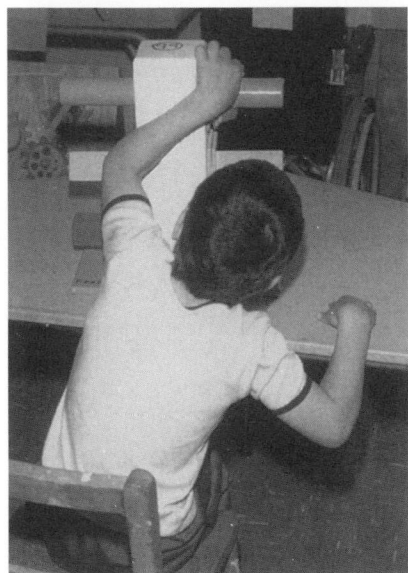

Fig. 8.125 Absence of counterpoising the arm. This may lead to a scoliosis. The table is too high. The object is too high for child.

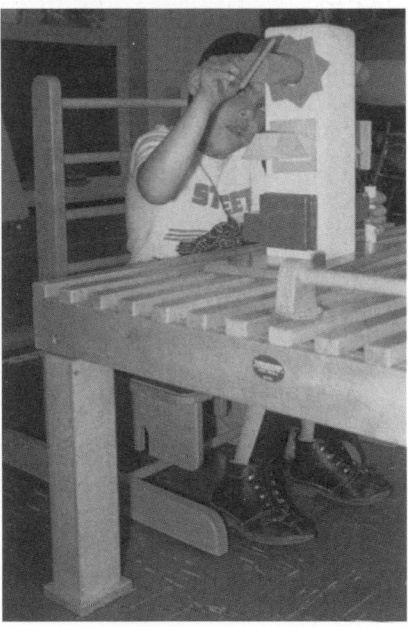

Fig. 8.126 Use of grasp for support and lower table to assist until counterpoising develops for arm elevation.

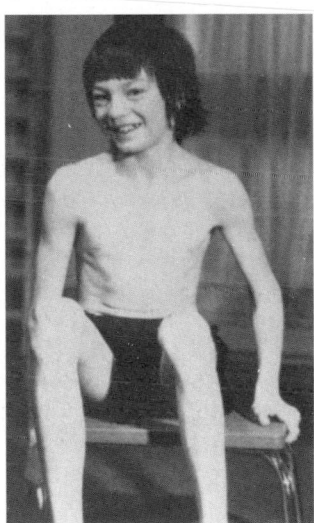

Fig. 8.127 Leaning on more affected arm during counterpoising improves stability of that arm as the more skilful arm is used. However, develop arm movements of the more affected arm so that counterpoising is activated on each side.

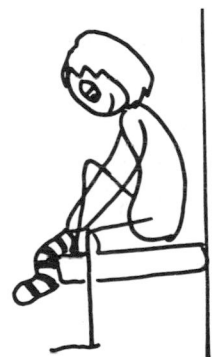

Fig. 8.128 Counterpoising during daily living activity.

leg up in the air to receive a shoe or sock, kick a ball or place foot on the seat of a chair. Sitting balance is best maintained without any back support, but *with* the child's own hand support (Fig. 8.128).

(4) See supine development, rise to sitting. Therapist may use baby gymnastics for head-trunk rising: to sitting from supine on mother's lap and astride sitting tipped sideways and raise to sit.

lish counterpoising (postural adjustment) (Figs 8.125–8.128).

(3) Use methods for sitting with the child using *one leg movement*, such as stretching one

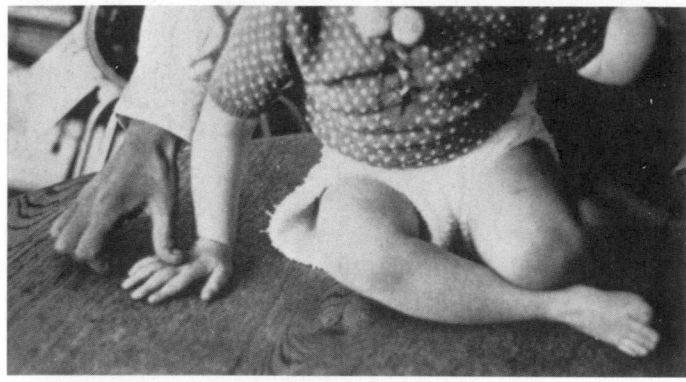

Fig. 8.129 Changing from sitting to side-sitting and back again. Change from side-sitting to four-point postures or to lying.

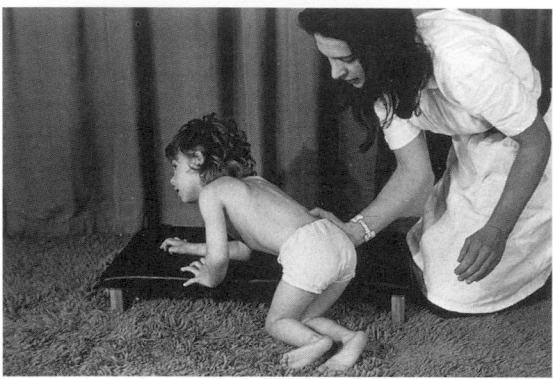

Fig. 8.130

(5) Give a child gentle pushes in all directions to train sitting control within his base.

(6) Encourage a child in sitting to look at or reach a toy of his choice and then re-erect himself to upright position. Help him tilt his pelvis for a forward reach, sideways and backward reach in the same direction as his arm motion.

(7) Upright sitting and looking behind with trunk turn is developed. However, this cannot yet be combined with reaching to side and behind him or he will fall.

9–12 MONTHS NORMAL DEVELOPMENT LEVEL

Common Problems

Delay in acquiring sitting steadily (for about 10 minutes) without support, on the floor and on a normal chair, sitting and playing without loss of balance, sitting, turning and reaching out or up without falling; changing from one sitting position to another or to lying, to crawling or pulling up to standing. Delays in sequences of any change of position, from and to reassume sitting. Delay in tilt reactions; Sit and pivot; Sit, reach across, side, up. Bottom-shuffle is delayed.

Abnormal performance as described in Abnormal postures in sitting, but carried out *without* support. Abnormal patterns of rising to sitting, and changing positions in stiff, jerky, unsteady patterns. Unusual patterns of rising devised by a child are acceptable if no other patterns are possible (Figs 8.70, 8.71).

Reflex reactions

(1) Expect: positive tilt reactions sideways, forward and backward – saving reactions of the arms in all directions including backward. If absent, sitting is insecure on any moving surface.

(2) Remnants of some infantile reactions may persist and be used for abnormal posturing or rising. A Moro reaction disrupts early tilt reactions.

Treatment Suggestions and Daily Care

Use methods in Figs 8.94–8.107 but encourage increased variety of arm patterns in play and

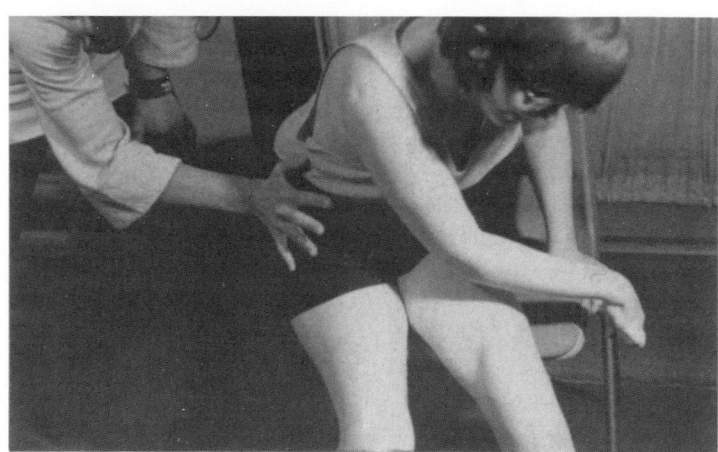

Fig. 8.131 Getting on and off chairs of various heights and widths.

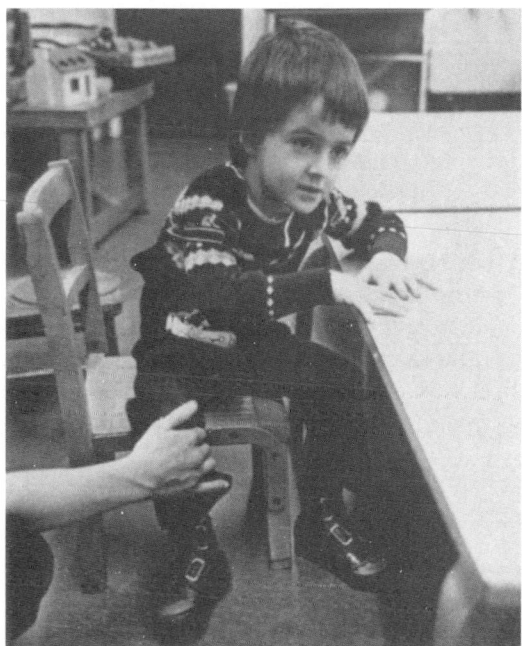

Fig. 8.132 Pivoting on a chair.

daily tasks, without supporting a child. Encourage his reaching overhead, across his body and behind his body. Use both arms simultaneously. Arm patterns are those used to correct abnormal trunk postures, e.g. the child's arm elevation corrects his kyphoscoliosis; his abduction and external rotation corrects any round backs. (See Hand function, Figs 8.190 and 8.192.)

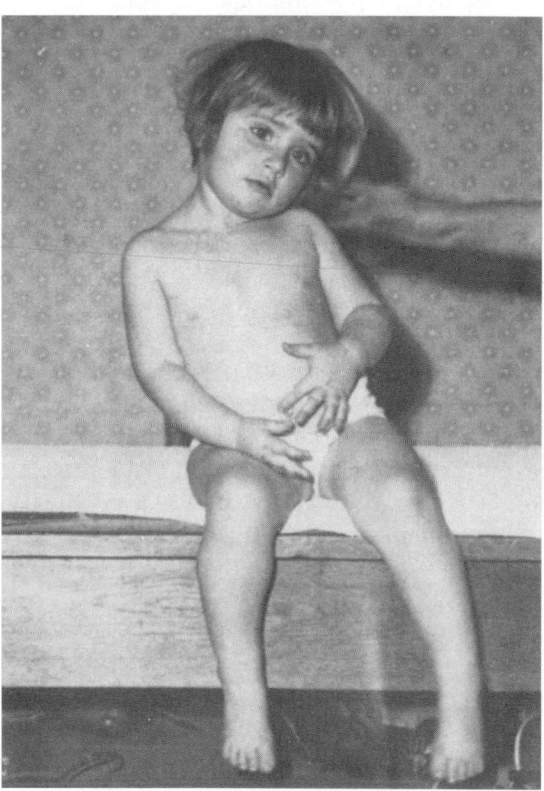

Fig. 8.133 Lateral weight shift stimulated by push off the vertical. A more vigorous push of a child's pelvis/hips well off the horizontal plane stimulates the tilt reaction. If the child falls, saving responses in limbs are activated.

Changing postures into and out of sitting position or rising reactions

(1) Rise into sitting from supine or prone (see prone development, supine development).

(2) Rise from sitting to standing up from a chair or the floor (see Standing and Walking development).

(3) Sitting on the floor with legs in front of the child, change to prone. The child either places his hands in front of him, between his legs or to one side and goes down to lying, or he places one or both his hands to one side of him, moves into side-sitting (Fig. 8.129) then change to prone kneeling (crawling position) and back again to sitting.

(4) Train the child to get on and off low wide stools (Fig. 8.130) and then chairs (Fig. 8.131). He often has to use his hands or grasp the arm rests to lean on the seat, the back of the chair or the table nearby.

(5) Train the child to get in and out of his wheelchair, in and out of a motor car, toy pedal car, tricycle and other apparatus.

(6) The therapist either moves his leg (or legs), and child pivots his body, or moves his arms, allowing child to pivot his body. Try pivot-training on each side so a child can get in and out of seats. Sitting on a chair and swivelling himself around on the chair is a useful motor ability which is well worth training (Fig. 8.132).

Enabling a child to achieve a variety of postural changes teaches separation of adducted legs, trunk control and arm extension, as his hand reaches out for the back of the chair or forward and sideways from floor sitting to lying, among other patterns. Body rotative patterns are used and these together with other aspects appear to reduce hypertonus, lengthen and strengthen muscle groups.

It is easier for a child to go down to lying from sitting first before having to learn how to lift himself up to sitting from lying *if* rotation is used. It is not so if straight patterns are used as lying down takes control or an individual would collapse into lying.

● Practise as many different sitting positions as possible: side-sitting (Fig. 8.129); sitting with one foot flat on the ground, the other bent or straight; sitting with both knees bent and feet flat on the ground (crook-sitting); sitting in various types of chairs of the correct size and in adult chairs if the child is correctly placed. Sitting with his legs dangling and no foot support is an advanced posture.

● Augment sitting with manual resistance given laterally, with rotation, anteroposteriorly (Fig. 8.107).

● Postural adjustment during weight shift as well as tilt reactions and saving reactions in the limbs are all stimulated by slow and by quick pushes (Fig. 8.133). Use rocking chairs, rocking horses, swings, see-saws, rocker boat or toys, and inflatable toys to help develop the tilt reactions and security in sitting. Play 'see-saw' games on parent's lap or body. Pony riding and horse riding stimulate tilt (Fig. 8.134) and a variety of postural adjustments within a child's base.

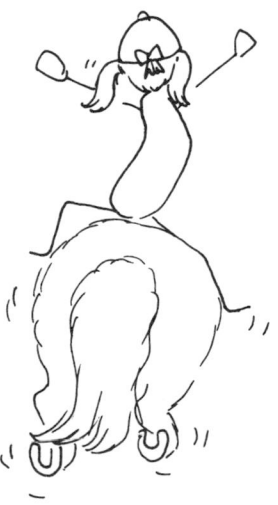

Fig. 8.134

DEVELOPMENT OF STANDING AND WALKING

The following main aspects should be developed:

Antigravity support or weight bearing on feet. Normally present at birth and modified at 6 months.

Postural stability of the head on the trunk (Fig. 8.135), trunk stabilizes on the pelvis in the vertical. Normally present by 9–12 months (see sitting).

Postural stability of the pelvic girdle in the vertical. Normally present by 9–12 months (see upright kneeling supported, and supported standing).

Counterpoising in the standing position when holding on (Fig. 8.136), i.e. normal at 9–12 months level, and without holding on, 12–18 months, becoming more varied in the second and third year of life. Example are: lifting an arm or standing on one foot, holding on at 9–11 months normally and much later on one foot,

and not holding on, at $2^1/_2$–3 years of age normally. Standing on one foot is a most important counterpoising action. The child can then take weight on one leg for long enough to allow the other to swing through and step. Prepare for one foot balance by weight shift from side to side.

Control of anteroposterior weight shift of the child's centre of gravity to initiate walking (propulsion) and to stop (retropulsion). Later in a diagonal direction and in turning (12–24 months normally).

Control of lateral sway from one foot to the other. Normally developed in cruising and walking each hand held laterally, and similar activities about 12 months of age. Lateral sway is very obvious in toddlers and becomes modified with development.

Tilt reactions in standing are anteroposterior and lateral. They are acquired after standing and walking alone. Tilt reactions are not important for standing and walking. However, children without tilt reactions will be unsure in the dark and on rough ground.

Saving from falling (Fig. 8.137). If tilt reactions fail, the child will take a protective step out to

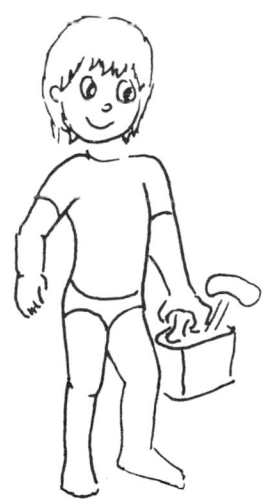

Fig. 8.136   Counterpoising a weight or movement of the arm.

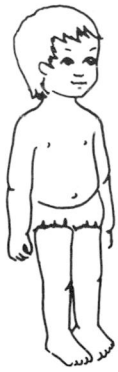

Fig. 8.135   Postural stability, head on trunk on pelvis and whole of child in standing.

save himself (staggering). He also flings out his arms in protective (saving) reactions. Normally these develop at 12–24 months of age. They are important as the child will have less fear of falling if he can protect himself, and may then become willing to walk.

Foley (personal communication) has described various abnormalities of gait associated with the absence of one or more of the above mechanisms. These problems are outlined and treated in the practical suggestions below.

Rising reactions (Fig. 8.138) from lying (prone and supine) to standing, from sitting to standing and from kneeling to standing. Some have already been discussed in the sections on supine, sitting and prone development. (See also Fig. 8.179.)

Prognosis. Montgomery (1998) reviewed seven studies identifying predictors of walking (ambulation). Walking was acquired between 3 and 9 years, and was unlikely afterwards. Sitting by 2 years and crawling by 2½ years were strong predictors but some who only sat by 4 years did eventually achieve walking. Children with *obligatory* primitive reflexes at 2 years were most unlikely to walk. Scrutton and Baird (1997) found that children not rising to sit and sitting alone by 2 years were less likely to walk by 5 years.

ABNORMAL POSTURES IN STANDING (see also Figs 8.151–8.154)

These may be due to:

Absence of postural stability. The child may be able to maintain equilibrium, even inadequately, by attempting an abnormal posture to compensate for this absence (Figs 8.151, 8.154). He may be:

(1) *Sinking* into hip flexion, knee flexion, with or without:
(2) Adduction-internal rotation of the legs.
(3) Lordosis may compensate for hip flexion.
(4) Round back and head flexion or head thrown back and chinpoking may be present.
(5) Feet in valgus or in overdorsiflexion. If overdorsiflexion is limited by tightness of ankle or plantarflexors, the child may stand on his toes.

Alternatively the child may fall or extend backwards and compensate by (Figs 8.152, 8.153):

(1) Hip flexion.
(2) Hyperextension of knees.
(3) Internal rotation of legs, occasionally.
(4) Valgus feet or normal feet.
(5) Rounding his back and jutting his head forward.

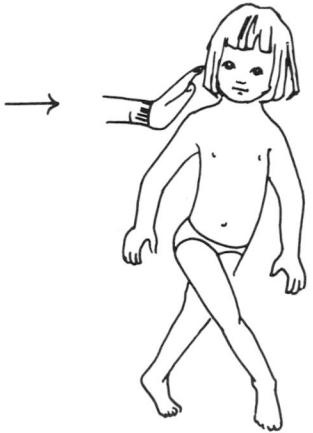

Fig. 8.137   Saving from falling with a protective step.

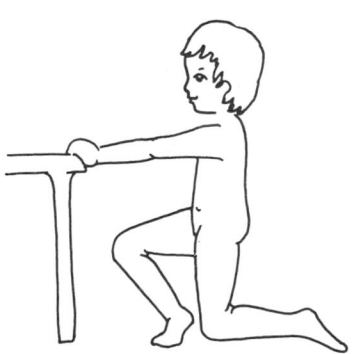

Fig. 8.138   Rising to standing.

Stages in the development of standing and walking

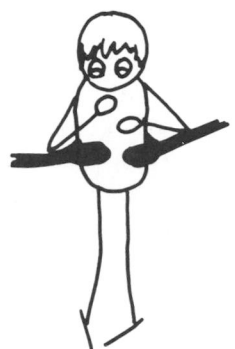

Fig. 8.139 Weight bearing on legs (supporting reaction) (*0–3 months*). Body held.

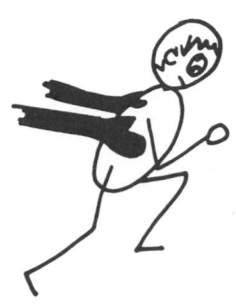

Fig. 8.140 Automatic stepping if infant is tilted forward, body held. (*0–3 months*).

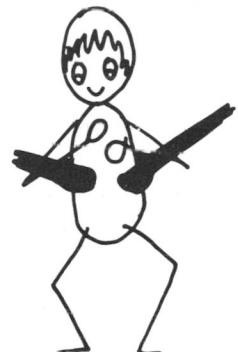

Fig. 8.141 Sinking or astasia (*3–6 months*). Head control.

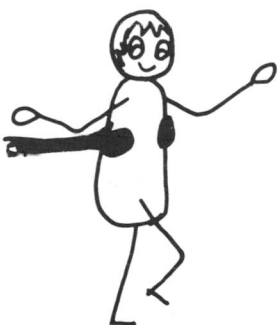

Fig. 8.142 Trunk supported standing and bouncing in standing (*5–7 months*).

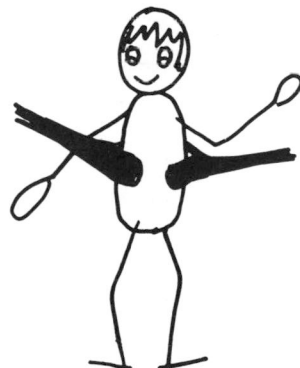

Fig. 8.143 Supported standing (*5–7 months*). Weight bearing of legs.

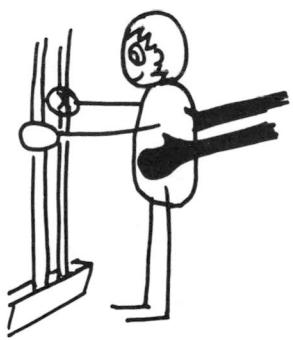

Fig. 8.144 Stand holding on to support with pelvic support (*7–9 months*).

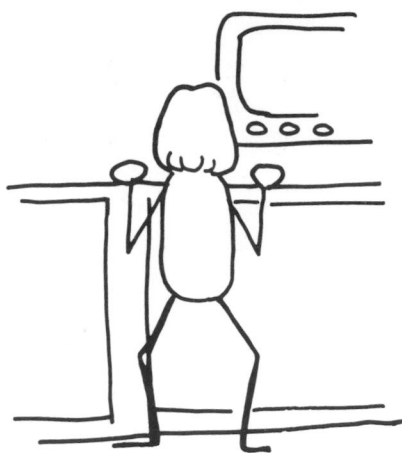

Fig. 8.145 Stand holding on to furniture (*7–9 months*). Begin weight shift.

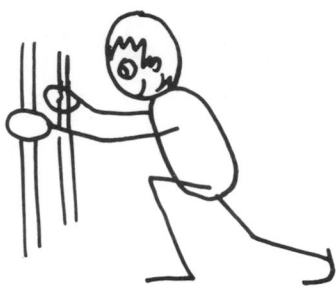

Fig. 8.146 Pull up to standing from various positions (*9–12 months*).

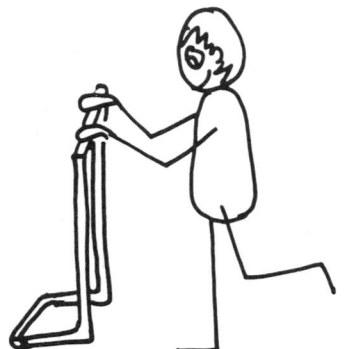

Fig. 8.147 Standing holding and lift one leg off the ground or one arm released (*11 months*).

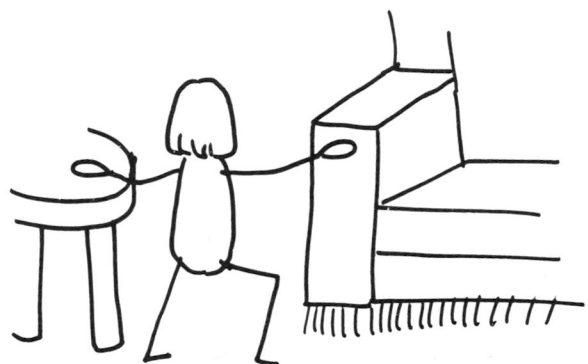

Fig. 8.148 Cruising (lateral stepping) (*9–12 months*).

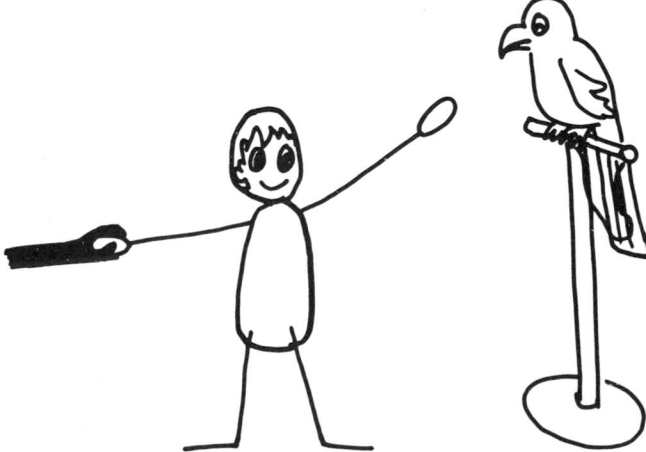

Fig. 8.149 Stand supported, reach in all directions (*9–12 months*). Weight shift.

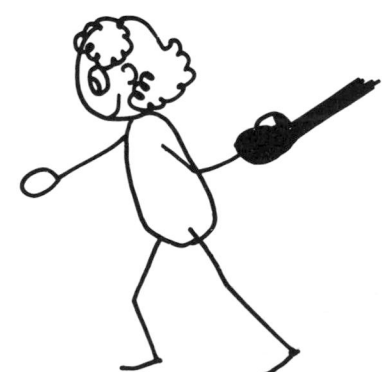

Fig. 8.150 Stand alone and walk with two hands, then one, then no hand support (*12–18 months*).

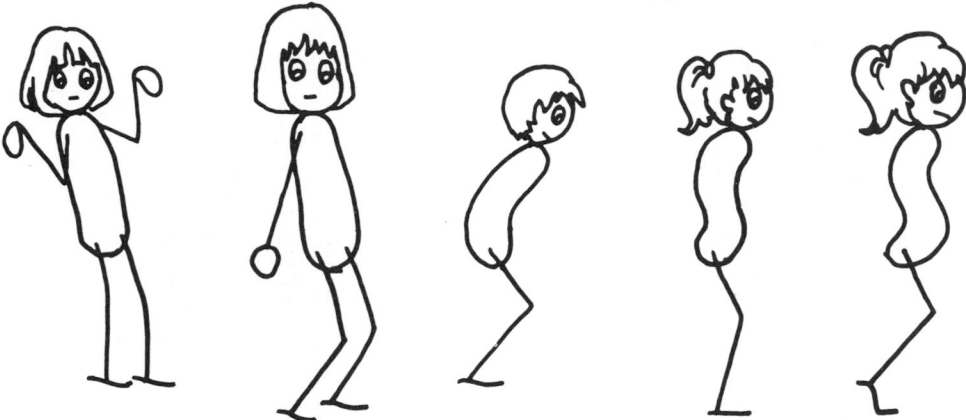

Fig. 8.151 Falling or extending backwards is compensated by hip and knee flexion and adduction, lordosis, valgus, over-dorsiflexed feet or plantarflexion.

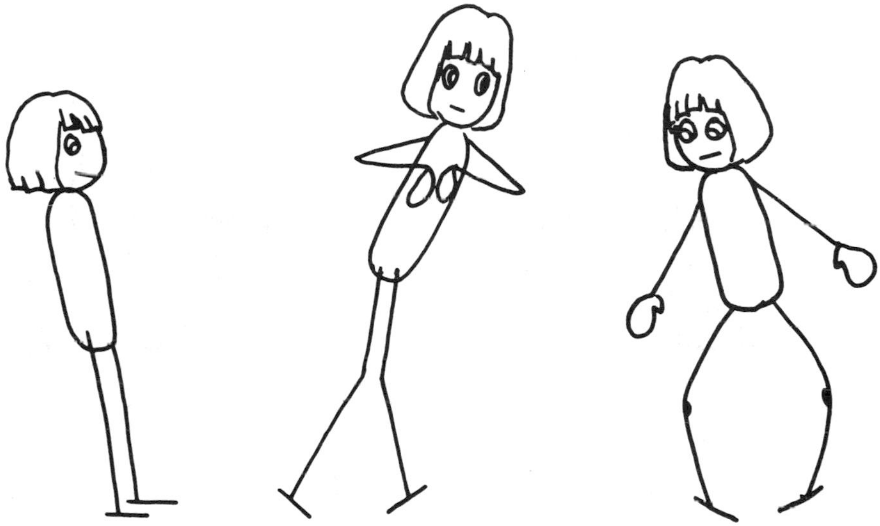

Fig. 8.152 Compensation for lack of postural stability (and thus falling backwards) by flexion-adduction of the hips and knees and pronation of feet, wide base, or by: hyperextension-abduction-internal rotation of knees, wide base, pronated feet.

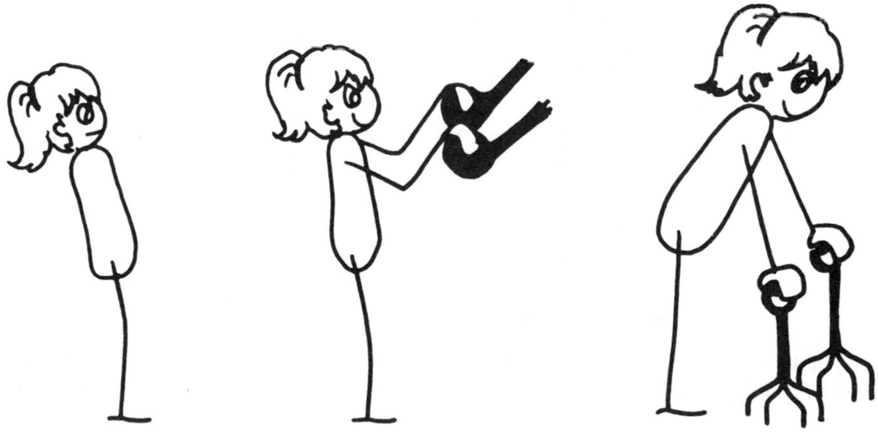

Fig. 8.153 Compensation for lack of postural stability and/or counterpoising in standing and/or standing on one foot by use of hand grasp or *walk on hands* for support. Children increase spasticity in their arms if they flex and grasp.

These postures, to maintain equilibrium under difficult biomechanical circumstances, are also seen in normal people on slippery surfaces or when first attempting ice skating or skiing.

If a child also has spasticity or rigidity with short stiff muscles, he may use that to prop himself up into the abnormal postures above.

If the child has *good* upper limbs or at least a grasp in poor upper limbs, he will use them for support. Such children *stand and walk on their hands* with walking aids (Fig. 8.154). They bear so much weight on their hands that fatigue of the good arms is common. Athetoid children are known to hold their shoulders and arms forward and together to stop the backward fall. Arms may even be held forward and up in the air to counterbalance the backward fall in standing.

Fear of falling is naturally appropriate when postural control is so inadequate. Fears exacerbate all these abnormal postures.

Asymmetrical postural fixation (stabilization) and counterpoising. The child will take weight on the better side and the leg with poor postural fixation will flex, adduct, internally rotate at the hip, flex at the knee and remain propped on the forefoot, or have no weight bearing. An athetoid child may have one leg *pawing* the ground with an involuntary motion.

Scoliosis may compensate for the body weight being distributed to one side only. This asymmetry may or may not also have been seen in other weight-bearing positions such as sitting, kneeling or four-foot kneeling. Sometimes, it is the postural fixation mechanism of the pelvis in standing only which fails, but which may be able to cope at lower levels of development, such as sitting and upright kneeling which provide a wider base or a lower base than standing.

The unaffected side in hemiplegia obviously takes all or most of the child's weight. The hemiplegic leg is usually rotated back from the pelvis. It may be abducted or adducted, internally rotated, knee flexed, straight or hyperex-

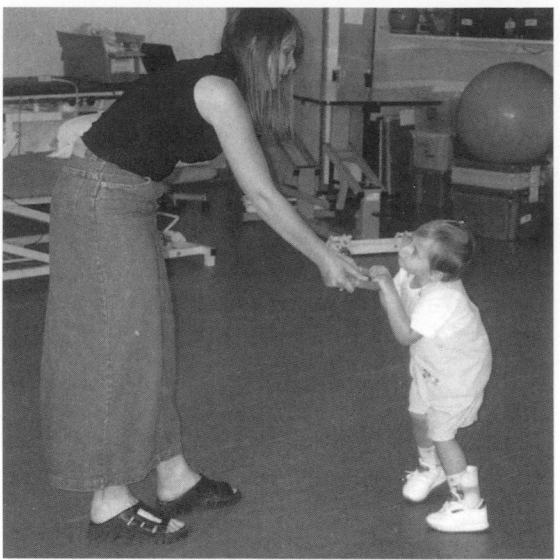

a

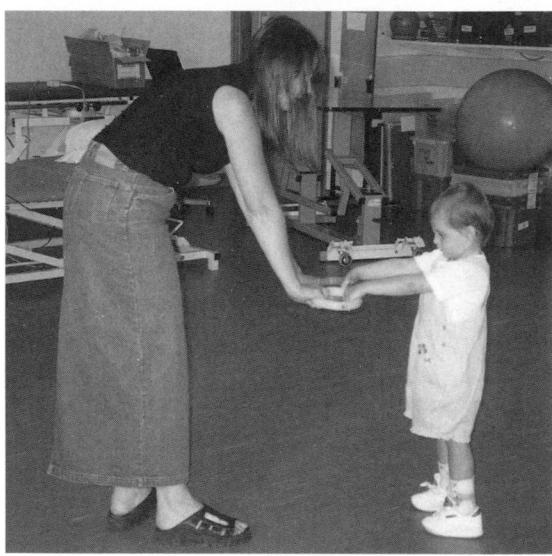

b

Fig. 8.154 (a) Standing with flexion and asymmetry, and poor postural control. (b) Correction with arms symmetrical elbows extended and both hands either grasping in front, below and in front, or at each side. Equal weight on each leg, head and trunk in midline, facing mother for motivation.

tended, and foot flat or in equinus, toes may claw the ground. If the young child's weight is taken on the hemiplegic leg and the good leg lifted, he may collapse or sink into flexion. Lack of counterpoise of one arm may lead to the child leaning abnormally to one side or on to the other hand for support. This creates asymmetrical postures. Presence of tilt reactions to *one* side only may be associated with scoliosis (Levitt 1984, p. 115).

Absence of protective saving reactions of arms or legs may delay standing and walking in some children because of a justified fear of falling. This absence of saving will create crouching postures as seen in normal people who fear falling. In addition, absent tilt reactions make them even more unsure and they will increase those abnormal postures which compensate for lack of postural stability and counterpoising (Figs 8.151–8.153). This is particularly obvious when they are on uneven surfaces.

Persistence of primitive reflexes and pathological reflexes. Unwitting constant stimulation of reflex stepping, excessive positive supporting reaction (Bobath & Bobath 1984), withdrawal reflexes increase abnormal leg postures. Repeated stimulation of one pattern of involuntary movement may increase tension in joint and abnormal posture may be seen. Persistence of abnormal reflexes on one side may be associated with abnormal supported standing postures, e.g. Galant's reflex on one side of the trunk, asymmetrical tonic neck reflex to one side only and the everted withdrawal reflex or involuntary motion in one leg in an athetoid child.

Growth of legs. Unequal growth of legs may be causing abnormal postures during standing, e.g. weight bearing on the longer side leads to an equinus on the shorter leg in order to reach the ground. Weight bearing on to the shorter side leads to the hip flexing or both hip and knee flexing on the longer side to tend to equalize the balance. Scoliosis to one side may occur to compensate for leg length.

Asymmetrical distribution of spasticity may be present and add to the abnormal asymmetry in postural control of weight bearing in standing (see below).

Use of spasticity for compensation. If there is no postural stability and counterpoising mechanisms and the child has a spastic type of cerebral palsy he will *use his spasticity* to *fix* him in the upright position. Thus if a child is *standing on spasm* he will collapse to the ground if his spasticity is removed by physiotherapy, drugs or surgery for spastic muscle groups. He may be left with straight legs but completely lose his independent standing or even his previous ability of stumbling around.

Some athetoid children have been observed to use an asymmetrical tonic neck reaction. The face turning to one side increases hypertonus in the weight-bearing leg on that side, so that they can then bear weight on it.

It is interesting that some workers called children with spasticity 'children with too much fixation' meaning postural fixation, and call children with rigidity 'children with too much postural stability' (Goff 1969). It is that they have *no* or poor normal postural fixation or stability and use hypertonicity to prop them up against gravity.

Biomechanics and spasticity. Spasticity may be greater in one group than another. If a resulting deformity is greater in one joint it leads to abnormal postures in the others to maintain a fairly upright position. These postures may also become deformities. For example:

(1) Hip flexion may be dictated by greater knee flexion.
(2) Hip flexion may be dictated by equinus in order not to extend and fall back.
(3) Knee flexion may be dictated by too much hip flexion to avoid falling forward.
(4) Hip flexion-adduction-internal rotation may be dictated by valgus flexed knees.
(5) Hip extension may occur by hamstrings flexing the knees and tilting the pelvis backwards. A long kyphosis or a flat back may be associated.

(6) Knee flexion or knee hyperextension may compensate for tight plantarflexors or equinus.

(7) Equinus may be secondary to excessive hip and knee flexion and the spastic plantarflexors cannot remain stretched by the mechanical overdorsiflexion.

(8) Lordosis compensates for hip flexion.

(9) Kypholordosis compensates for hip flexion.

Clearly, abnormal postures or deformities are rarely localized in one joint. Thus one spastic muscle group with its weak antagonists should never be considered alone in treatment, with or without orthopaedic surgery.

The child's abnormal posture may be different when he has to maintain his balance on his own. Thus abnormal postures are:

Supported standing

- Hip extension or semiflexion, adduction with legs together or crossing (scissoring), internal rotation.
- Knee extension.
- Equinus or *on toes*.

Later in unsupported standing

- Hip flexion, adduction-internal rotation.
- Knee flexion or hyperextension or normal.
- Feet equinovarus, varus (supination), valgus (pronation), sometimes heel may be down and forefoot everted.
- Toes may clench and evert.
- Lordosis, kyphosis, flattening of lumbar area or kypholordosis.
- Excessive pelvic tilt backwards is associated with flat back, pelvic tilt forwards with lordosis.

Perturbations of a child in standing. Nashner *et al.* (1983) have shown in their studies that the sequence of muscle activation in a cerebral palsied child differs from that of an able-bodied child. Nevertheless, such a child with cerebral palsy does not fall over.

Arm and Head Postures

These are similar to the abnormal postures seen in the lower levels of the child's development. However, if the hands are grasped by an adult or the child holds on for support he may use an abnormal pattern in arms and hands. The child with the spastic type of cerebral palsy usually increases flexion-adduction in shoulder, shoulder hunching, flexion-pronation in elbow, palmar flexion with or without ulnar deviation in hands, adduction of thumbs. Increase in flexion in the arms often seems to increase flexion in the legs and aggravate the abnormal postures of the whole child, and vice versa. Increase of abnormal shoulder extension often associates with hip extension. Children who have dyskinesia may abduct and hold their arms up excessively and with dystonia. This aggravates their backward fall or lean. The child may flex his head or *poke* his chin forward in standing.

ABNORMAL GAIT

The problems in standing will affect the gait, therefore walking should not be 'pushed' if standing is absent or very abnormal. Fears of falling may increase abnormal gait patterns in such cases.

Delay or abnormal walking patterns may be due to:

Poor or absent stability and counterpoising or asymmetrical ability to counterpoise. The child may *waddle* from side to side without counterpoising each leg, that is he 'falls' from foot to foot as he cannot maintain posture for any length of time on one side. There may be excessive trunk sway from side to side. The pelvis and trunk may rotate forward on the side of the swing-through (stepping) leg instead of counterpoising on to the weight bearing leg in an upright position. The child may have a better postural mechanism on one side, most obviously seen in hemiplegia or asymmetrical tetraplegia or triplegia (asymmetrical ability). A limp on to the good side is then characteristic of the gait.

Children with dyskinesia may *run headlong* as they cannot bear weight long enough on each side for a step. Children with dysknesia or ataxia stumble about and were thought to be drunk by some members of the public. Children with intellectual impairment as in the case of cerebral palsy may not wish to walk, show fear of walking and hang on to adults excessively and on to their walking aids. Excessive arm flinging movements or emphasis of the saving reactions in the arms come into play to help the child balance on each unstable leg. 'Sinking' patterns of standing and compensation for falling back are seen as in standing (see Figs 8.151–8.153). Involuntary motion of a child's arms observed in dyskinesia can also throw him off balance.

Absence of anteroposterior shift. This makes it impossible for the child to *start* walking. A walking aid on wheels may start him off. Stopping is also difficult if this mechanism is not operating. He may also *mark time* and then stop, as he is unable to stop or reverse the anteroposterior shift. Some children only stop by a collapse onto their bottoms.

Absence of lateral sway. This is obvious in the athetoid pattern of running headlong and other children pushing wheelwalkers. In treatment, lateral sway is helped by training standing on one foot (counterpoising), and is also developed in cruising sideways and other activities which promote lateral weight shift from leg to leg.

Lack of tilt reactions in prone, supine, sitting, upright kneel and standing rarely delays walking. This training in walking should not be delayed if these reactions are not yet acquired. Martin (1967) found that labyrinthectomized adults could walk although tilt reactions were not possible without their labyrinths. Similar observations have been noted in children who walk but have absent or poor tilt reactions. Nevertheless, tilt reactions should be included in the programme as it makes the child more steady in changes of terrain and in the dark. As Dr Foley puts it, 'you cannot walk across a ploughed field at night if you do not have tilt reactions' (personal communication).

Saving or protective reaction (arms and legs). These must be trained to prevent the danger of the child falling on his face, and giving him confidence to walk. Remember that the protective step in falling is not the same as a voluntary step which the child takes as he is being trained to walk. Foley observed the presence of voluntary stepping without the presence of protective stepping and vice versa (personal communication). Therapy must therefore train both of those stepping movements. Excessive saving reactions in arms or legs may occur to compensate for the absence of the other mechanisms. It is most noticeable in ataxic children and athetoid children. The *drunken walk* may be excessive staggering reactions in the legs. Children with dyskinesia cannot *stand still* but take little protective steps. A wide base is used for better balance by children with dyskinesia or ataxia and by those who are only motor delayed without cerebral palsy.

Forssberg (1985) and Leonard *et al.* (1988, 1991), among others, have contributed studies on abnormal gait patterns compared to normal children's walking.

Abnormal Gaits in the Spastic Type

All the problems above will be included with the addition of the pull of short or stiff spastic muscles and associated weakness. There may be abnormal postures which are associated with each other, as described in the section on Abnormal postures in standing.

Hips and Knees

Hips may adduct and legs cross when the child is supported, and adduct-internally rotate and flex when the child is walking independently. Excessive flexion occurs as the leg is swinging through and/or on weight bearing (stance).

Knees may overflex on swing-through and on weight bearing. Hip and knee flexion may occur to allow a plantarflexed foot (or toe pointing foot) to swing and clear the ground, and once on the ground hip and knee flexion occur to push the heel to the ground. *Toe first* and not the normal heel strike is common in spastic types of cerebral palsy.

Lack of heel strike after swing-through may be compensated differently.

In hemiplegia, diplegia and tetraplegia the hip alone may flex with hyperextension of the knee to press the heel to the ground. This is usual with extensor patterns or excessive antigravity support as the forefoot strikes the ground.

A wide base is used with flexed adducted (valgus) knees as the child cannot balance on the small base created by adduction of the legs.

Feet

Walking on the toes is seen if the child is supported and later when he walks alone. There is not only weight bearing on the toes but the toes are brought down first for weight bearing (see above).

Walking on the toes may become walking on a pronated-everted (valgus) foot in the child's efforts to compensate for spastic plantarflexors.

Walking on toes may be accompanied by slightly flexed hips and even straight knees or slightly flexed in younger or milder cases.

A rare *normal ballerina walk* has been observed (Holt 1973). Hips and knees are straight and flexible. I have also observed this in toddlers with severe visual impairment without any cerebral palsy. Rising onto toes may be a response to a forward fall seen in leg protective reactions. It is also seen in normal unstable toddlers.

Pelvis and Trunk

The pelvis often rotates abnormally in 'spastic gaits'. The rotation may be backwards so the leg appears *retracted* and behind the other. Usually the front, better leg may take more weight, as in hemiplegia. However the back leg may take more weight and allow the forward leg to step, take its momentary weight and then transfer on to the back leg, which only has time to take a small step and *cannot* get in front of the forward leg.

Pelvic tilt is also backwards with flattening of the lumbar area, or pelvic tilt forwards with a lordosis of the lumbar area. Kyphosis of the thorax may occur with flat back or lordosis. Scoliosis may be present due to unequal weight distribution, leg length and other reasons already given for asymmetry in standing and sitting.

If the child takes a step, his spasticity may be so great that he has to lean back to push his leg forward. He has an anteroposterior *waddle* or jerky walk. Lateral waddle is associated with spastic adductors and weak abductors. It is also involved with inability to stabilize the pelvis or to adjust the trunk when counterpoising in standing on one leg. The trunk and head may lean forward to help overcome spasticity as well as maintain balance. This usually *increases* toe walking as the child cannot put his heels down in this pattern.

Arms

Excessive arm swing up, arms held up in the air, or excessive saving reactions may occur in the arms. Therefore, normal reciprocal arm swing may be absent. Abnormal postures of arms may be seen as in earlier normal motor development. The retraction of the shoulder may accompany retraction of the pelvis and hip. (See Figs 8.165–8.171.)

Summary

Abnormal features of gait for therapy

Excessive (1) Hip and trunk sway from side to side or a pelvic waddle.

(2) Hip and trunk sway antero-posterior and jerky gait.

(3) Asymmetry of weight bearing and unequal steps.

(4) Abnormal postures of head, trunk, pelvis, knees and feet.

(5) Abnormal stepping patterns, e.g. walk on toes.

(6) Athetoid *running gait*; *drunken gait* in ataxia or dyskinesia (athetosis); *high stepping gait* or *scissoring gait* in spastic or dyskinetic types of cerebral palsy.

(7) Overactive arms to maintain balance, *tightrope walking* or abnormal arm postures and lack of reciprocal arm swing. Excessive involuntary arm motion seen in dyskinesia.

TREATMENT SUGGESTIONS AT ALL LEVELS OF DEVELOPMENT

Practical Points

Train standing (stability and counterpoising) with weight shift and postural alignment *first*, *and also* in phases of gait for a child learning to walk or already walking alone with an abnormal gait. The abnormal gait may be compensation for poor postural control in standing. Therefore concentrating on postural stability and counterpoising one foot stance improves gait. All the abnormal gaits discussed above will be treated in a programme concentrating on:

(1) Equal distribution of weight on each foot.
(2) Correction of abnormal postures.
(3) Building up of the child's stability by decreasing support.

(4) Delay training in standing and walking if the child is not ready.

(5) Continuing to develop head, trunk and pelvic postural stability and weight shift with counterpoising in mainly upright postures, such as sitting, as well as in standing.

(6) Weight shift leading to stepping.

(7) Training lateral sway (weight shift), cruising and walk holding support each side.

(8) Training stopping and starting, turning (pivots), walking on uneven ground, on different surfaces, and using stairs and inclines.

(1) Equal distribution of weight bearing on each foot. Supported and later unsupported standing according to developmental level.

(a) Check this by having child standing on two weighing scales and help him correct this as you read the *equal* weight borne on each scale. Also, biofeedback with force plates and visual display for training an older person (Hartveld & Hegarty 1996).

(b) Head and trunk in midline supported and then unsupported after 9 month level of normal development.

(c) Teach weight shift on to the side that bears less weight. Do this by asking and assisting the child to move himself on to the leg. If possible, ask the child to move against your hand placed firmly against his lateral hip and maintain trunk alignment.

(d) Use a mirror for both you and the child to see that he is in correct alignment with his weight on both feet. A white stripe on the mirror gives added visual cue for his alignment.

(e) Use a wide base and then bring both feet together for standing, then stand with one foot in front of the other.

(f) Correct any deformities, especially of the feet, such as equinus, so that there are *two* plantigrade feet for equal weight bearing. Equinus may be secondary to other deformities, see below.

(g) Check length of legs in case of growth asymmetries and raise shoe if there is more than $1/2$-inch (12.5 mm) difference.

(h) Remember to keep the child's weight forward over both feet and help him avoid any twist or lean backwards. Try *not to have a child lean back* against the wall, standing apparatus or an adult. This aggravates the tendency to fall backwards.

(i) Practise standing him in a corner with a stable chair in front of him to help him overcome fears of falling. He then also actively and equally sways laterally from wall to wall and anteroposteriorly towards the chair and to midline, posteriorly to wall and back to midline.

(j) Whenever possible face a child. He uses your presence as motivation to stand in correct postural alignment with gravity and initiate weight shifts forward (to greet you/touch you in a game).

(k) Stand on different surfaces, e.g. carpet, sponge rubber, rough ground with (and later without) support.

(2) Correct abnormal postures or deformities
See correction of abnormal postures in sitting and use the same methods for kyphosis, scoliosis, hip adduction and internal rotation, feet deformities. See standing frames (Fig 8.156c, d, e).

(a) Place the child's legs apart in standing, hips and knees turned slightly outward with head, trunk, pelvis upright and hips straight, knees slightly flexed varying with extension for control of posture. Keep feet flat on the ground, facing outwards. Stand him like this over a roll, inflatable toy, sponge rubber or large stuffed toy. You can hold him like this when you are seated on the floor and the child's legs are abducted over your thigh or legs. Hold the child's knees and thighs facing apart and outward (in external rotation). The toy he straddles needs to avoid valgus knees by keeping both his *knees and feet* apart. Press his heels to the ground by pushing down through his knees to his heels (joint compression).

(b) Equal weight distribution and weight forward over feet will correct many abnormal postures. Symmetrical postures and head in midline corrects asymmetry. Motivate and facilitate child's arm reach behind at shoulder level or overhead to overcome a rounded back or bent hips and knees (Figs 8.166, 8.165).

(c) Splints and orthoses. If abnormal positions cannot be actively corrected by the child *in every joint*, at the same time, splintage or bracing should be used for one joint whilst the others are actively corrected by him. For example, correct abnormal adduction with abduction splint, as child actively stretches his knees and keep his heels down with his weight taken towards the external surface of his feet. Another possibility is to correct bent knees with the knee gaiters/splints, whilst the child actively corrects the position of hips and feet. Yet another possibility is to correct the feet in below-knee orthoses or in plaster casts whilst the child actively corrects hips and knees, head and trunk.

Lower limb orthoses are used for standing and walking depending on assessment of joint ranges, muscle action and biomechanics. They are used for support, alignment, prolonged stretch of hypertonic muscles and as part of the whole functional programme. A physiotherapist works closely with an orthotist and/or an orthopaedic surgeon. Gait analyses are used in research and clinical work for the most effective designs for individuals. However, the following orthoses are commonly used with clinical assessments when gait analyses are not available.

(1) Hip abduction with trunk brace for correction of hip deformities and pelvic and trunk deformities in lying, sitting and standing

positioning equipment and/or SWASH orthosis (Fig. 8.155e).

(2) Knee gaiters or splints correct and support knees in standing and weight shift so that trunk and hip control and some foot adjustments can be practised. This can also be managed in standing frame when supports/straps are removed for training and for periods of the day (Fig. 8.156c; see also Appendix).

(3) Ankle foot orthoses are of a number of designs and can also correct the hip and knee. These consist of the following designs used within shoes, trainers or boots.

- Solid ankle foot orthosis (AFO) (Fig. 8.155a) of moulded thermoplastic material. It is often set at 2–3° dorsiflexion to counteract the plantar flexion deformity. The range of motion in the ankle with knee straight should be neutral or other parts of the foot especially at the subtalar joint will compensate and become hypermobile while the planter flexion can persist and may become a contracture. There will be rubbing by the orthosis which will alert the therapist that the fit is incorrect. Inhibitive plaster casts for such ankle limitation or surgery will need to be used before the AFO is recommended. The stability in standing is enhanced but gait patterns remain in a rigid pattern.

- Hinged ankle foot orthoses (HAFO) (Fig. 8.155b). The hinge at the ankle allows some dorsiflexion so that an individual can use correct biomechanics in rising from sitting, from squatting or from half-kneeling to standing. Weight shift forward is better and improves the gait. An HAFO in a hemiplegic condition may allow more symmetry. Orthotists may adjust a hinge to allow minimal plantar and dorsiflexion. The solid AFO sometimes leads to weakening of push-off by plantar flexors in gait.

- Dynamic foot orthosis (DAFO). This is a moulded orthosis for calcaneous, mid-tarsal joint and toe flexors inhibiting hypertonus. Longitudinal and transverse metaphalangeal arches are corrected. DAFO can be small above the malleoli when ankle control is needed with minimal tibial forward travel. The DAFO can be incorporated with a tibial component. A plantar stop is usually included (Hylton 1989).

- Ground reaction (Floor reaction). Ankle over-dossiflexion may increase a crouch hip-knee flexion posture or not overcome hyperextended knees. Range of motion test of ankle and knee needs plantigrade at the ankle with a straight knee,

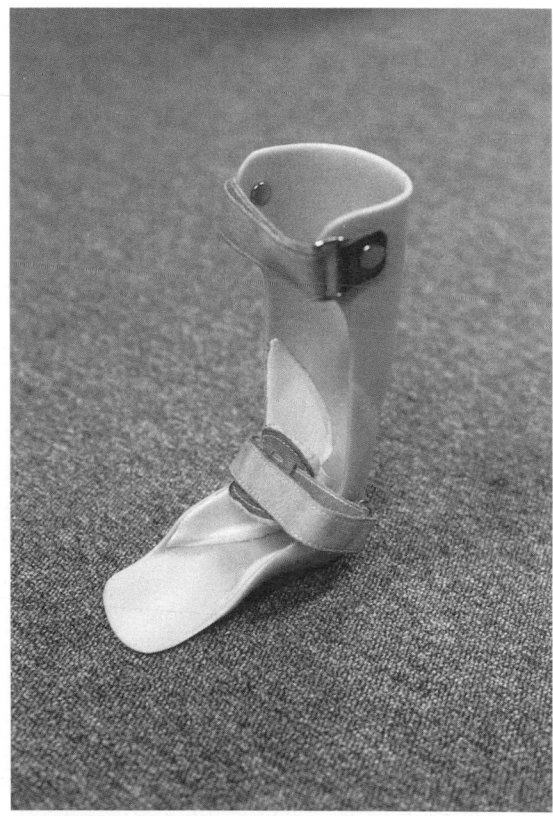

Fig. 8.155a Solid ankle foot orthosis for dorsiflexion and moulding foot.

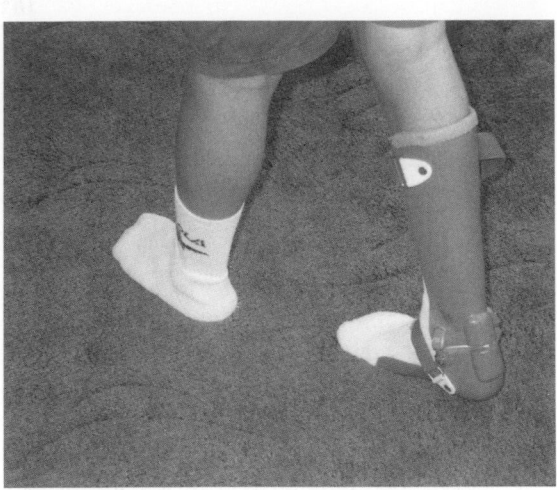

Fig. 8.155b Hinged ankle foot orthosis allowing dorsiflexion for gait, stairs, half-kneeling and sit-to-stand. Minimal plantarflexion for push-off in gait.

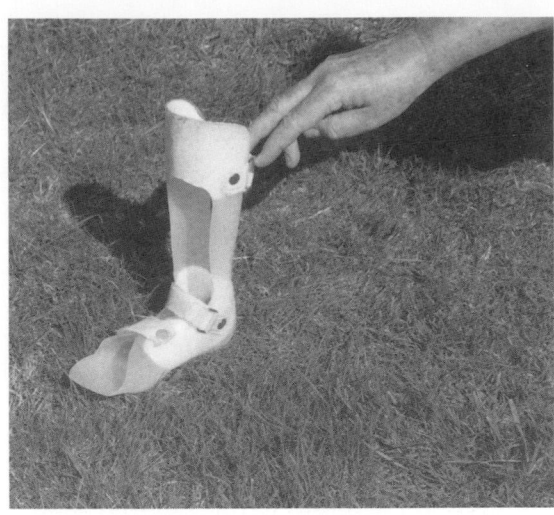

Fig. 8.155c Ground reaction ankle foot orthosis limits excessive dorsiflexion. Knee element maintains knee extension.

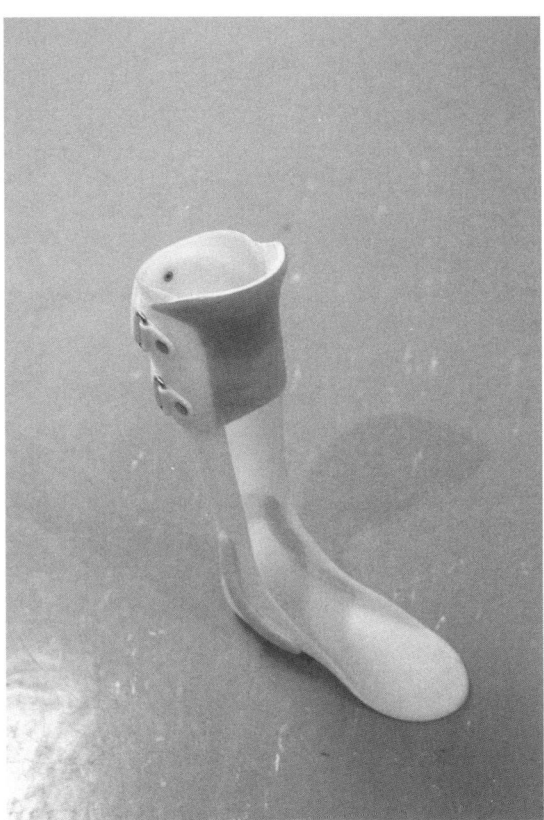

Fig. 8.155d Ground reaction ankle foot orthosis with stiffening at ankle and with extended sole to correct flexion of toes. Front can be moulded to the lower leg in severe crouch-walk.

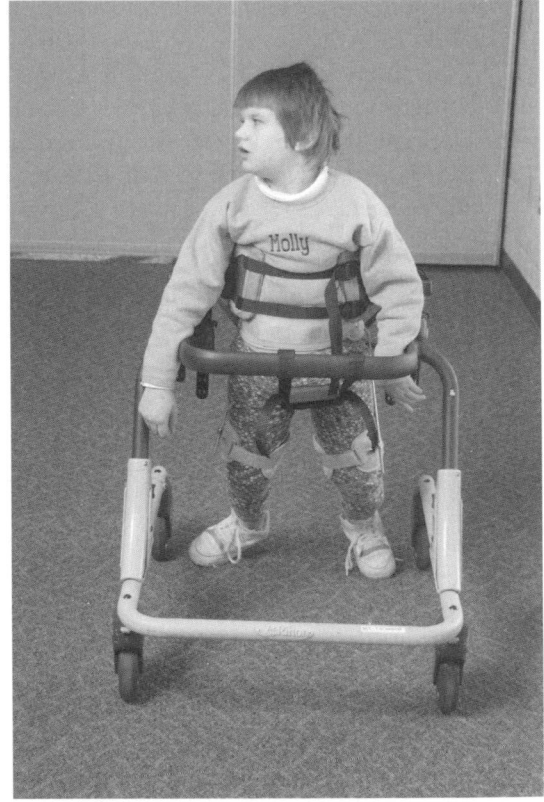

Fig. 8.155e The SWASH (Standing, Walking And Sitting Hip) Orthosis, with variable hip abduction, dynamically corrects adduction and/or hip dysplasia. May need trunk support. Image from Camp Scandinavia.

preferably assessed in standing. The orthosis is moulded to the front or sides of the lower leg to limit ankle dorsiflexion. A knee element or knee piece is necessary to increase knee extension. As the heel touches the ground there is an associated reaction of knee extension which also improves hip extension. A posterior walker is best used for extension (Fig. 8.155c).

Hyperextended knees decrease if they are compensations for plantar flexor tightness. However, increasing the set of an AFO to 5–7° into dorsiflexion increases the knee flexion so that midline of the knee is promoted. A hyperextended knee needs assessment to confirm that it is not due to the quadriceps.

- Night-splint ankle foot orthosis can either be a solid AFO, bivalved plasters or a hinged ankle foot orthosis with adjustable straps to grade the amount of dorsiflexion over time. This prolonged stretch is used for spastic plantar flexors during sleep. However, positioning lying equipment for postural management includes such correction during rest.
- Inserts or foot orthoses. These correct heel position in footwear. However, the forefoot often also needs correction so that the heel-cup is extended to include correction of longitudinal and transverse arches. The sides of the inserts may be raised for extra support, the forefoot moulded or sponge and leather inserts included. The flat foot of early walking is seen in able-bodied children under 3–4 years of age and may be present in delayed walkers with cerebral palsy. Discussion with orthopaedic surgeons is advisable as orthoses can prevent the activation of small muscles during weight-shift which corrects flat feet during standing and walking.

Shoes should be checked for correct fit and support for all children whether worn with or without orthoses. Slow range of motion and stretch are useful before orthoses or shoes are applied.

Research studies showing the value of ankle foot orthoses continue, as well as those by Mossberg *et al.* 1990; Butler and Nene 1991; Butler *et al.* 1992; Radtka *et al.* 1997. See critical review, Morris (2002). Different materials are being developed as well as modifications of designs based on studies and experience, and the important reports by parents, children and older individuals. Comfort, temperature and pressure points and ease of application as well as parents' and individuals' understanding of the purposes of orthoses are important considerations for cooperation. Studies have shown prevention and correction of deformity, reduced plantar flexor hypertonicity, greater stability, improved gait and less energy expenditure in walking.

(d) Botulinum toxin, baclofen and other drugs as well as orthopaedic surgical procedures aim to correct abnormal hypertonic postures. Physiotherapy precedes and follows these procedures with the methods above. (See Chapter 10.)

(3) Building up child's own stability by a decrease of support given to him
Carry out methods with trunk or shoulders supported by your hands and selected standing frames. Progress to support of a child at his waist, then hips, then thighs and knees. This is equivalent to developmental levels 0–9 months. At 9–11 months his own hand grasp is spontaneously used for support, but before this, the child's hands will have to be placed on to bars for grasp. Hold his hands on a bar by gently pressing down on his wrists. To overcome any fears let a child tell a therapist when she should 'let go' so that he can balance with less or no support. *Combine methods.* See 9–12 months development level for manual resistance.

Note: weight bearing and stepping are not walking. Children who are able to bear weight and step needing trunk support for balance are really at 0–6 months normal developmental level. These children are frequently the ones who need support on chest and lower trunk in walking frames. Some children with dyskinesia will use a walker on wheels to run headlong, but are unable to stand alone, having not yet developed the postural stability of head, trunk and pelvis of later developmental levels. Children with ataxia often use wheel-walkers to stagger in all directions. The training of standing and walking in such children should concentrate on the next levels of development which build up trunk and pelvic control.

(4) Delay the training of standing and walking in the following instances:

(a) Abnormal weight bearing, without the trunk and pelvic control of 6–12 months developmental levels, are seen in severe cases of much older children as well as in young children. If excessive antigravity reaction of hip adduction (scissoring)-internal rotation, hip and knee extension, toe standing occurs when the child is held in standing and this cannot be corrected, or only corrected with difficulty, by the therapist, then the training of standing should be *delayed*. This is frequently a problem with the spastic type. Treatment in these cases should concentrate on lengthening short muscles, practising rising, arm support and upright trunk control with activities in prone, supine and sitting development. An inclined *prone stander* with control of feet, knees and hips with an abduction wedge may be appropriate so that a child can be placed at eye level with his peers who are standing. This incline is adjusted to 30° for correct weight-bearing (Miedaner 1990).

(b) Delay standing and walking in the case when the excessive antigravity reaction (supporting reaction) is only controlled at the cost of *abnormal overflow* of muscle activity despite positioning the legs and trunk correctly. There may be more unwanted hypertonus or

involuntary motion of head, arms and hands, or trunk. Check whether this *overflow* can be corrected as soon as possible. If not, although the development of standing may proceed, there will be a loss or decrease of hand function or increase of deformity in the upper limbs and trunk. Thus, treatment suggestions for standing should be followed when the child is more able and ready to respond to them. This will be after a period of training the postural mechanisms. Development of these postural mechanisms does seem to decrease excessive hypertonus during weight bearing on the feet when these children are finally placed in standing.

(5) Continue training of head, trunk and pelvic stability and counterpoising in all vertical postures as well as standing.
Train this control mainly in upright postures, in sitting, knee walking (sideways, forward, backward), half-kneeling and upright kneeling. *Do not use upright kneeling* if the child has hip or knee flexion tightness or lordosis.

Points (1) to (5) relate to all developmental levels below. Points (6), (7) and (8) are discussed in the developmental level 9–12 months, below, as well as in later development.

Make standing training interesting with, say, songs, tables of toys, biofeedback (Winstein *et al.* 1989) and praise for child's own efforts when he attends to any specific control of his standing.

0–3 MONTHS NORMAL DEVELOPMENTAL LEVEL
Common Problems

Delay in taking weight on feet, when fully supported. Poor head control, round back with pelvic posterior tilt is delayed development.

Abnormal performance. See Abnormal postures in standing, supported.

Reflex reactions

(1) Excessive antigravity response, see Abnormal postures in standing.
(2) Persistence of automatic stepping after 1–2 months (reflex stepping).
(3) Various abnormal stepping reactions such as *athetoid dance*, when each leg jerkily withdraws outwards with eversion on sole contact with the ground. Sole contact may also include grasping reflex of the ground. Some athetoid individuals on sole contact 'conflict between grasp and withdrawal reflexes' (Twitchell 1961). One leg may exhibit a *pawing* repetitive involuntary motion.
(4) Excessive *crossed extension reflex* seen in a jerky high-stepping pattern, with the other leg rigidly extended as its sole contacts the ground. This is similar to automatic stepping above.
(5) Withdrawal reflex of both feet on contact with the ground, as opposed to alternate withdrawals of each leg.

Treatment Suggestions and Daily Care

Increase weight bearing on both feet which counteracts delay as well as the various abnormal reactions to foot contact with floor. Trunk support or trunk and pelvic support is needed at this stage. Manual extension of a child's legs assists his weight bearing. Stimulate head control.

(1) Use of knee gaiters, knee splints, long leg orthoses or braces.
(2) Periods of weight bearing in apparatus, e.g. standing frames with tables at upper chest level: for support (Fig. 8.156a–e).
(3) Joint compression through hips and pelvis or through knees (Fig. 8.156f).
(4) Desensitize soles of feet by weight bearing on feet with heels pressed down in sitting, squatting and then in standing. Use shoes and various floor surfaces, sponge or a

trampoline etc. to find which the child can tolerate. Inclined *prone stander* allows partial pressure of child's weight on his feet to assist toleration (Fig. 8.156d).
(5) Prone standers are used to correct postures of trunk and legs. Select support and correct positioning elements for each child (Miedaner 1990).

Correct abnormal postures. Stimulate head control

Prone standers or inclined frames do not train standing itself, but correct postures and desensitize soles of feet. Upright positions are needed to train standing (later stages).

3–5 MONTHS NORMAL DEVELOPMENTAL LEVEL

This is the level at which the normal body does not take weight in standing but sags (astasia). The next level of development should be attempted from time to time until there is a flicker of response, then work at 6–9 months level on the development of standing.

6–9 MONTHS NORMAL DEVELOPMENTAL LEVEL

Common Problems

Delay in weight bearing with flexible knees, if supported, active *bounce* when held in standing, alternate stepping (not automatic high stepping), if held with hip flexion, knee extension and heels down on the floor and beginning to stand alone grasping a support. Delay in achieving upright pelvis, straighter trunk.

Abnormal performance. See abnormal posture in standing, supported, above.

Reflex reactions. Those expected to develop at this level are:

(1) Parachute or saving reactions in the arms on falling forward or sideways (see Development of sitting, Figs 8.76 and 8.133).

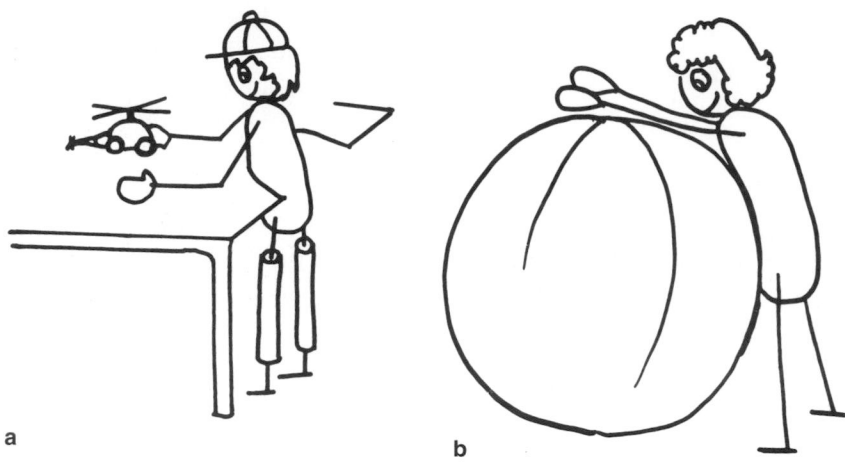

a   b

Fig. 8.156a,b,c Child's arms symmetrical, head and trunk central, weight equal on each foot. Keep child's weight forward on to his feet. Trunk is supported by a roll, a large ball, table, high couch or the body of the therapist behind him. Also use a high couch, ordinary table with padded, rounded edge or cut-out table. Later remove the trunk support and use his hand grasp on support, or lean only on forearms, lean on hands on low table (9–12 months level). Legs are apart and externally rotated, hips flexed or extended, knees straight, feet flat on the ground. Use orthosis or abduction splint, knee splint, foot supports according to the child's difficulties. Later remove knee splints. Rhythmically shift the knees into semiflexion to avoid rigid infantile stance and if the knees also hyperextend. Later shift weight from foot to foot.

(2) Propping reactions in the arms to *break* the fall (see sitting, Fig. 8.84).

(3) Tilt reactions in sitting which may make standing more secure if not directly related to its acquisition.

(4) Presence of toe clenching in supported standing until about 9 months level.

(5) Persistence of reflex reactions from 0–3 months is abnormal.

Physiotherapy Suggestions and Daily Care

See Fig. 8.156a–f and 'Treatment suggestions at all levels of development' with support.

9–12 MONTHS NORMAL DEVELOPMENTAL LEVEL

Common Problems

Delay in standing, holding on and releasing one hand. Standing may be stable but become unsteady if reaching with one hand, and turning

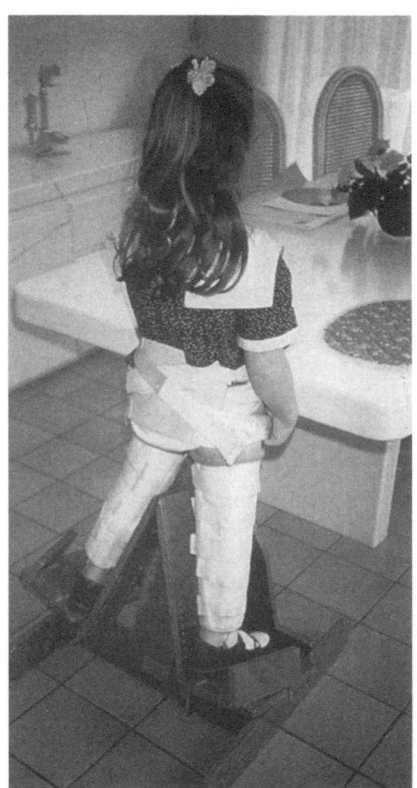

c

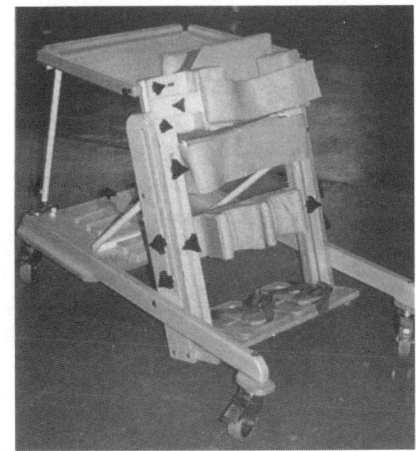
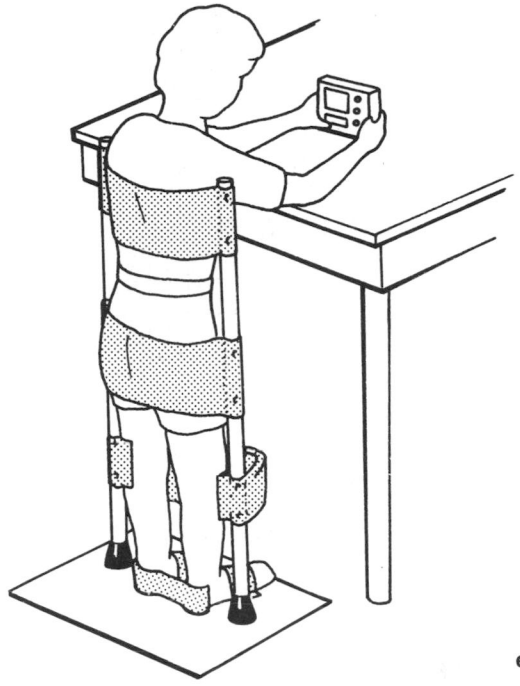

Fig. 8.156d,e (d) Prone stander. Height and angle are adjusted so that pelvis is aligned without hyperextension of back or head. Lateral adjustment of pelvic band with derotation and adjustment of knee blocks obtains symmetrical weight bearing. Incorporate foot block if legs are of different lengths. Table is adjusted for hand function and for head control with chin in. Table may be angled or horizontal. Time in any stander needs supervision so that excessive use does not increase hypertonus or fatigue (30–60 minutes). (With acknowledgement to James Leckey Design, Dunmurry, Northern Ireland.) (e) Standing frame, supporting chest, hips, knees and feet.

to look behind him without reach. Delay in holding on and standing on one leg, stepping sideways or cruising. Inability to stand alone momentarily, step two-handed support, one-handed support. Delay in rise from prone or supine to standing with help given in the transitional positions of either sitting, kneeling on all fours and half-kneeling. Delay in pulling himself to standing from kneeling holding on, from sitting or from hands and knees. Delay in standing on narrower base in line with hips. Delay in pelvic tilt forward with normal lordosis. Weight shift forward/back, laterally is delayed when standing holding on and later with less support.

Abnormal performance of standing posture, see abnormal posture in standing, supported and unsupported (above); abnormal gait, above.

Excessive toe grasping, inadequate base for balance and arms held up in air (highguard).

Reflex reactions. Those expected at this level are the saving reactions in the arms if falling backwards as well as propping on hands to break the fall (see Development of sitting, Figs 8.76 and 8.133).

Physiotherapy Suggestions

Remove support from child's trunk, and later from pelvis.

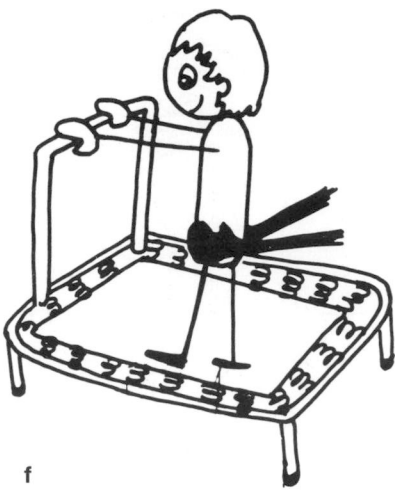

f

Fig. 8.156f Joint compression through hips, later through knees. Child may stand on floor, but trampoline, sponge rubber, inflatable mattress may be used if posture is kept corrected, and *bouncing is restricted*. The trunk may be supported by his own grasp or holding your shoulders (9–12 months level) or if his trunk requires more support (6–9 months level) lean child against table, roll, couch, large stuffed stable toy, or large ball. Head and body alignment must be well over straight legs and feet on the ground. Avoid hyperextension of knees and any abnormal postures.

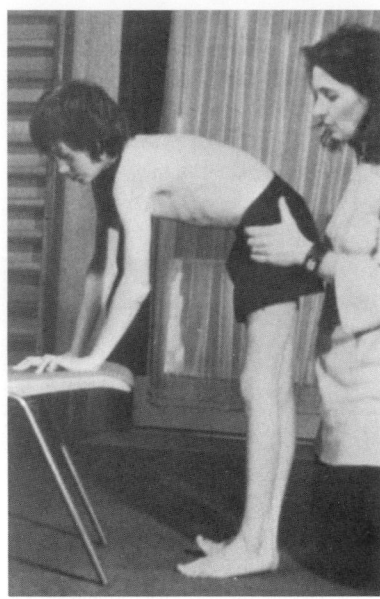

Fig. 8.157 Stabilization on hands and feet, then more upright. Lateral sway, anteroposterior weight shift.

Improve stability with the following techniques: the child stands, holding on or alone. Apply manual pressure at his hips or shoulders, pushing him off balance; he must actively maintain his upright standing – 'Don't let me push you over'. Do this laterally and also anteroposteriorly (Fig. 8.157). Do this with rotation – 'Don't let me turn you'. Another way of using manual resistance is to ask the child to push against your hands placed in positions on his hips or shoulders or on one hip and one shoulder – 'Push against my hands'. Resistance should not be *so great* that the child twists his limbs into abnormal positions, or increases involuntary movements, or even falls over!

Once standing is present, practise standing with blindfold and with a veil or in light subdued by sunglasses worn by child.

Stand and sway (Figs 8.157–8.159). Train lateral sway with legs apart then together. At first the child is swayed from side to side, then shifts his weight along or against your hand on his hip, shoulder, or hip and shoulder. Augment weight shift against your hand offering resistance. Carry this out initially with support to child's chest or having him lean on his forearms, on hands, or grasping a support with elbows straight. Encourage his own active sway between two stable chairs or parallel bars, lateral and anteroposteriorly.

Child's grasp should be forward, sideways at waist and at shoulder level. Lateral grasp on poles is preferable to parallel bars as it improves symmetrical weight bearing, back and head position and trains supinated grasp. Lateral sway prepares child for cruising and is part of gait training. Motivate a child to lateral weight shift and reach well to his side to obtain a desired toy. See 'Equal distribution of weight bearing' for methods at all levels.

Sway child *forward and back* (anteroposterior shift) (Figs 8.160 and 8.161). Child shifts

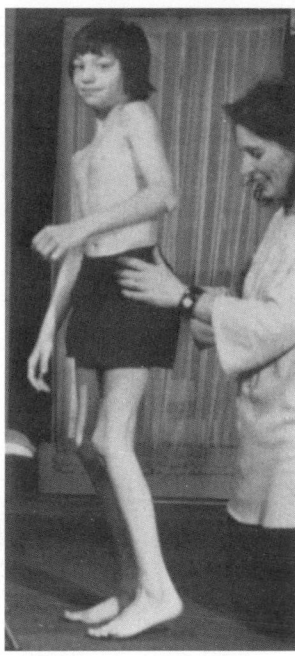

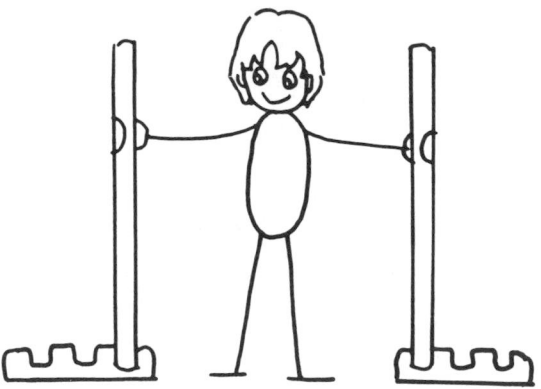

Fig. 8.159 Lateral sway practised with lateral grasp for trunk and hips extension. Use externally rotated arms.

Fig. 8.158 Activate an individual's own lateral sway against manual resistance and 'pushes' for postural adjustment. Active sway by person/child is the next stage.

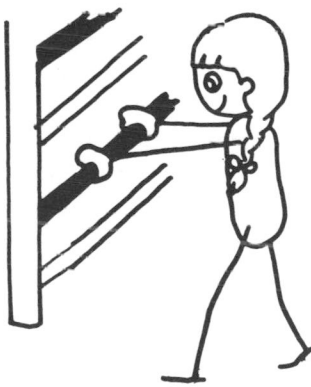

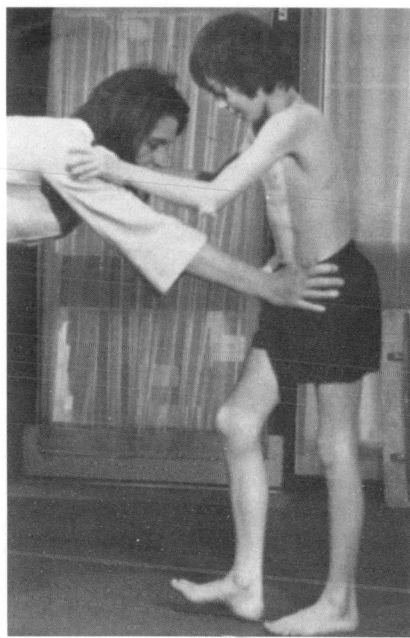

Fig. 8.160 Anteroposterior sway in preparation for step.

Fig. 8.161 Anterior weight shift with step taken against therapist's manual resistance. Note activation of dorsiflexion.

his weight forward and back. Child shifts his weight against your hands placed first on anterior-superior iliac crests or on his gluteii. Weight shift forward initiates stepping. *All these actions can be done to rhythm and song*. Lateral

sways can become steps included in a simple dance routine.

Standing and counterpoising (Fig. 8.162). The child stands holding on with both hands, then

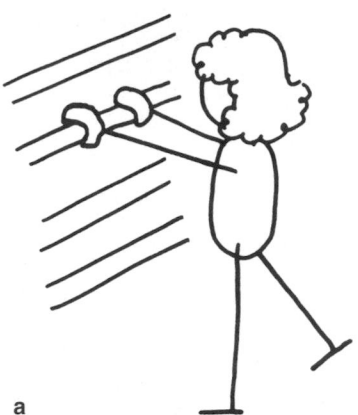

a

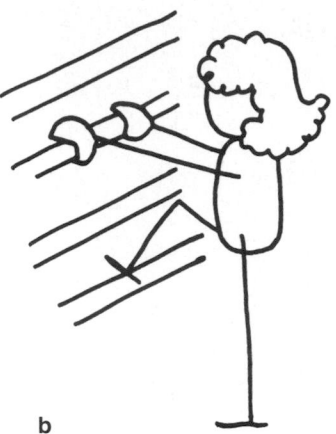

b

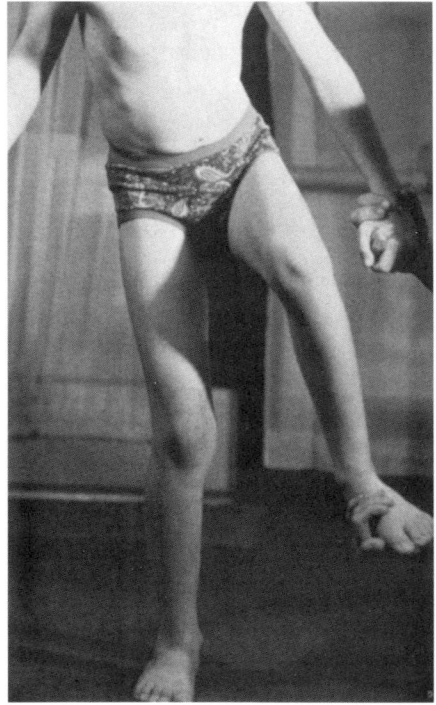

c

Fig. 8.162a,b,c Counterpoising exercises for walking and climbing stairs as well as for putting on and off socks, shoes and trousers, and for washing and play activities.

one hand, whilst lifting one leg to different heights on the bar or in the air. He could lift one of his legs up in front, to the side and backward, on to bars, box step, a beachball, onto your hand, or to have his shoe put on or off. He could also stand and reach in all directions for toys offered to him, and stand supported, bend down and fetch an object on the floor or low box. He could also walk hands down the bars, and fetch a toy hung on the bottom bar or on a high bar. Later increase demands with tasks such as stand and pick up a cup of water and place back on table or on stools of different heights.

Train standing and counterpoising using the facilitation of arm and leg patterns. The child stands grasping support; it may be necessary to maintain alignment and therefore hold his weight-bearing leg in external rotation, while he moves the other leg using various patterns (Figs 8.163 and 8.164). Facilitate the patterns against resistance by holding correctly as *must be shown clinically.* Heavy objects may be managed with different desirable arm patterns carried out by a child.

A child is shown leg patterns and weight bearing in his phases of walking in parallel bars or in stationary walker. Leg patterns that may be used are flexion-adduction-external rotation (stepping pattern) from and to extension-abduction-internal rotation (push-off pattern), the knee extended and foot dorsiflexed in *stepping*. Hold toes and forefoot in dorsiflexion in *push off* and to prevent extensor thrust.

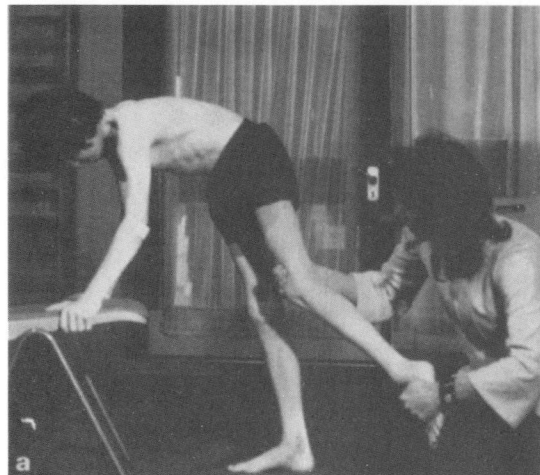

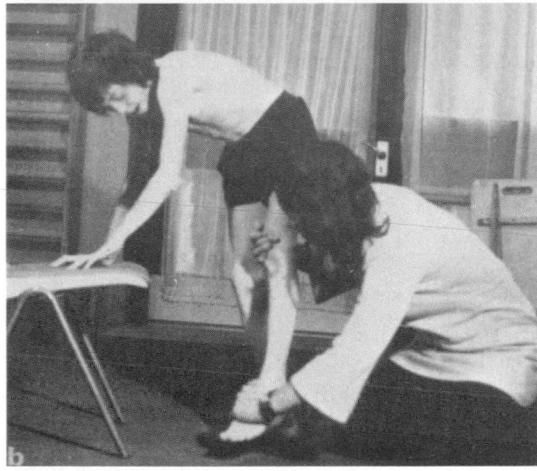

Fig. 8.163 Correction of stepping pattern, i.e. facilitation of leg flexion-external rotation, knee extension with dorsiflexion. *Push off* pattern, a. *Heel strike* pattern, b. Progress to use within stepping while pushing chair/ladder or in parallel bars.

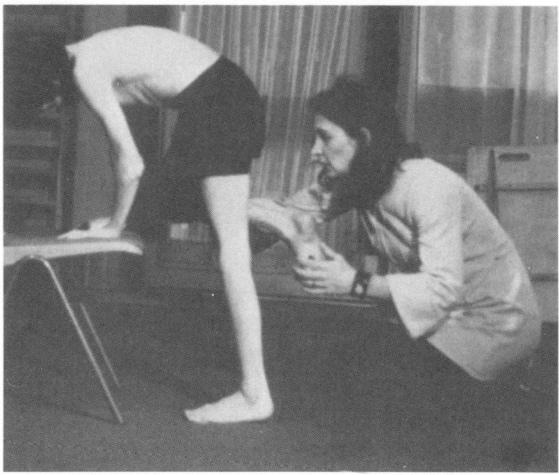

Fig. 8.164 From this hip-knee flexion-abduction-internal rotation pattern facilitate *stance* of extension-adduction-external rotation in his right leg.

Arm patterns for function are shown to a child in the context of reaching for an object or daily care activity. Arm patterns should also be used in the following ways. With the child standing holding a support with one hand or leaning on one hand, correctly facilitate the other arm into elevation-abduction-external rotation against resistance or in assisted or active reaching for a toy overhead. He could also stand while 'walking' his hands up the wall, sliding up the wall up a soapy mirror or other play activities. Also facilitate all other arm patterns in standing. Use objects that interest a child to encourage reaching out in all directions.

Note. Use leg and arm patterns *without* giving resistance if excessive overflow of spasticity cannot be controlled and if methods are not skilfully carried out.

Correction of abnormal postures. The arm and leg patterns are not the only ways tasks are managed but selected to activate counterpoising and to correct abnormal positions of arms and legs. In addition rotation of the pelvis and trunk with the arm or leg movements appears to decrease hypertonus and improve postures (see Basic arm and hand patterns for all levels of development).

Correction of some common abnormal postures in standing and walking. These are from approximately the 9 month developmental level (supported) to over 12 month developmental level (unsupported).

(1) Flexion and *sinking* posture (Figs 8.165 and 8.168).

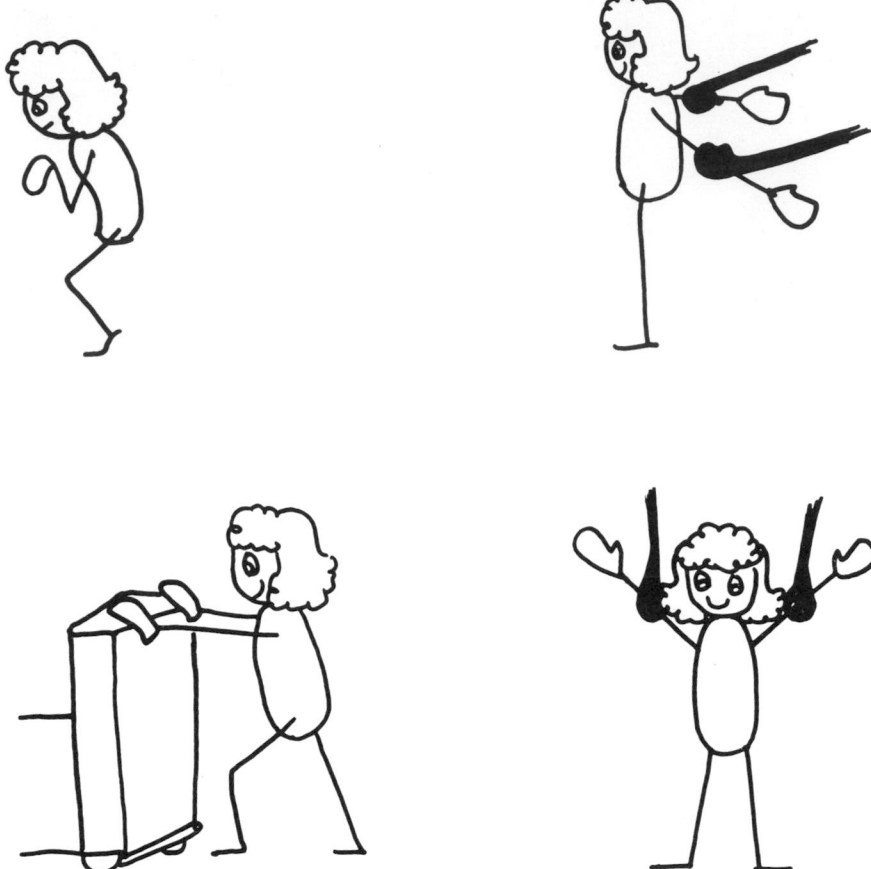

Fig. 8.165 Correction of a flexed child whose limbs may also adduct and internally rotate, in standing or in walking. *Keep child's weight forward as in these exercises there is a tendency to lean too far backwards.* Arms are extended and externally rotated. This corrects head, trunk and legs. Hold child's shoulders, elbows or wrists. Encourage weight shift from side to side by tipping child from your hold on his arms. Stand and walk by pushing walker at shoulder level. Open hands overcomes too much flexion. Keep elbows straight, elbow splints (gaiters) may be needed. Knee splints to maintain extension of knees and/or to get heels down if required. Calipers or back-slabs for knees may be needed in older children. Slow walk and a long lunge forward when stepping and pushing truck helps to stretch tight heel cords and tight knee flexors.

(2) Asymmetrical posture (Fig. 8.166).

(3) Internal rotation of legs (Fig. 8.167).

(4) Hip extension, knee flexion, plantarflexion, arm flexion also for arm abduction-extension in the air, elbow flexion, wrist palmarflexion (arms in *high guard*) (Figs 8.168 and 8.169).

(5) Hyperextended knees and lordosis (Figs 8.170 and 8.171).

Correction of a waddling gait or running headlong must include training of lateral sway and this is also developed in cruising around furniture. The 9–12 months level of development includes the important cruising.

Cruising or stepping sideways. The child holds horizontal bars and takes a step sideways. Avoid steps with hip flexion, rather emphasize abduc-

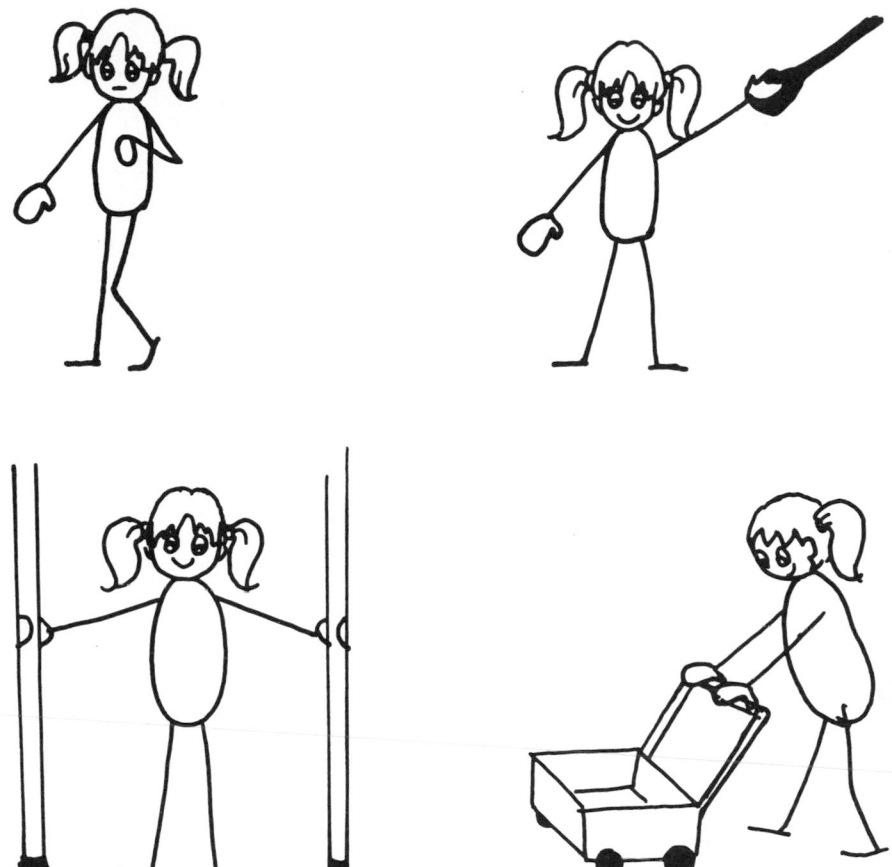

Fig. 8.166 Activities to increase weight bearing on to more affected side or on to hemiplegic side. Hold arm in position to counteract arm flexion-adduction-internal rotation. Bring arm forward if shoulder retracts. Symmetrical grasp, or *both* hands open and pushing truck. Use elbow splints to maintain elbow extension. Weight distributed equally on feet. Shift weight to more affected side. Child tries to grasp with his arms apart and turned out or with his arms abducted in mid-position but not with shoulders turned inward.

tion in lateral step. At first give support and then expect him to keep his pelvis and/or trunk upright, so that he takes weight through his standing leg. Improve this activity by joint compression through the standing hip or knee whilst manual resistance is given to the abduction movement of the stepping leg. Some children respond to resistance without the joint compression through the weight-bearing leg. Others may require you to correct any abnormal positions of hip, knee and foot by holding the thigh and knee extended and externally rotated, and the child's weight on the outside of the foot. In *walk holding*

two hands below use technique to train weight shift sideways which also helps cruising. Observe that a child's pelvis is symmetrical and in vertical alignment. Manually correct any retraction on one side and tip the pelvis upright.

Walk holding two hands or one hand. This developmental level of walking (normally about 12–13 months) is the level at which children are functioning when they walk with walking aids of many different types. The walkers stimulate locomotor reactions of initiation of stepping and lateral sway.

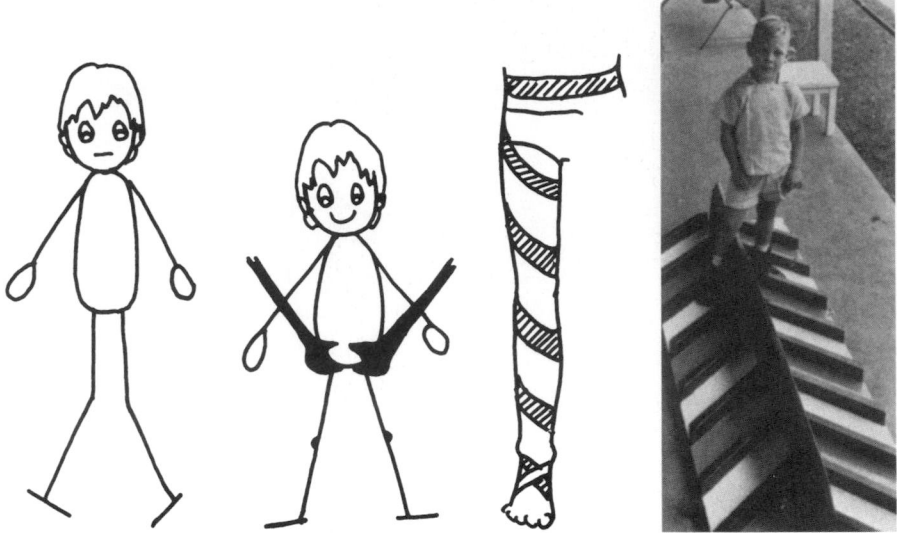

Fig. 8.167   Correction of internal rotation of the legs. Hold child's pelvis and rotate the leg outwards as he takes a step. Trunk at first is aligned and supported by your body and later unsupported. After step press down on that hip to augment weight bearing in external rotation. In milder cases, try using *twisters* to pull leg into external rotation. Child tries to repeat this on his own. *Point feet out.* Also methods in Fig. 8.165.

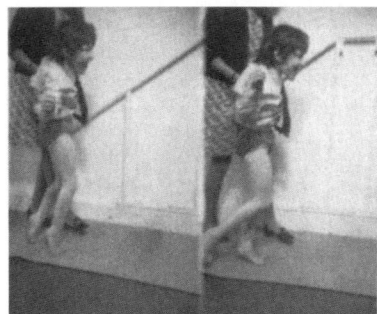

Fig. 8.168   (*left*) Hip extension, knee flexion, plantarflexion. (*below*) Correction of hip extension, knee flexion, arm flexion, plantarflexion (toe walk). For arm abduction-extension in the air, elbow flexion, wrist palmar flexion.

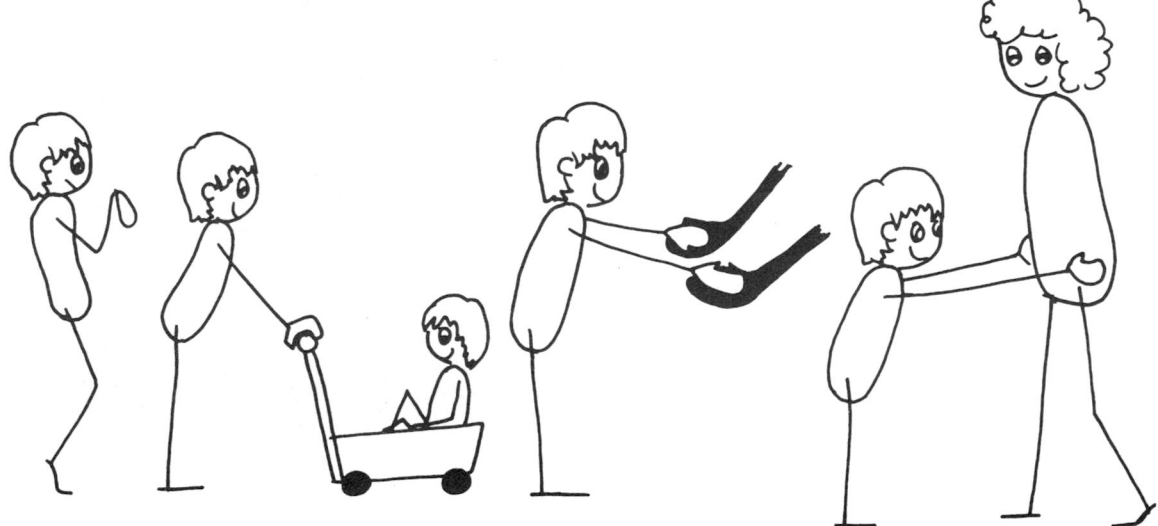

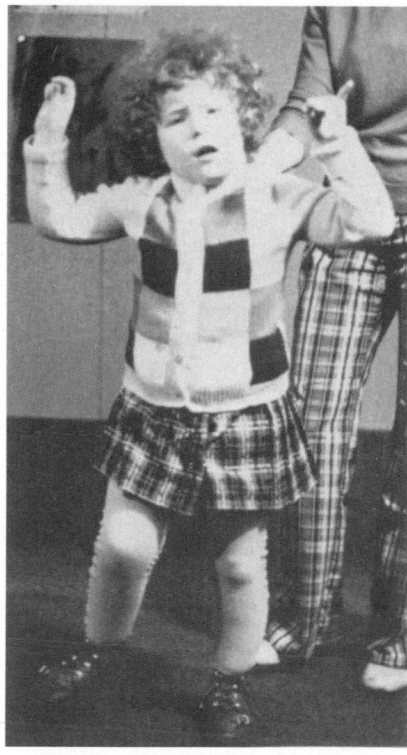

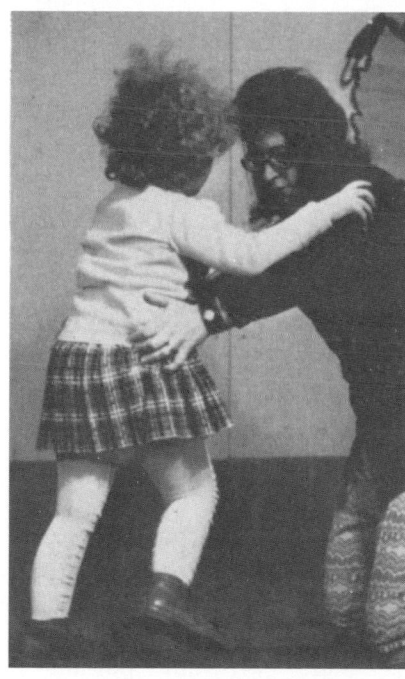

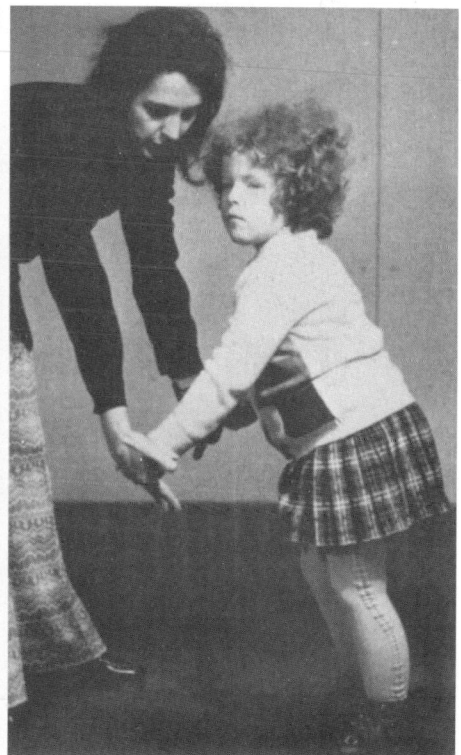

Fig. 8.169 Methods to gain correction of hip extension, knee flexion, arm flexion, plantarflexion (toe walk). For arm abduction-extension in the air, elbow flexion, wrist palmar flexion.

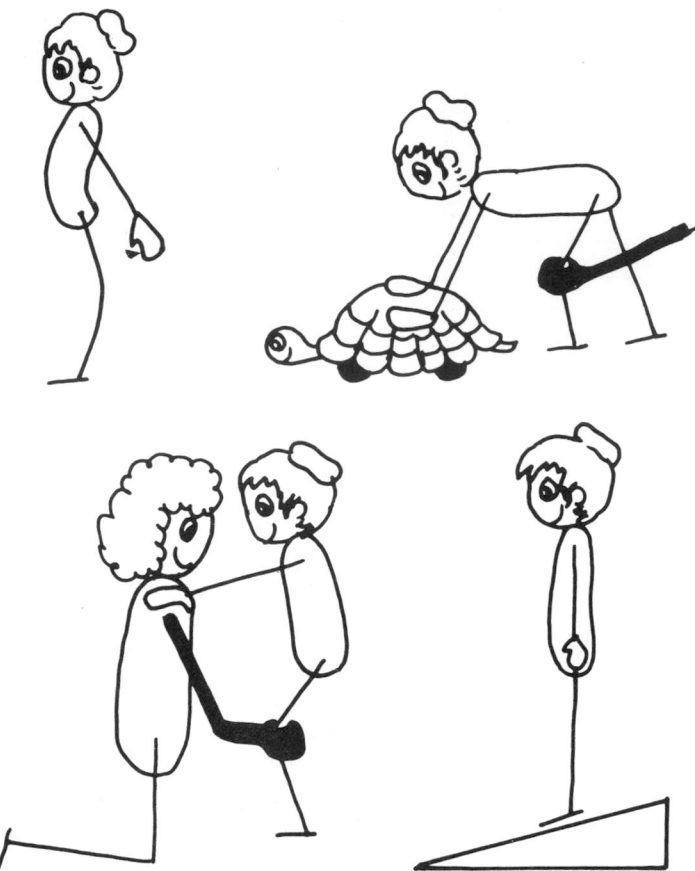

Fig. 8.170 Correction of hyperextended knees and lordosis. Check tightness of plantar flexors and stability of pelvic girdle.

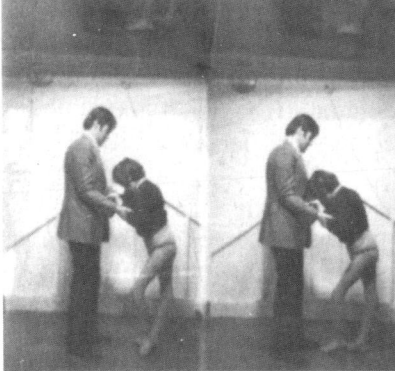

Fig. 8.171 Hyperextended knees.

(1) Walk holding parallel bars or parallel ropes. If the child has not yet achieved grasp and release, a felt cuff or moving hand grip which slides along the bar may be used.

(2) Walk with a walking frame grasping in front or at the sides. Progress from using walkers (Figs 8.172a,b, 8.173, 8.174a–c) to having the child grasp a horizontal stick which is held at each end in your hands. He may hold a small stick in each hand which you grasp at each side of him. Decrease these hand supports further by having him grasp tenoquoit rings lightly held in each of your hands or both of you hold on to a large ball (netball size) simultaneously as you step. Always ensure that his weight is well forward over his base.

(3) Walk holding someone's hands on either side or in front of him.

(4) Walk pushing a weighted doll's pram, another child in his wheelchair, a child's chair, a kitchen chair, a chair on wooden

skis or with set of runners, or a metal walker on four points which slide.

(5) Walking using crutches, elbow crutches, tripods, quadripods or sticks.
(6) Walking using vertical poles at either side with thick rubber bases (Fig. 8.166).

When using walking aids consider the following

Grasping a support at the side of the child tends to train lateral sway for walking. However, if the support involves elbow flexion this may be contraindicated as the grasp-elbow flexion and hunching of the shoulders increases spasticity in individuals and may also overflow into the legs. The child's grasps need to be low down and slightly in front with straight elbows (Figs 8.172–8.174). Use elbow gaiters to assist extension. You may instead hold both his elbows straight as you bring his weight within and slightly in front of his base.

Grasping the hand support in front helps to train the anteroposterior shift needed to start walking. Once again avoid shoulder hunching and excessive arm flexion, so that use of elbow gaiters to assist in reminding child to keep elbows as straight as possible is advisable. A posterior walker may be more effective if a child has an anterior weight shift and is ready to step with hip-trunk extension (Fig. 8.174). Normally early walking uses hip flexion to maintain balance. It may also be helpful to press a child's wrists down to improve his grasp. Try having him lean forward and down on to open hands

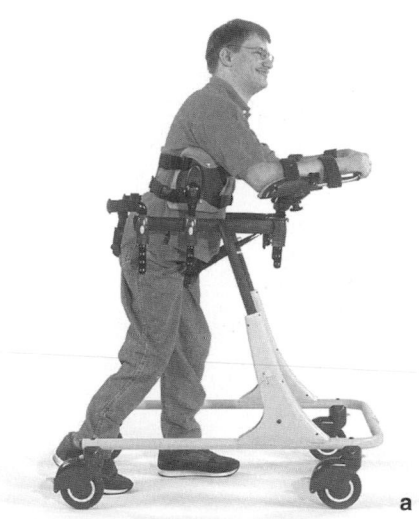

a

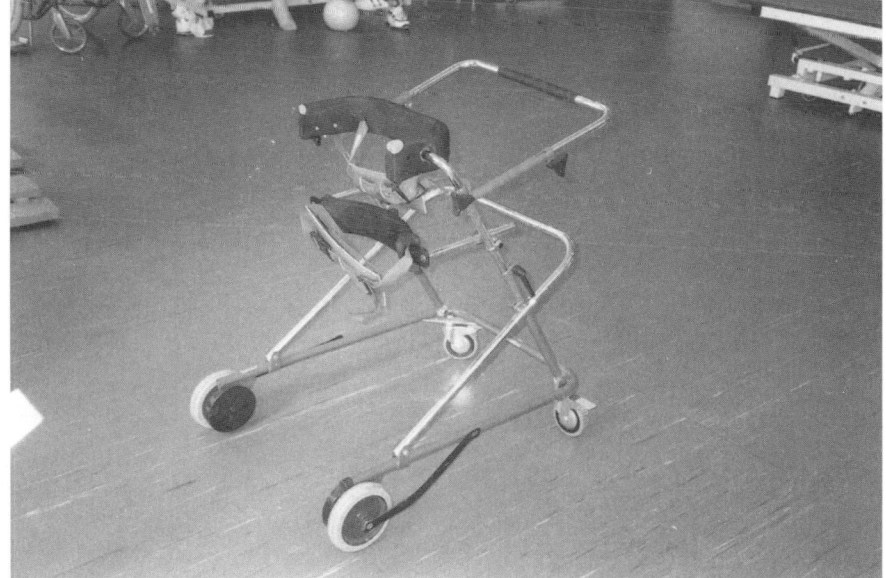

Fig. 8.172 (a) Walker for a person needing chest support. It can be adjusted forward or upright. Forearm supports assist symmetrical shoulder stability and grasp. (Acknowledgement to Rifton for Rifton Pacer Gait Trainer.) (b) The Orlau Walker for a person needing chest support and symmetrical elbow extension with grasp. A similar walker is the Arrow Walker (Pony).

b

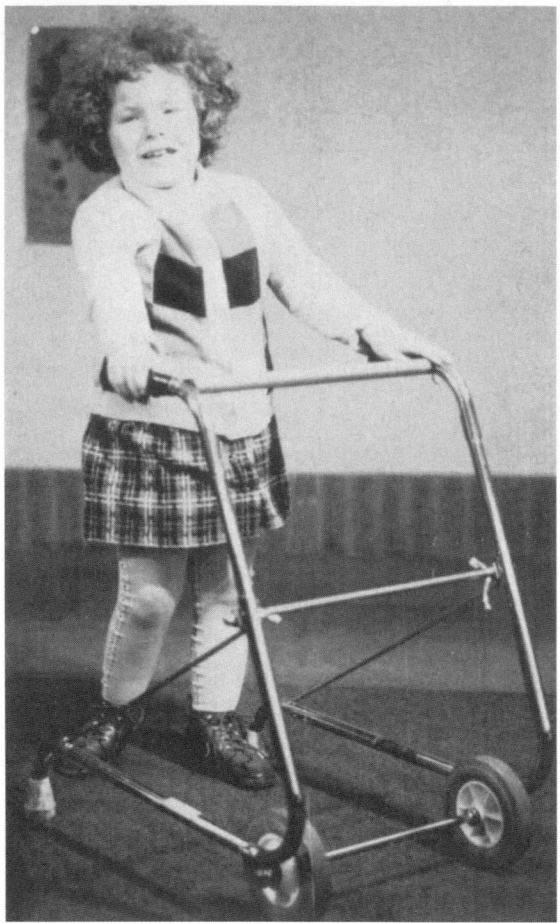

Fig. 8.173 Rollator.

or forward onto his grasp. This is most effective in training the initiation of stepping and continuation of stepping. In Fig. 8.169, note the open hands of the therapist allowing the child to press down and forward to initiate stepping. Although Logan *et al.* (1990) prefer posterior walkers, this is an individual assessment which does not apply to all children.

Inadequate hand use for walking aids. Some athetoid movements or poor grasp ability with weakness interfere with a child's maintenance of grasp. Children with severe intellectual disabilities or perceptual problems may not manage to use walking aids as well as concen-

trate on balance and stepping. Hold these children's hands on to the bars directly or by pressing through their wrists as they grasp. Use particularly stable walking frames, weighted trolleys or doll's prams. The ladderback walker or chair on padded wooden skis is often helpful. Avoid walkers with castors or wheels, which run too quickly for a child. Later, crutches with weighted bases may be managed by some children.

Do not use baby walkers or walkers with a body ring and canvas sling or seat with castors. These mass-produced walkers are not safe for any baby as they tip over easily and lead to other accidents. The wheels on all four corners create undesirable postures and prevent a child from taking weight within his own base and keeping his feet plantigrade. Development of independent and better patterns of walking is prevented as standing and weight shift by the child himself is disrupted by the wheels. The child will therefore sit into the canvas or hang on to the rim of the walker and clutch it with tense bent arms and may hyperextend onto toes. However older children do use walking aids which suspend a child from an overhead bar in a parachute design between his legs. Weight bearing is taken through both plantigrade feet and, as some of the suspension lifts the child's weight off his feet, there is less hypertonus and better weight shift, e.g. treadmill walking.

Children who run headlong are most likely to hang on the rims of any wheel walker and run dragging their feet. Their walkers should be weighted or a brake applied to the back wheels or, perhaps, remove all wheels. Remind these children to walk more slowly and in a stationary walker practise standing still with feet together or as little apart as they can manage.

Grasping with one hand is usually a progression from walking holding on with two hands. However, if the child takes weight abnormally through one side more than the other or if there

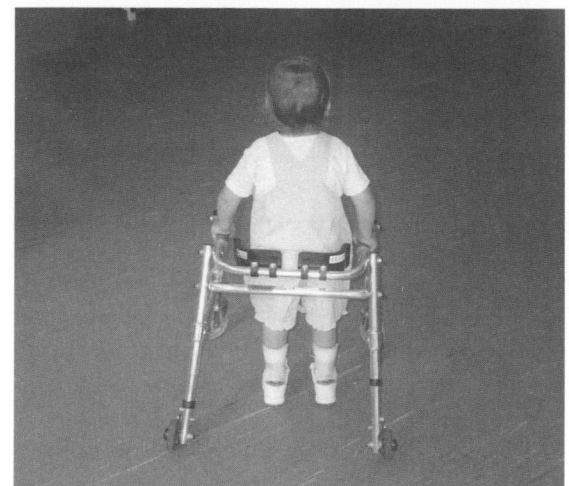

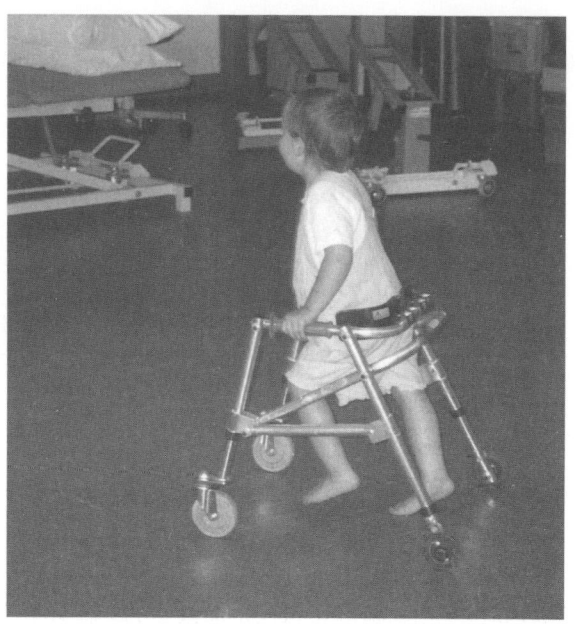

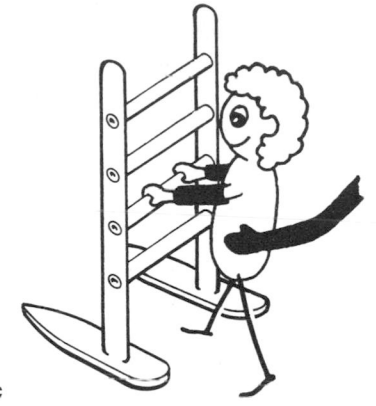

a

b

c

Fig. 8.174 Walkers to promote extension.

are asymmetrical postures, then *two* aids need to be used, until he walks alone. Some children progress to grasping one *clumper* or quadruped stick in the centre and in front of them, instead of using two aids.

A child 'walking on his hands' and 'handing on his armpits' in walking aids so that he hardly takes weight on his feet needs to be discouraged from doing so. If not he will step in this way for years and his independent walking will not have any opportunity of developing. Give extra training in all aspects of head, trunk and pelvic stability in both standing and sitting development for these children.

Abnormal postures of the head, trunk and legs need to be corrected as much as possible (Figs 8.165–8.174). If correction is not possible with a particular walking aid then a better one should be found, or perhaps walking with aids not trained at all. In such cases rather train the earlier levels in the development of standing or walking more thoroughly. Offer trikes or wheelchairs for mobility until control of posture improves, or instead of walking in severe cases.

Note. Pushing a trolley with handles which are too low or sticks and other walking aids which are too low may increase head and back rounding.

Walking aid giving too much aid. Reassess walking aids regularly to monitor the child's own ability to weight bear, step, control head, trunk and pelvis, and grasp. Select or omit walkers according to each individual so that too much aid is avoided. However for longer distances, poor weather conditions or unfamiliar environments, more aid may be indicated. *Other forms of mobility* should always be available for people who need them, for social and exploratory reasons, to counter fatigue and for a sense of control.

Rising to Standing (0–12 months)

Prone to standing (Fig. 8.175). At earlier developmental levels the child has learnt to roll over and get on to his hands and knees or rise from prone on to hands and knees (0–6 months). Train him to rise to half-kneeling then to standing (6–12 months); see Prone development (Fig. 8.179). Some individuals may rise onto hands and feet to standing. Avoid the pattern of dragging legs into extension-adduction, on toes, in a rise to standing.

Supine to standing. Rising from supine to sitting into squatting on both or one foot and pulling up to standing may be preferred by a child, rather than using the half-roll pattern. Help him to develop this by taking both his hands when he is sitting on the ground. Stabilize his foot with your foot and wait for him to pull himself forward over his feet and then extend his legs. From crook-sitting or squatting assist rising if child actively can stretch his legs. Use a hoist on his trunk if he is tall or heavy. The full rising can be carried out from supine to squatting and up to standing by holding the child's hands and feet flat on the table. Hemiplegic or asymmetrical children can be encouraged to take weight on the more affected side as they squat and rise (see Supine development; see also Fig. 8.177). Rising from the ground using squatting is a necessary skill in cultures where people use floor activities in daily life.

Sitting to standing. Rising from sitting on a chair (Fig. 8.176) or from squatting to standing (Fig. 8.177) can be carried out with manual resistance applied on the top of the child's thighs. The child's thighs are carefully kept apart and in external rotation by the therapist who is either behind or in front of the child. If the therapist sits on the ground in front of the child she has the advantage of making sure that his weight comes forward and well over his feet. Teaching a child to bring his weight forward or *nose over his toes* is important or he will not become independent in rising. He will tend to use an extensor thrust or get up abnormally by

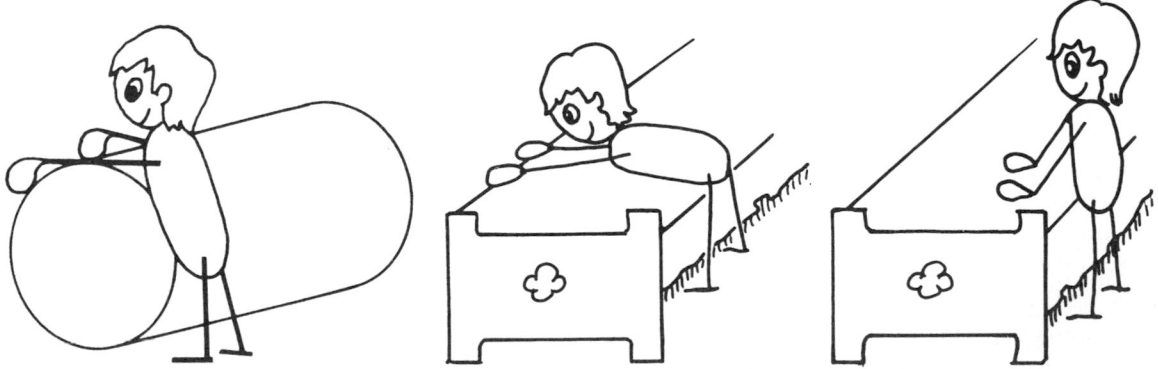

Fig. 8.175 Assume standing from prone lying across a roll, large ball or bed. Check that heels are on the ground, knees and hips straight and, if necessary, turned outward.

pushing on his feet, leaning backwards and grasping your hands, being totally dependent on you in order to rise to his feet. He may learn to bring his own weight forward over his feet if he is also told to reach forward and down to the floor and *raise his bottom* off the chair. In some children resistance may be given at the lumbar area to augment this movement. Rising from the floor and from a chair to standing can be taught by careful verbal instruction. For example, rising from a chair involves: 'Put your feet flat on the ground, bring your nose over your toes, lift your bottom, stand up'. Teach getting up to standing from kneeling (Fig. 8.178), holding crutches or other walking aids. Other rising problems have to be solved. Rising from bed to sit/stand must be included. Figure 8.179 gives various sequences for rising reactions. Supine lying to squatting then to standing is only learnt by people functioning at the 3–5 year developmental levels, which involves a straight lying-to-stand pattern with no/minimal rotation. Slow rising and hold prepares for attainment of squatting in next stage. Individuals use a momentum to rise from different postures, as postural stability in each transient position is not necessary for independence. However, train slow rising sequences to augment stability in the transient postures, and establish safety.

12–24 MONTHS NORMAL DEVELOPMENTAL LEVEL

Common Problems

Delay in walking alone, improvement in walking pattern, e.g. narrower base, arms coming down from being held up in abduction, steps more rhythmical, equal, smoother, standing alone and play in standing, rising to standing completely on his own, starting and stopping his walking, stair ascent and descent, use of inclines and walk on rough ground improves until second and third years.

Abnormal performance. A variety of abnormal gait patterns in the walking child, see the section on abnormal gait above.

Reflex reactions. The following are expected at this level:

(1) Saving from falling by staggering (protective) reactions in lower limbs, forward,

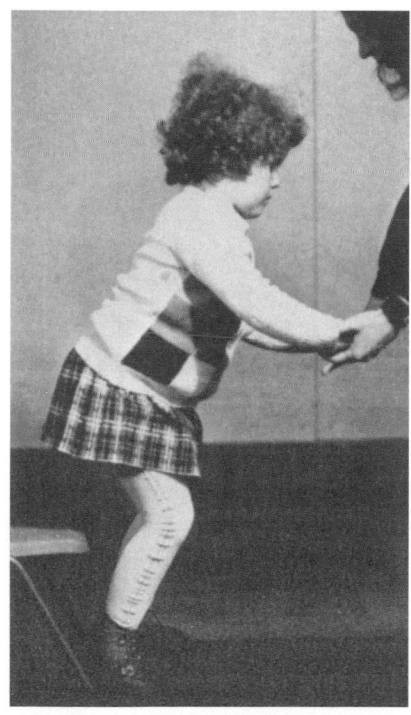

Fig. 8.176

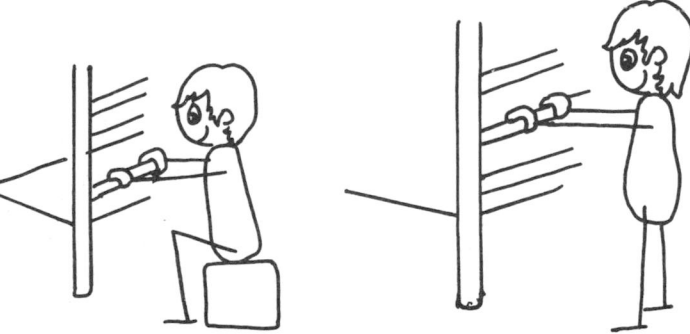

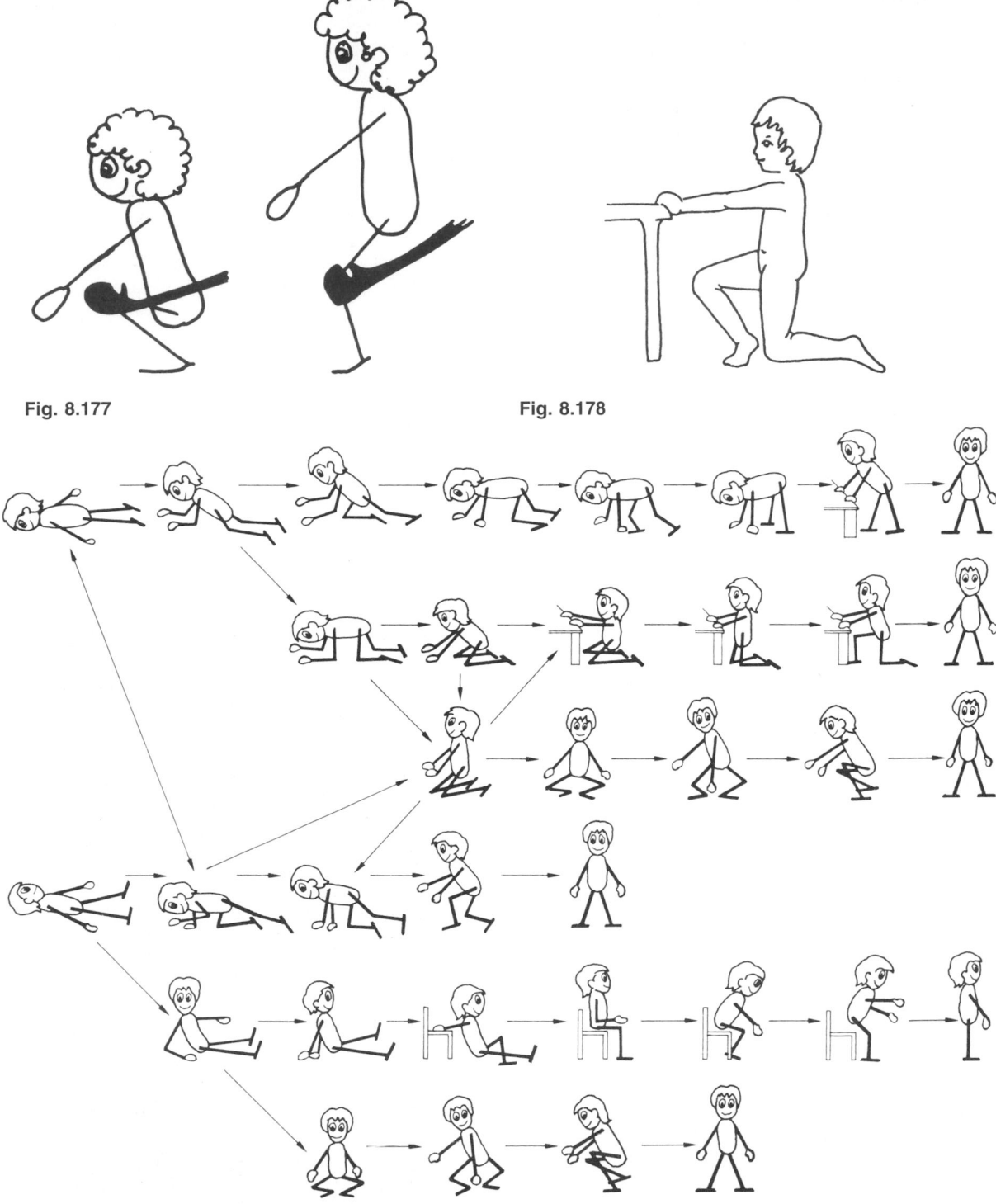

Fig. 8.177   **Fig. 8.178**

Fig. 8.179   Some patterns of rising to standing (see Appendix – wheelchair transfers).

sideways, backward, crossing over and hopping.

(2) In standing, tip child backward resulting in trunk flex forward with or without dorsi-flexion of feet – forward results in back extension, with or without a rise onto toes, laterally results in trunk incurving towards the upright, inversion of one foot, pronation of the other. If the tip (push) is slight, only feet respond symmetrically. A tilt board is also used to activate tilt reactions.

(3) Rotate child in standing, feet apart, results in one foot inversion to the rotated side, the other foot in pronation.

(4) Arm saving reactions become more established in all directions.

Treatment Suggestions

Gait. See Figs 8.165–8.169, without support.

Other techniques. See 9–12 months level without walking aids. Self-correct gait and balance.

Stair climbing is also dependent on standing on one leg long enough for the other to deal with the step. This should be trained on and off a low box, progressed to higher boxes as well as staircases, pavements, and wall-bars or stable ladders. Use of bannisters, two hands, one hand and independent stair climbing is achieved by 3–4 years developmental levels (see Tables 8.1, 8.2).

Train walking and stop, walk and turn, walk between and around objects, walk on different terrains. Walk backwards. Run holding child's hand. Stoop, stand, pick up toy, re-erect; stand, kick and throw balls.

Train a person to pivot in standing by assisted trunk turn while he moves his legs in steps to turn. Once achieved, pivoting is usually valuable for transfers and turning in small spaces.

Train staggering reactions. Hold child's arm and push and pull him in all directions to stim-ulate staggering or hopping reactions (Fig. 8.180). One foot may be held instead and the child pushed forward and a protective step provoked. Also hold hips and sharply rotate child to provoke a protective step.

Tilt reactions (Fig. 8.181). Tilt the child back, sideways or tilt him at his hips (Fig. 8.182) or tip (push) slightly at shoulder/trunk.

- In order to stimulate tilt response, tip child well off the horizontal to develop a safe postural control. A child also tries to sway himself forwards and backwards using an active postural adjustment to maintain balance. Later try this laterally with supervision.

- To provoke reaction in his feet. See also Chapter 10 on the treatment of valgus feet.

Carry all these out against manual resistance – 'Don't let me push you'.

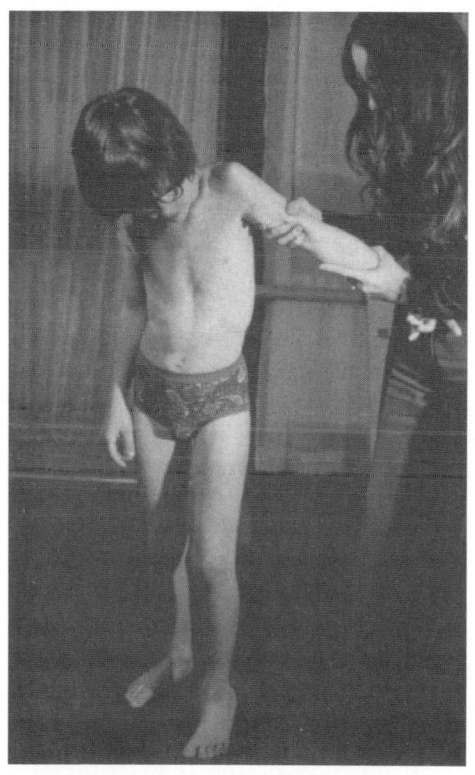

Fig. 8.180

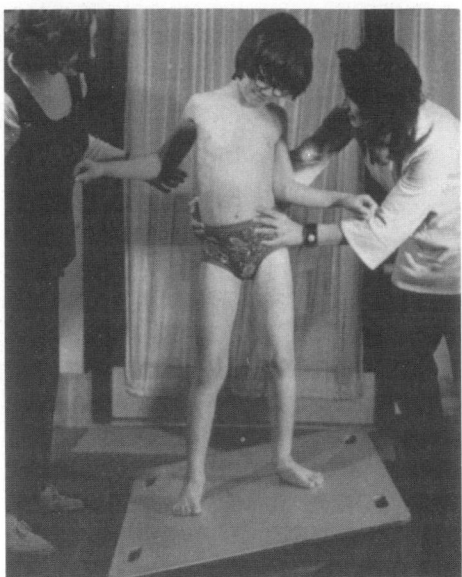

Fig. 8.181 Tilt reaction sideways.

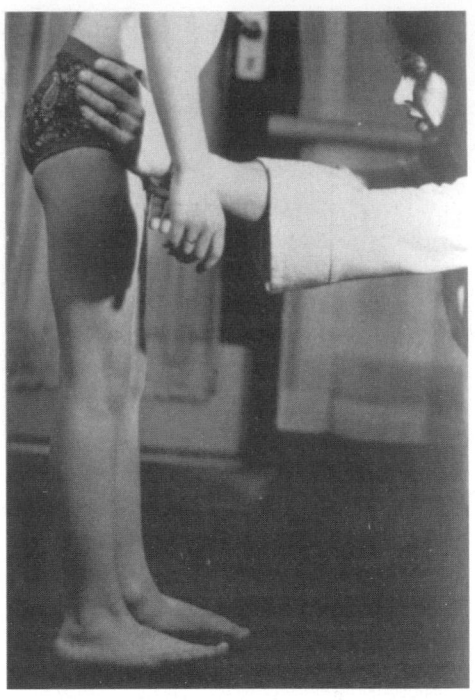

Fig. 8.182 Tilt reaction backwards using hip flexion with dorsiflexion. Slight push activates dorsiflexion only.

More advanced counterpoising on one foot is shown using a scooter (Fig. 8.183a) and when stepping over benches or toys of different heights (Fig. 8.183b) as well as in activities such as climbing and kicking balls (see Tables 8.1–8.3).

2–7 YEAR LEVELS (Tables 8.1–8.3)

Train tricycling (Fig. 8.184), hop, skip and jump and the variety of activities at the different developmental levels described in the work of Gesell and others (see Table 8.1).

DEVELOPMENT OF HAND FUNCTION

The development of hand function not only depends on the motor control of the shoulder girdle, arms and hands but also on visual, perceptual, perceptual-motor and cognitive development.

The *main motor aspects* of hand function involve the type of grasp, the pattern of reach, the pattern of reach-and-grasp and the pattern

of release. These aspects may develop independently of the gross motor activities in prone, supine, sitting, standing and walking development. Such development of upper limb function depends on well-supported lying, sitting and standing postures. Postural control can therefore be at different motor levels. Although this discrepancy of motor levels appears, it is essential to develop this fine motor ability as:

(1) Use of hands is helpful for perceptual development, cognitive development and for the emotional satisfaction of the child.

(2) Use of hands is particularly important for a child with motor disabilities so that he can use them for support on open hands or grasp in order to support himself to sit, stand, walk or pull himself into any position.

(3) Hands can be used to help establish shoulder girdle stability which is fundamental to

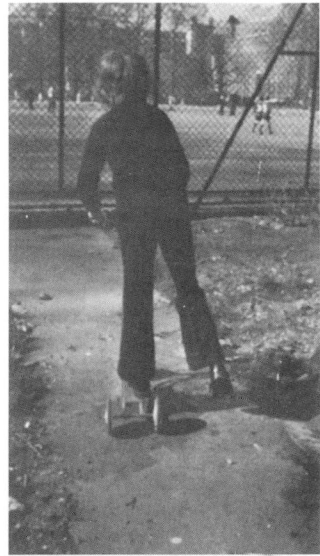

a

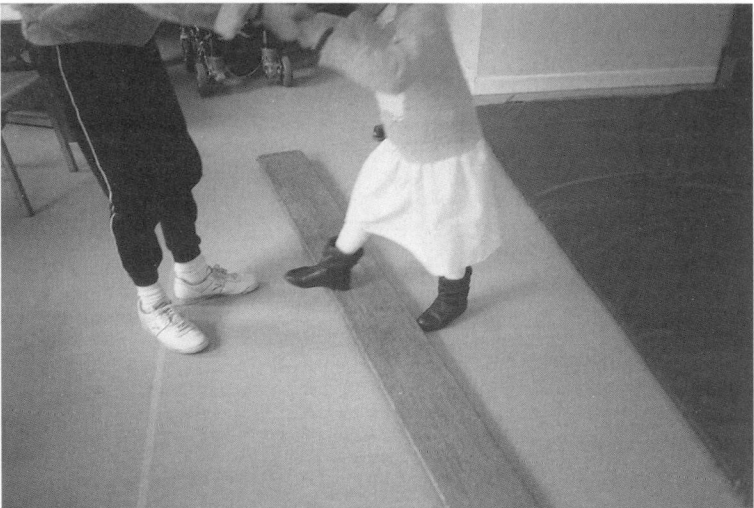

b

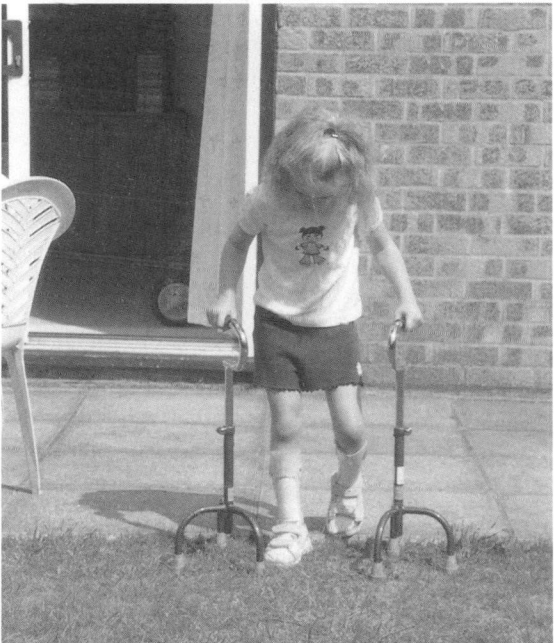

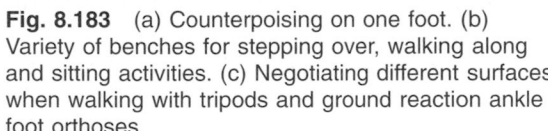

c

Fig. 8.183 (a) Counterpoising on one foot. (b) Variety of benches for stepping over, walking along and sitting activities. (c) Negotiating different surfaces when walking with tripods and ground reaction ankle foot orthoses

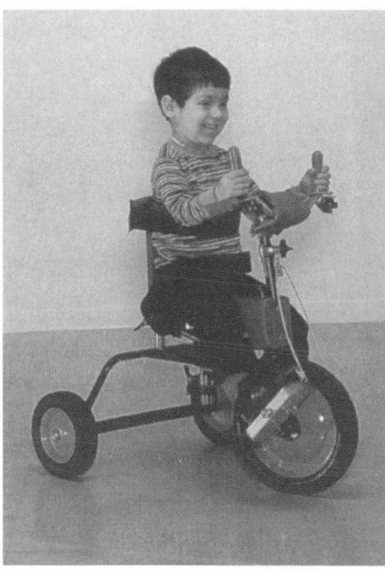

Fig. 8.184 An adapted tricycle for handgrips, trunk support, knee extension-flexion and dorsiflexion (acknowledgement to Rifton Tricycle).

many of the fine and gross motor skills. This distal to proximal control is a modified normal development and also a variation in able-bodied babies.

Hand function can develop if a child is well positioned and appropriately supported at his trunk and pelvis. As arm and hand actions activate the anticipatory postural adjustments it is unwise to omit unsupported trunks in a hand function programme. See prone, supine, sitting and standing development for

Table 8.1 Motor developmental stages, 2–7 years (based on Cratty 1970; Gesell 1971; Sheridan 1975).

2 years
Climbs on to furniture
Pulls wheeled toy by string
Ascends and descends stairs holding on, two feet per
  stair
Gait pattern changes from wide base, short, flat foot
  steps to narrower base, more heel–toe action
  established by 3 years
Arms held in abduction during gait come down to relaxed
  flexion at child's sides
Legs change from external rotation to facing forward
Walk, run and stop alone
Avoids obstacles while running or walking, steers
  wheeled toys
Throws ball without good direction and excessive effort
Arms held out when asked to catch a ball
Walk backwards, sideways, between obstacles
Walks into a ball to attempt kick

2·5 years
Jumps two feet together
Ascends stairs, holding on, alternate feet
Descends holding on, two feet per stair, ascends two
  feet no hold
Steers tricycle while 'walking' his feet on ground
Stands and kicks ball with one foot
Stands on tiptoe by imitation

3 years
Ascends stairs, no holding on alternate feet
Descends stairs usually two feet per stair, no holding on
Jumps from bottom stair or pavement
Climbing furniture, apparatus well
Runs and turns, runs and pushes large toys
Walks on tiptoes, on heels, heel–toe action in walk up
  inclines, uneven ground
Balances on one foot alone, momentarily, enough to
  walk on line unsteadily

Pedals tricycles and pedal cars
Imitates movements, e.g. wiggles thumb, asymmetrical
  arm position unless very complicated

4 years
Throws and catches ball with more control, less effort,
  more direction and does not need to place arms out to
  catch
Bounces ball, picks up ball or object with bend from
  waist
Walks on wide balance beam, near ground, walks heel
  to toe on line steadily
Stands on one foot 3–5 seconds alone
Hops on right or left foot increasing distance
Imitates finger plays including fine pincer actions
Gait pattern now with arm swing, as adult: stops
  suddenly; turns on the spot

5 years
Climbs trees, ladders, apparatus
Expert at sliding, swings, 'stunts'
Dances, hops and skips to rhythms
Throws and catches ball in various directions, smaller
  balls
Kicks ball on the run
Counts fingers by pointing

6 years
Wrestles, tumbles
Roller skates
Jumps rope, begins skip with rope
Stands on one foot with eyes closed
Bounces and catches balls

7 years
Walks on narrow and high balance bars
Throws ball about 30 feet
Begins team sports

Movement development shows improvement in speed, precision and decrease of effort or extraneous movements. Increase of endurance. Perception of space, timing and rhythm become integrated with many of the motor skills, see physical education literature for further details and for patterns of performance.

interaction of postural control with limb function/movements.

Upper limbs and the postural mechanisms

(1) Establishment of head control is important for hand/eye coordination.
(2) Establishment of postural stability of the shoulder girdle is obtained when leaning on elbows or on hands in various gross motor

activities in prone, supine, sitting, standing and walking development. This contributes shoulder stability for reach, reach-and-grasp, and assists coordination of manipulation or activities such as pouring liquids.

(3) Establishment of head, trunk and pelvic postural stability, weight shift and counterpoising in sitting and standing allow arm and hand function in postures other than in lying or only if the child is firmly held sup-

Table 8.2 Character sketch of developmental stages, 1–7 years. (With acknowledgements to Dr P.M. Sonksen from her thesis (1978) for MD entitled: *The neurodevelopmental and paediatric findings associated with significant disabilities of language development*, The Wolfson Centre Library, University of London, Mecklenburgh Square, London WC1.)

Item	Stage by age (years)	Stage 1	Stage by age (years)	Stage 2	Stage by age (years)	Stage 3	Stage by age (years)	Stage 4	Stage by age (years)	Stage 5
Gait in walking	1·6	Early toddler	1·9	Late toddler	2·3	Young child heel strike	6·0	Adult. Heel toe push off		
Upstairs	1	Creeps on hands and feet	1·9	Walks 2 feet/step + hand. Exaggerated foot lift	2·3	Walks 2 feet/step + hand. Economical foot lift	3·0	Walks 1 foot/step and hand	4·0	Walks 1 foot/step. No hands
Downstairs	1·3	Sitting bumps or creeps backwards	2·0	Walks 2 feet/step + hands (giving much support)	3·0	Walks 2 feet/step + hand	4·0	Walks 1 foot/step and hand	4·6	Walks 1 foot/step. No hands
Tip-toes	2·0	Balances momentarily but lowers heels to floor before walking	2·6	Walks on toes but with much ↑↓ movement of heels which touch floor often	3·6	Walks well on toes with no ↑↓ movement of heels	4·6	Runs well on toes		
On heels	2·0	Toes raised when standing but lowered to floor before walking	2·6	Walks with toes raised and whole forefoot off floor only for some steps	3·0	Able to walk on heels with forefoot only occasionally sinking	3·6	Walks well on heels		
One foot balance	2·0	Tries but unable (may *cheat* by holding on to something)	3·0	Momentarily succeeds 0–2 seconds	4·0	3–9 seconds	5·0	10–12 seconds	6·0	12–16 seconds
Hopping	2·0	Unable – may jump up and down 2 feet together	3·6	1–4 hops	4·0	5–8 hops	5·0	9–12 hops	6·0	Over 12 hops

Note   Ages given are in years and months.

ported with straps of a special chair/wheelchair. Thus decreasing manual or other supports in developmental stages, especially in sitting, standing and upright kneeling, needs to be associated with arm and hand func-

tion. If not, anticipatory postural adjustment essential for daily function remains dormant (Fig. 8.185).

(4) Development of rising reactions. Hands and arms are used to help in the change of

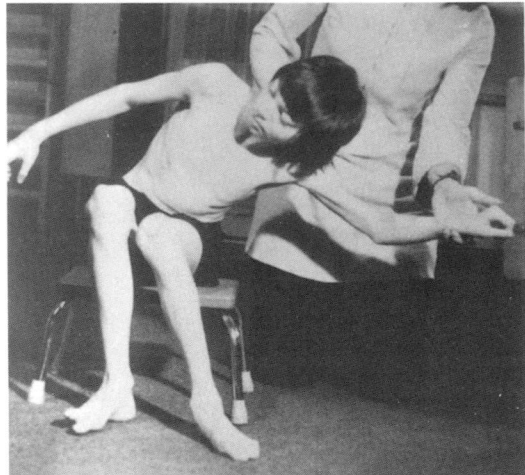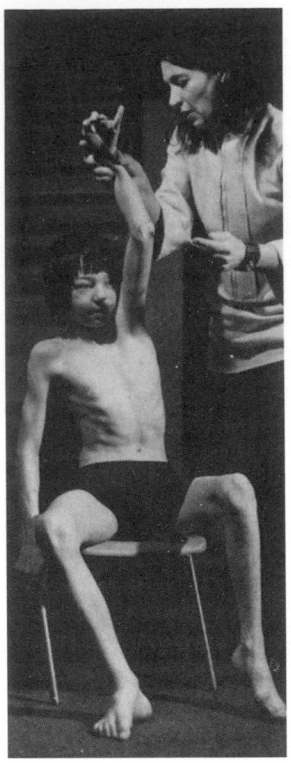

a   b

Fig. 8.185 Training reach (strength, synergy and postural control). (a) Absence of counterpoising in the trunk leads to child falling over the arm during its movement. *Note* attempts to counterpoise with the better arm or by grasp or arm support by child is used initially and progressed to trunk adjustment without arm support or grasp. (b) The trunk is counterpoising the arm movement. Patterns of arm movements should be trained together with counterpoising, in all positions. *Note* the height of the chair controls the position of the legs. A lower chair should be used to prevent any extensor activity in legs, to stabilize the child or to diminish athetosis.

various postures or the assumption of posture in gross motor development. A child also needs to assume a position in which he will carry out his chosen task in various environments.

(5) Development of saving reactions in the arms. The upper limbs are thrown into various patterns involving active contractions of the muscles in synergies (patterns), to save and prop the child as he falls off balance. Although the hands and arms participate in *automatic* saving and propping reactions as well as in various rising reactions, these will not necessarily contribute to *voluntary* movements. Voluntary movements of reach, grasp and release have to be

specially trained in fine motor activities, and, may find a variety of synergies necessary.

(6) Some of the arm synergies trained in gross motor function are those used in voluntary reach (Fig. 8.186). However, these patterns need to be practised in the context in which they are used in daily tasks.

Upper limbs and abnormal motor behaviour

(1) Abnormal postures of the whole child include abnormal postures of the arms and hands (Figs 8.187–8.189). Correction of the whole child often corrects the arms. Also correct arm patterns improve the rest of the child (Fig. 8.190). Deformities are mini-

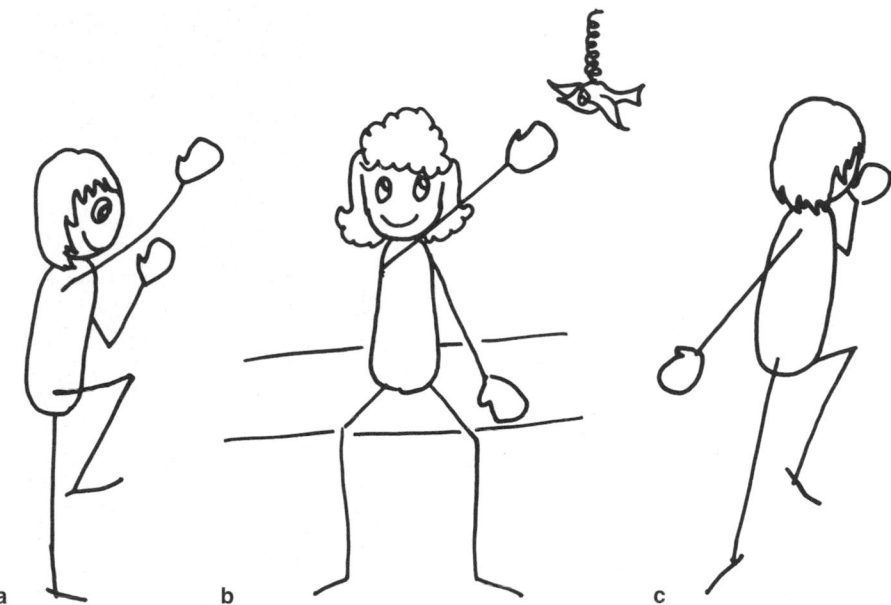

Fig. 8.186 (a) Arm pattern of shoulder flexion-adduction-external rotation trained within training of rolling. (b) To reach a toy in lying or sitting. (c) Arm pattern of shoulder extension-adduction-internal rotation within rolling prone to supine, or within creeping pattern in prone, may be used in reaching back and behind child as, say, in putting on a coat.

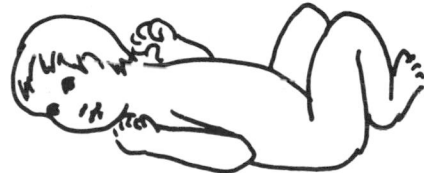

Fig. 8.187 Shoulders protracted or retracted with arms flexed-adducted and hands clenched in a predominantly flexed child similar to the newborn. Inability to reach out or can only reach near his body. Problems of release occur if hands flex or clench excessively. Asymmetry may exist with visual input only available from hand on one side.

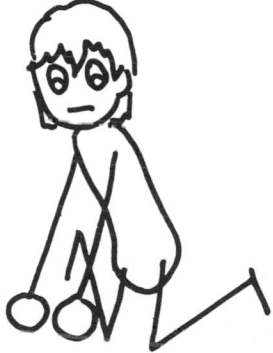

Fig. 8.188 Arms flexed-adducted and internally rotated with elbows flexed and pronated, wrists flexed or mid-position and hands clenched or open. Shoulder flexion-adduction-internal rotation may also occur with elbow extension-pronation. Shoulder flexion-adduction may also occur with elbow supination and flexion in children with dyskinesia who *fold their arms in* towards their bodies.

mized by corrective actions so that a secondary problem of such deformity does not block function.

(2) Involuntary movements in the hands or whole arm disrupt hand function. These involuntary movements may stem from the whole body. There may be involuntary motion in another part, say the 'kicking about' of legs only, which disturbs the use of the hands.

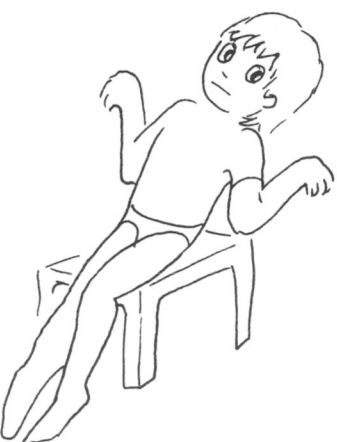

Fig. 8.189 Arms held up in the air in abduction-external rotation, elbow flexion and supination with palms facing toward the child. Elbows may also be flexed and pronated with palms facing outward. Hand may be hanging down or clenched; this is also called the *bird-wing position* and is seen in supine, sitting and standing positions. This may alternate with an asymmetrical tonic neck reaction or other asymmetry. There is inability to reach forward, bring hands together and develop *hand regard* and bring hands down for support.

(3) Asymmetries. For example, one side only is used; fisting of one hand is greater. Various visual problems affect one side.

(4) Inability to rotate trunk or shoulder to reach across midline.

BASIC ARM AND HAND PATTERNS FOR ALL LEVELS OF DEVELOPMENT

Although one should not be dogmatic about the pattern in which a child uses his arms and hands to achieve his goal, it is important to select corrective patterns below in treatment because (a) abnormal patterns of a limited repertoire are easier for cerebral palsied children but are not suitable for tasks in different situations. Their repetition tends to create deformities which often makes movement ineffective; (b) the child may have no idea on how to move and needs training in basic neuromuscular patterns. He

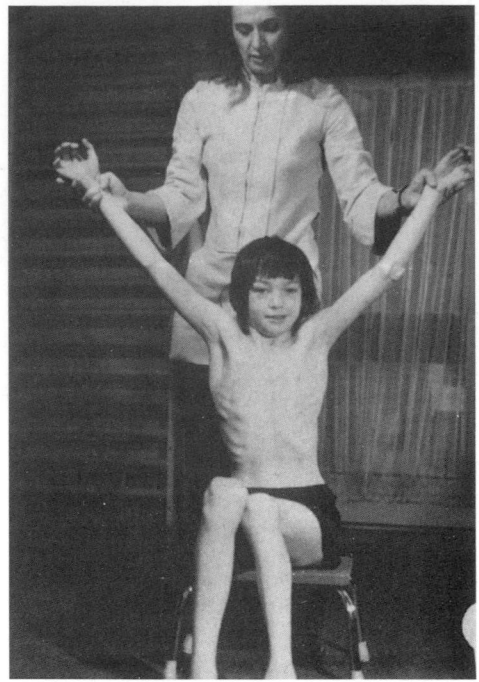

Fig. 8.190 Correction of asymmetry of arms, flexion-adduction-internal rotation and other abnormal postures of the arms also corrects abnormal postures of head and trunk (kyphosis, kyphoscoliosis) and vice versa. *Note* child tries to maintain postural fixation in vertical alignment and not fall backward against the therapist. Use arm elevation for dressing, ball play and other activities.

may later modify these patterns within his individual development and what he finds is his most effective hand use through experience and learning.

Abnormal Arm Patterns and Reaching Actions Treatment Suggestions

Although various arm patterns, or individual joint motions, can be found for correction of abnormal synergies, select those which can also be directly related to the use of the arms *in function*. Basic arm patterns which do this are:

(1) Shoulder flexion, elbow extension, pronation, hands open or grasp (Fig. 8.191).

Table 8.3 Developmental stages of the kick, 1–8 years (after P.M. Sonksen).

Stage I: boys <1–2·6 years/girls <1–3 years
The child walks, runs, or *straddle-toddles* towards the ball, and then walks into it, displacing the ball rather than actually kicking it. Some children who are standing near the ball or have come to a stop near it, lift up one foot and then step on to the ball. Children at this stage sometimes overbalance and fall.

Stage II: boys 1·6–>7 years/girls 2·6–>7 years
From a standing position the child propels the ball forward by flexing the leg at the hip and maintaining his balance on the other leg. If the child has run to the ball, he will stop just in front of it, adjust himself and/or the ball, and then kick the ball.

Stage III: boys 1·6–>7 years/girls 2·6–>7 years
The child can now run towards the ball and kick it whilst running, propelling it forward with some force and good direction. He anticipates the kicking position and brings the supporting leg at the side of the ball before swinging the kicking leg forward. The latter leg is not kept fully extended throughout the kick, but is kept slightly flexed during the swing and then fully extended for the actual kick.

Stage IV: boys 4–>7 years/girls 5·6–>7 years
The child and the ball are moving towards each other, and the running child can now kick the oncoming ball with good direction and force. He can anticipate the slight modification of the ball's position moving towards him as he brings himself to the kicking stance, and he hits the ball end on, suddenly reversing its trajectory towards the examiner.

There are *many variations* on the basic patterns described above. However they do not reinforce the patterns already used in cerebral palsy, but offer variety as well as correct deformity.

Practical Points

Positions. Carry out the above patterns in all positions of the child's gross motor levels, i.e. at normal developmental levels of:

0–5 months   use arms reaching in side-lying, supine, prone on elbows.

5–7 months   arm reach in prone, supine, rolling and then reaching, or arm reaching to roll, sitting propped on hands and reach with one arm.

7–9 months   arm reach on hands and knees, upright kneeling, support one forearm on table.

9–12 months   arm reach while sitting independently, upright kneeling or standing *holding* on with one hand.

Over 12 months   arm reach in standing.

Reach, grasp and release are also practised in these positions. Trunk rotation with reaching must be included, especially if resistance is given to the child's arm movement. An individual may find hand function easier in well-supported positions. Start with the successful position and progress to others.

Direction of reach is first low down in front of child, forward at shoulder level, to the side, above him, and then behind him. This progression is easiest for most children.

Facilitation. These patterns can be facilitated with:

(1) Touch, pressure stretch and resistance and good rotation of the child's shoulder girdle and/or trunk.

(2) The therapist may manually rotate the shoulder girdle, pull shoulders forward or backward to initiate automatic arm pattern (see section on Creeping patterns in prone development, 0–3 months stage).

(2) Diagonal, shoulder elevation-abduction-external rotation, elbow extension or flexion, supination, hands and thumbs open (Fig. 8.192).

(3) The opposite diagonal to (2) is down into adduction-internal rotation, elbow pronation, hand closed (Fig. 8.193) or open.

(4) Diagonal flexion-adduction-external rotation, elbow supination, flexed or extended (Figs 8.194 and 8.195).

(5) The opposite diagonal to (4) is arm extension-abduction-internal rotation (Fig. 8.196), elbow pronation, hand closed, or open (Figs 8.196 and 8.197).

Table 8.4 Development of hand function and eye–hand coordination.

0–3 months
Eye-to-eye contact (parallel eyes)
Fixes eyes on light; eyes follow object to midline
  (1 month), to past midline (2 months), over 180°
  (3 months), down, then up eye movement
Hands opening from closed posture
Reflex reactions: Tactile grasp; stretch grasp; blink; doll's
  eye reflex. Moro, ATNR, reflex hand flare open

3–5 months
Grasps with his eyes when interested in object
Hand regard or studies his hands, brings hands together
  in midline, clutches and unclutches hands
Visual exploration of environment, visual directed reach
  begins
Clumsy reaching, bilateral; corraling an object
Clutches clothes, touches body, mouth, face
Grasps object placed in hand; adducted thumb
Reflex reactions: Moro, ATNR disappearing, absence of
  grasp reflex

5–7 months
Reaching successfully in all directions, depending on
  trunk balance
Bilateral reach, unilateral reach; excessive MP/finger
  extension
Grasps feet in supine and sitting – bilateral then
  unilateral; thumb pressed into opposition
Maintains grasp (grip) on stationary object
Ulnar grasp changing to palmar grasp; wrist flexed
  becomes straight
Mirror movements of grasp in the other hand
Moves head to see things, eyes converge and focus on
  pellet at 10 feet; smaller pellets seen by 9 months
  (Stycar tests); rakes pellet with flexing-adducting
  thumb
Continues to mouth everything, hand to mouth
  movement with object
Reflex reactions: Saving and propping downward,
  forward and beginning laterally; posteriorly later (12
  months)

7–9 months
Transfers object from hand to hand
Unilateral reach and grasp; wrist extends
Radial grasp, beginning use of fingertips with opposed
  thumb
Holds one block while given another
Offers cube, but cannot release it; drops objects
Releases cube by pressing it against a hard surface
Bangs two objects together; compares them
Pats, bangs, strokes, clutches, rakes, scratches – pats
  mother's face, pats image of face in mirror; thumb
  abducted or opposed

9–12 months
Protrudes index finger, pokes objects with finger, other
  fingers flexing
Grasps between fingers and thumb, then one finger and
  thumb (crude to fine pincer grasp)

Pick up and place in and out of large containers; places
  lids
Reach and grasp possible in all directions, with
  supination and other improved control of arm;
  appropriate anticipatory grasp
Release with gross opening of hand, then more precise
  until places small objects in jar, peg in hole, for
  appropriate anticipatory release
Looks for fallen toy (permanence of objects); casts toys
Reflex reactions: Saving and propping backwards behind
  child; lateral and oblique

12–18 months
Casting of toys stopping; mouthing stopping
Watches small toy moved across room up to 12 feet
Builds tower of two cubes; places pellet into bottle
Pushes and pulls large toys
Drinks alone from cup, often spills

18 months to 2 years
Delicate pincer grasp and release
Takes off shoes, socks, vest, hat
Turns pages of book
Strings large beads, later smaller beads
Scribbles with pencil; whole hand grasp, supinated
Feeds self clumsily
Hand preference more obvious

2 years
Pencil grasp, pronated fingers, wrist deviates
Throws ball inaccurately
Unwraps sweet
Screws and unscrews lids, toys
Imitates vertical line; scribbles and dots

3 years
Takes off all clothes, puts on most clothes
Feeds self completely, using fork
Copies circle; static tripod pencil grasp
Draws a man simply
Cuts with scissors
Washes alone

4 years
Draws simple house, more detailed man
Brushes teeth, dresses alone except for buttons and
  laces
Constructive building, including three steps with cubes
Matches and names four colours
Copies cross; static tripod grasp modified

5 years
Copies square, triangle, letters; dynamic tripod pencil
  grasp
Matches 12 colours
Drawing and copying improved
Uses knife and fork
Dresses and undresses completely

Note Assessment measures of detailed hand function interwoven with conceptual, perceptual and ADL development are
carried out by occupational therapists and psychologists. (See also the Physical Ability Assessment Chart in the Appendix, and sections on Developmental stages, Feeding, Dressing, Play and Perception in Chapter 9.)

(3) The child can be taught to reach to grasp/touch food, for toys or take part in a play activity selected to activate the use of specific arm patterns (Fig. 8.191). This is preferable in all activities.

(4) The child can be asked to concentrate on the arm pattern, e.g. 'stretch your arm up and back', 'stretch your elbow'. However only draw his attention to the pattern once he is clearly working towards his goal, i.e. his chosen task.

(5) The daily activities of feeding, dressing, washing, bathing may use many desirable arm patterns including those described below, if activities are carefully designed and of interest to a child or older person.

Vision and arm patterns. It is important to stimulate the child's visual development and to associate it with development of hand func-

tions, e.g. encourage child to look at hands or object he is reaching for during facilitation of arm patterns.

Unilateral and bilateral arm patterns need to be included in the programme. For example:

(1) Unilateral patterns such as moving on side only; leaning on one hand and move with the other; grasp a support with one hand and move the other (asymmetrical work) (Figs 8.192–8.197). Apply during daily tasks to obtain action of each limb in normal asymmetry.

(2) Bilateral patterns with both a child's arms in the same direction (bilateral and symmetrical) for support and for motion. This takes place to counteract abnormal asymmetry during function, involving the whole body (Figs 8.198–8.200, see also Fig.

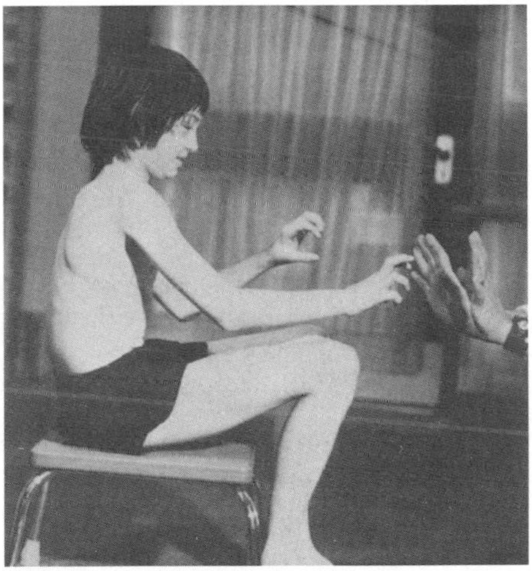

Fig. 8.191 An individual boy attempting basic pattern of bilateral shoulder flexion with elbow extension and dorsiflexion of the hands. This pattern not only corrects many abnormal patterns as in Figs 8.187–8.189 but is functionally useful, e.g. shoulder flexion-elbow extension hands flat or grasping support for sitting and standing well; in movements to reach for shoes or socks down at his feet, in pulling off a jumper over his head, reaching down to pull up pants or to push them down to his ankles. Note hands in poor anticipatory action.

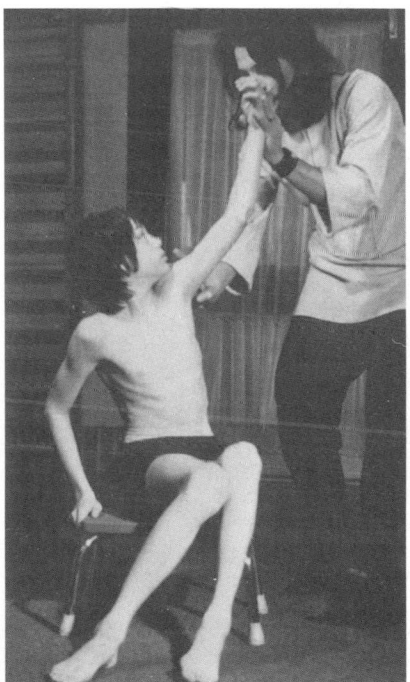

Fig. 8.192 Arm elevation-abduction-external rotation corrects abnormal patterns in Figs 8.187–8.189 and is used to reach out for an object, to dress or brush hair (elbow flexion/extension).

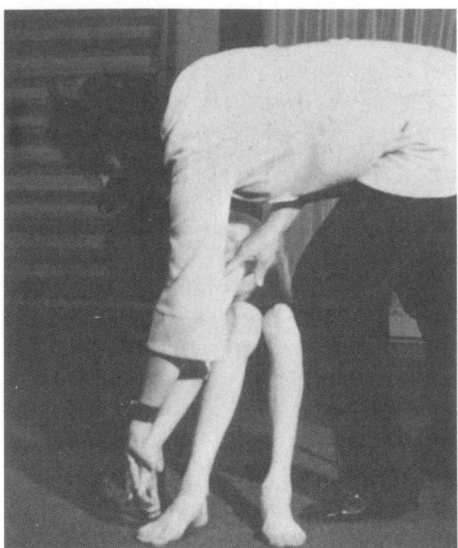

Fig. 8.193 Arm pattern adduction-internal rotation corrects abnormal arm pattern in Fig. 8.189 and is used to reach down for an object, dress, wash and other functions.

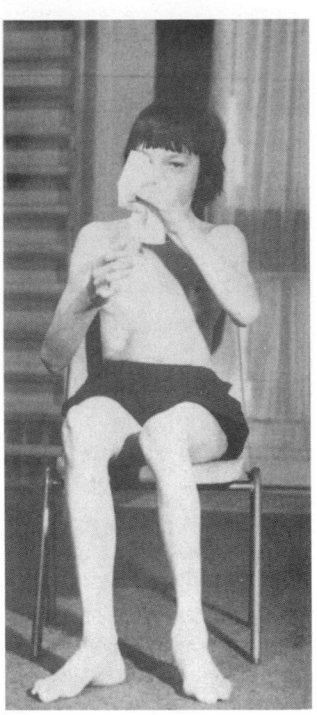

Fig. 8.195 Arm pattern in use for wiping nose or face. From Fig. 8.194.

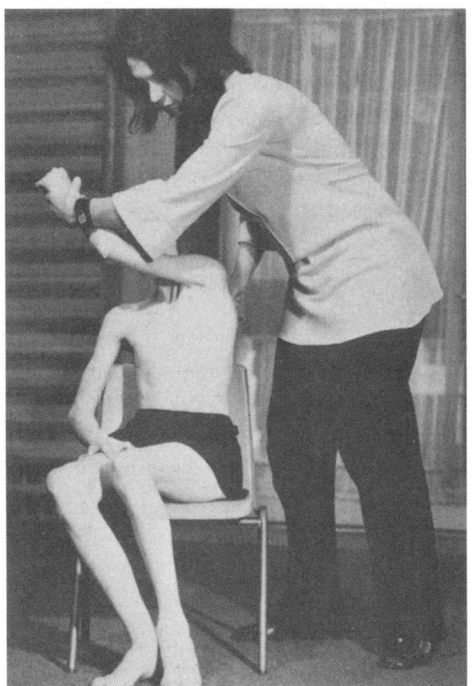

Fig. 8.194 Arm pattern flexion-adduction-external rotation corrects arm patterns in Figs 8.187–8.189 and is used to reach for an object, touch own face, blow nose, dress or eat.

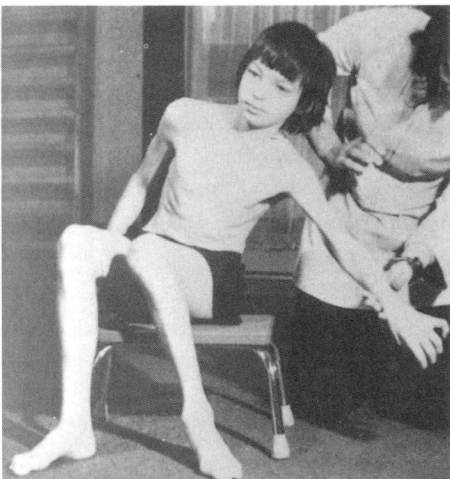

Fig. 8.196 Arm extension abduction-internal rotation corrects arm patterns in Figs 8.187–8.189 and can be used for dressing, reaching out and pulling trolleys in play.

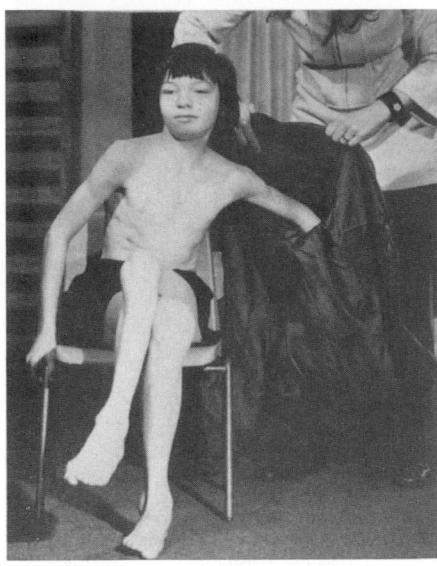

Fig. 8.197 Arm pattern in Fig. 8.196 in use for putting on a jacket.

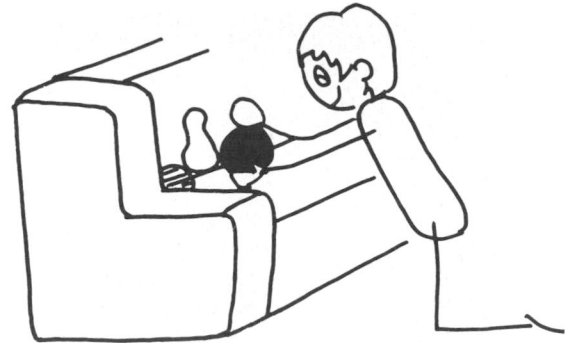

Fig. 8.198 Both arms stretch towards toys and palms face inwards to hold toys. In this way elbow extension, supination is encouraged and simultaneously corrects abnormal motor patterns. *Note* the rest of the body is also in better alignment associated with a better arm pattern (synergy). Use of *both* arms corrects asymmetry particularly in hemiplegia.

8.190). Use of less affected arm together with affected arm often activates it better.

(3) Bilateral patterns with each arm, in opposite directions (bilateral and reciprocal). This takes place in creeping, reciprocal arm swing, or motion using play equipment, pulleys or hand pedals.

(4) Bilateral patterns with each arm in a different direction, e.g. one sideways, the other forward (bilateral and asymmetrical), which is used in advanced perceptual motor training and for highly complicated counterpoising activities and hand skills.

Abnormal Hand Grasps and Treatment Suggestions

(1) Abnormal grasp may be present in association with the total abnormal posture or only with the arm posture and synergies of movement when the rest of the body functions well.

(2) Limited joint motion, weakness and problems with isolated finger, thumb movements are all found in abnormal grasps.

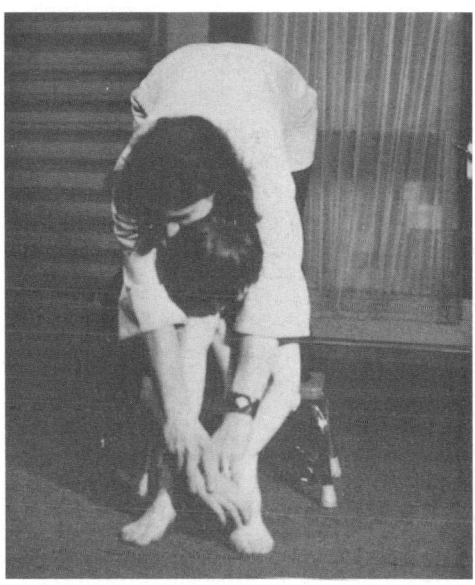

Fig. 8.199 Bilateral arm patterns against appropriate manual resistance in diagonal patterns. Use to reach feet or floor for daily activities. Postural mechanism is also assisted.

(3) Grasp may appear to be abnormal because it belongs to a lower normal level of development. This is motor delay.

(4) Anticipatory grasp is distorted by inability to open clenched hands and by intellectual

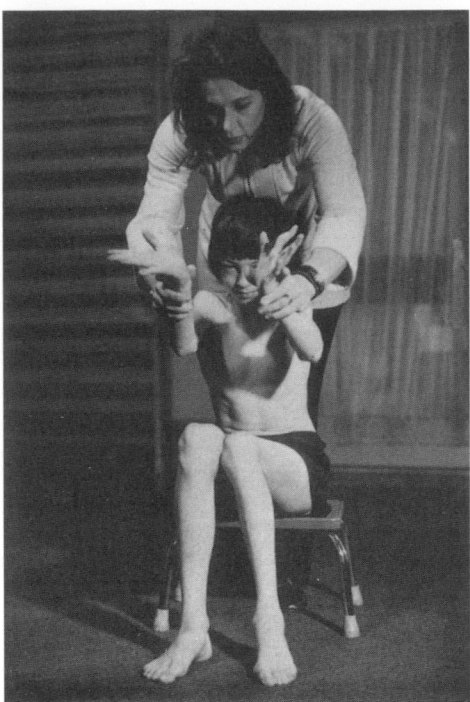

Fig. 8.200 Bilateral arm patterns against appropriate manual resistance in diagonal patterns. Note facilitation of wrist extension.

delay. Lack of experience in hand use also causes such delay. Perceptual and cognitive abilities are essential for shaping a hand during reach and for fingers' force to be regulated according to different objects.

Treatment suggestions for some abnormal grasps

Grasp only possible in one position of the child's arm. Train grasp within all the corrective arm patterns (above, in different directions, and body positions). Movements to increase range, weakness and isolated finger and thumb exercises may contribute to hand grasp and release. However, activities directly related to tasks are more important and may well treat these problems at the same time.

Wrist flexion with palmar or pincer grasp or inability to grasp in this position (Fig. 8.201).

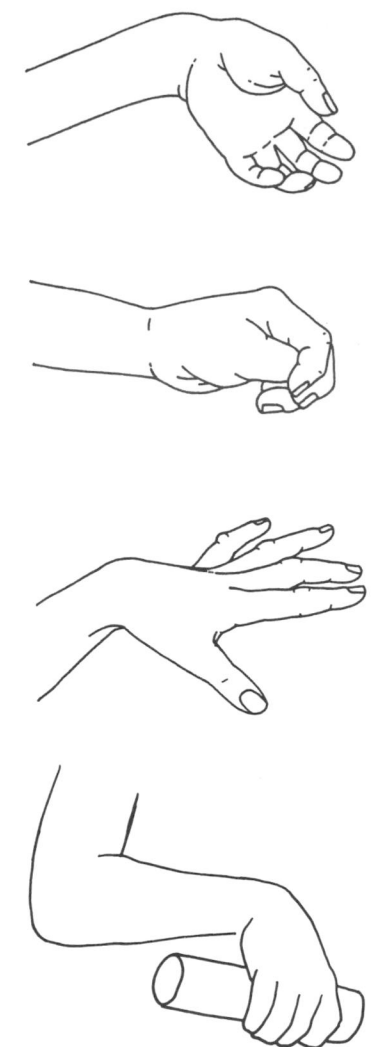

Fig. 8.201 Common abnormal patterns of arm, wrist and hand.

Press the child's wrist down as he tries to grasp; place the object above the level of his wrist; ask him to lift his hands to the object, see Figs 8.200 and 8.203. Some children may need a wrist splint to train grasp with wrist in midline or extension (dorsiflexion). In some children with hypertonus, the wrist extension should only be to the midposition as there is excessively tight finger flexion with full wrist extension. This also prevents the child from

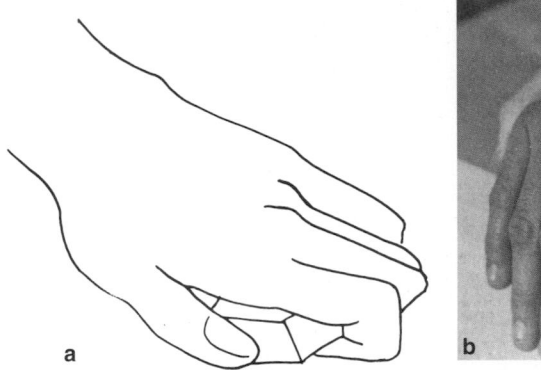

Fig. 8.202 Abnormal grasp with excessive finger flexion and no flexion or even with hyperextension of metacarpophalangeal joint is being corrected by the therapist in **b** during grasp and release.

opening his hands to release the object held. The Lycra hand and wrist splint, or arm splint and a flexible splint encouraging midline and dorsiflexion, is used to decrease excessive palmar flexion. See hand and arm splints below.

The use of glove puppets, hammering, lifting dowels out of holes, rings off a stick and similar activities may help to obtain active wrist extension for grasp and release. In some cases, grasping with the wrist in extension may be achieved at the cost of opening the hand in this particular position.

Excessive finger flexion in grasp. With or without hyperextension of the metacarpophalangeal (m-p) joints (Figs 8.202 and 8.203). Place the child's hand over thick, larger objects such as bars and handles. Avoid the hand clenching onto squeezy toys. Hold the dorsum of the child's hand, lift his m-p joints and he or you can then press his fingers straight over the large ball, box or square bar. This may be done with the child's m-p joints pressing on the edge of a table as he tries to hold on to the edge, or the solid edge of a truck or box. Counteracting this abnormal grasp will prepare him for grasp with his fingers straight, using finger tips later. Grasping edges of cards or lids is one way of training this straight finger grasp.

Adducted thumbs and ulnar grasp. The adducted thumb may grasp or be useless. It can be seen with ulnar grasp (Fig. 8.201). In some

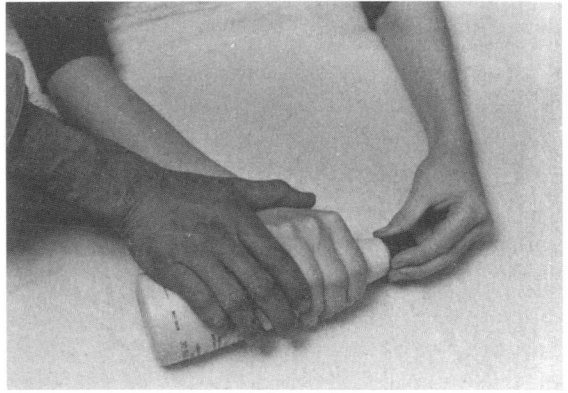

Fig. 8.203 Overcoming excessive wrist flexion, overflexion of fingers by the task selected and the therapist pressing the wrist down. Press on a child's wrist as he grasps bars of walkers, spoons, cups and other tools.

children the ulnar grasp may result when the child tries to compensate for or avoid the adducted thumb. When the thumb is abducted a radial grasp may occur. In other cases, the child grasps his fingers in midposition with an adducted thumb. Adducted thumbs may also accompany palmar flexion, or excessive finger flexion with hyperextended m-p joints. The child should be encouraged to move his hand towards the thumb side, for example he pushes rolling toys away towards the radial side; brings a spoonful of food towards his mouth and other activities which encourage him to move his hand towards the thumb side. He may not manage this unless you hold his hand in

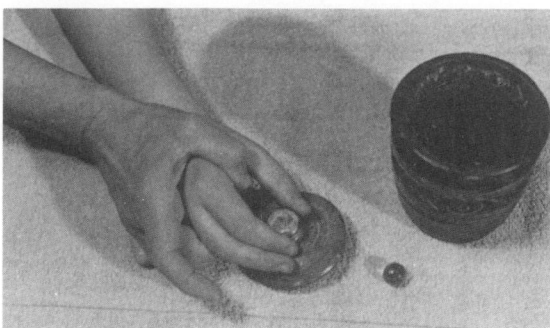

Fig. 8.204 Guided abduction of thumb and pincer grasp.

midline during grasp. Hold the child's hand between his thumb and forefinger on one side and hold down the ulnar side as he grasps (Fig. 8.204).

The little finger and ring finger may be bandaged if the child does not resent such a procedure. Training grasping of objects with the radial side is then encouraged. Check that the child is not given handgrips on walkers, handles and other supports which encourage an abnormal ulnar grasp. The handles at the sides of rollators or on crutches may do this. Avoid the angled spoons for children as they create an ulnar grasp. The child's adducted thumb may be abducted-extended if he tries the above suggestions. Also use techniques for hand opening in the developmental levels below.

Adducted thumbs may be held out with thumb splints made from soft, firm pigskin or other splints made from a variety of materials. To take an adducted thumb out of a fist or hand, never pull it by its tip or you may dislocate or sublux the m-p joint. Sometimes the other fingers flex more as you do pull on the thumb. Rather turn the whole arm or forearm to face palm up to the ceiling and abduct the thumb out from its base. It is important to accompany this procedure with placing the child's hand over a toy, so teaching him a palmar grasp or later a radial grasp. See 'Opening of hand' techniques; hand splints below.

Anticipatory grasp. The methods to reduce tight fingers and thumb contribute to opening of the hand to anticipate the size of object for grasping. More experiential learning is still needed for practice with different sizes and weights of everyday objects (see developmental levels 7–9 months).

Inability to use both hands simultaneously. Although this is normal in many children under the 6 months developmental level, it may also be due to:

(1) Lack of head control in midline so the child uses the hand that he can see; lack of midline head control is seen in persistent head turning to one side, which occasionally improves spontaneously.
(2) Asymmetrical tonic neck response to one side which is 'used' to reach to that side and when head turns away to grasp the object on the occipital side.
(3) Hemiplegia or greater involvement of one arm in any diagnostic type.
(4) Excessive spasms or involuntary motion on one side, rare hemiathetoids.
(5) Sensory loss on one side especially astereognosis two-point discrimination in the hand or visual field defect, usually found in some hemiplegia and tetraplegia.

Inability to grasp on one side will often be associated with *inability to use both hands together* or to hold with one hand and carry out an action with the other. During training of prone, supine, sitting and standing development check that both hands are given objects to grasp simultaneously or to grip for support. Use play activities which require two hands, e.g. play in water and washing, sand, clay, dough, larger toys, handles on bowls, rolling pins, sieves, sticks with dangling bells, broom, bicycle pump, toy concertina, small cymbals, maracas or toys which make a noise if pushed at both ends. See developmental level.

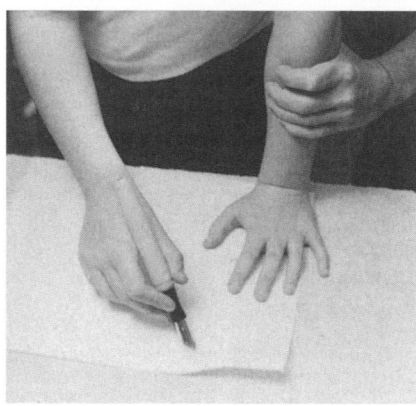

Fig. 8.205 Support on more affected hand pressed open whilst child uses more skilful hand. Affected hand stabilizes the paper or toy during use with the other hand.

Associated grasping or clenching on the affected side when grasping with the unaffected or the less affected side. This is usually seen in the spastic type; associated *mirror* movements of the hand not in use are normally seen in very young children but disappear on normal development. If these mechanisms persist they can prevent the child's transfer of objects from hand to hand and holding with one hand while using the other hand. Hold the more affected elbow straight with hand flat on the table while the other hand grasps. Have the child lean on the more affected hand held open, with the weight on the elbow or hand. Carry out joint compression to facilitate support on this hand as the other hand is used actively. Practise activities which include each hand in a different action, e.g. hold toy with one hand, carry out action with the other, winding a bandage or hold support with one hand, and use a variety of movements with the other (Fig. 8.205).

Other parts of the body may also tense or assume abnormal postures during grasp. Check that these associated reactions or excessive activity are controlled by the therapist and as much as possible by the child as well. Correct positioning of the rest of the body during hand function will help to control this. Motor tasks too advanced for an individual can increase excessive activity in the whole child.

Practical Points in Training Grasp

(1) Use of the eyes needs to be associated with development of hand function. Follow the developmental levels below.

(2) Normally the grasp reflex and hand clenching disappear before voluntary group develops. Do not wait or work on total disappearance before putting the object in the child's hand to grasp. Use techniques (below) to open the hand just before methods to develop palmar grasp, in the same session.

(3) Children should avoid a grasp in association with any of the abnormal arm postures shown in Fig. 8.201, e.g. grasp with wrist and/or elbow flexed, shoulder adducted and flexed. Use the arm patterns suggested in 'Basic arm and hand patterns' for all levels of development. Check that the rest of his body does not assume abnormal postures as he grasps.

(4) Have the child hold objects with his hand in pronation, then later in midposition and still later in supination. However, some children with dyskinesia may start with grasp in supination and then midposition and finally in pronation.

(5) Make sure that the child looks at the object in his hand. Talk about the object at his comprehension level. Encourage his speech before and later during the use of his hands if this does not distract him. Later draw attention to the properties (soft, hard, heavy light, size) of an object so that he develops an appropriate anticipatory grasp.

(6) Check that he is interested in the object placed in his hand. Always have him choose from an array of objects which help his function.

Abnormal Release and Treatment Suggestions

Total inability to let go of an object placed or grasped with excessive flexion by the child after 5 months developmental level (see treatment for hand opening below).

Release only possible if wrist is palmar flexed. The child may use his other hand, his chin or even his forehead, or a hard surface to press the back of his hand to obtain palmar flexion. Teach release with wrist in midline using a splint, manual support and active control by a child.

Release object against a hard surface after 11 months of age. These problems of release are discussed in the appropriate developmental levels below.

Release with thumb adducted and flexed in palm. Train a release with child's active hand opening together with thumb abduction following supination of the forearm by the therapist. Sometimes external rotation from the shoulder is indicated. Thumb splints may help. Isolated thumb abduction and extension is very difficult and is best acquired using larger objects placed in the hand.

Release with ulnar deviation can be improved if objects are released into container or dowel holes on the radial side of the hand.

Release with excessive splaying of the fingers, i.e. hyperabduction with hyperextended metacarpophalangeal joints. A similar but less pronounced pattern is also seen in normal babies casting objects at about 11–15 months of age. In addition this pattern is seen in excessive avoiding reactions in the hands of children with dyskinesia. There may also be plantar and/or a visual avoiding reaction with the avoiding reaction in the hands caused by tactile and visual stimuli respectively. Grasp smaller objects and train release into a defined area or container. Hold the ulnar side of the child's hand and train release on the radial side and later with thumb and finger. Training a more precise release is closely allied with the training of pincer grasp (Fig. 8.204).

Hand and visual avoiding reactions can be helped if one introduces the object slowly into the child's visual field and into his hands. Encourage him to maintain his grasp on a desired object to gradually assist him to become less sensitive to the stimuli. Avoid hand-over-hand method to maintain his grasp if he is sensitive. This is particularly unwise if a child is severely visually impaired and can lead to marked avoidance of touch on his hands.

Conflict between grasp and release. This problem is seen in dyskinesia, when a person attempts to grasp an object but immediately withdraws his hand, splaying it open. This presents itself as a repeated involuntary motion in the hands. This conflict between the grasp reflex and the avoiding reactions was described by Twitchell (1961). To break this disabling conflict, it is advisable to reinforce the child's active grasp or grip using your hand placed over his hand, or pressing an object gently against his palm with his wrist fixed on the table. Encourage maintained grasp for as much of the day as possible on bars, handles, in front, at his side, above or below him in his various situations during the day. When he is sitting in classrooms, toilets, at meals, in a buggy, place his hands to grasp bars. Frames or manual supported standing and walkers need to have bars for grasp. Independent walking with a rod/stick/tenoquoit grasped in hands give practice for maintained grasp.

Other involuntary motion disrupting hand use. Train conscious control of manipulation. With practice the involuntary motion is mastered by a child to a greater or lesser degree. Help the child by having him use his hands while leaning on his forearms, or reach for toys through a thin padded hoop which limits the excursion of the involuntary motion. Wide upright poles also limit his involuntary motion as he reaches between them for toys or objects.

Note. It is important to carry out all the training of reach, grasp and release at an individual's particular developmental levels. Abnormal patterns may not be due to spasticity, athetosis or ataxia. The arm and hand patterns can be normally seen at an early age of development and not at the chronological age of the individual child or older person. These are outlined below and treatment suggestions for them are sometimes the same as those for the abnormalities of cerebral palsy discussed above.

All the patterns of grasp and release are also disrupted by visual loss, any sensory loss in the hands, cognitive delay, and by lack of visual, perceptual or perceptual-motor development as seen in intelligent 'clumsy' children (developmental coordination disorder, dyspraxia).

Sensory loss of two-point discrimination in children predicts inability to adapt fingertip force to texture in manipulation (Lesny 1993; Yekutiel *et al.* 1994).

0–3 MONTHS NORMAL DEVELOPMENTAL LEVEL

Common Problems

Delay in eye focusing, visual fixation, visual following of an object. Clenched hands; thumb still held in palm. Opening begins and continues into next stage.

Abnormal performance, see abnormal patterns of arms and hand above. Hypersensitive hands.

Reflex reactions Grasp reflex, Moro reaction, tonic neck reaction, sudden flexor or extensor spasms.

Treatment Suggestions and Daily Care

Eye focus and following (hearing and vision)

(1) First offer visual interest in the midline and help the child keep his head in midline. You may need to hold both his shoulders forward, occasionally backward to allow him to keep his head upright (see sitting development, vertical head control; prone development, head control).

(2) At first place your face or toys close to the child's eyes, about 8 inches (20 cm) from him. Then gradually move further away with encouragement to follow you.

(3) Eye-to-eye contact is of first importance before interest in objects. This is best done at the child's eye level whether he is in side-lying, supine, prone, supported sitting or supported standing.

(4) Associate vision, hearing and head control with face-to-face singing, talking. Vary tones of voice. Encourage a smile and general communication as he attends, follows and looks for your *voice*.

(5) Help him to look at and follow your face and then shiny, moving, colourful noise-making mobiles, toys, fishes in a tank, marble runs, a torch light. Use coloured ribbons, Christmas decorations, shiny bottle lids and also objects which do not make any sounds. Following a visual lure on its own is more difficult for some children.

(6) Use red, yellow or primary colours, and black and white pictures.

(7) Use jingling noises and not high-pitched or sudden loud noises as the child may still have a startle reflex.

(8) Hang tinkling bells, jingling beads or mobiles in the window or doorway so that they make a sound as the wind blows. Guide any visually directed early arm reaching with full body support of child (von Hofsten 1992).

(9) Put him in different positions, but start with well-supported upright sitting as well as lying on his back, side or stomach to carry out active looking and listening activities.

Also see. Opening of hand, treatment suggestions at next stage but begin at this stage. Hands open in prone, supine, side-lying channels of development. For example:

(1) Hand may open within the arm pattern of elevation-abduction-external rotation, or extension-adduction-internal rotation in techniques of creeping, rolling and reaching out in lying, and fully supported sitting at this developmental level.

(2) Weight bearing on elbows and/or on hands decreases hand clenching, see prone, sitting, standing development which include leaning on elbows or hands.

(3) See correction of whole child's postures in all developmental levels – as these also correct arms and hands.

3–5 MONTHS NORMAL DEVELOPMENTAL LEVEL

Common Problems

Delay in hand regard, visual exploration; bringing hands together and to mouth, touching self. Delay in active grasp of an object placed in his hand, grasp and shake toy, no clumsy reaching for objects. Grasp is normally on ulnar side at this level. The clutching of child's hands on clothes on himself or mother may be delayed. Hands fully opened is expected by this stage.

Abnormal performance

(1) Asymmetrical bringing of hands to midline; reach or grasp on one side only.

(2) Touching with semiflexed or closed hand.

(3) Abnormal patterns in reaching (see abnormal patterns, arms and hands above).

(4) Abnormal grasp (see above) except ulnar or lateral grasp, at this stage.

Treatment Suggestions and Daily Care

Hand regard and bringing hands to midline and early guided reach:

(1) Place the child in side-lying or lying equipment, or in well-supported sitting, with shoulders brought forward and arms placed in front of child's eyes. Have a child sitting and leaning with his body against the table with arms along the surface for easier movement with such support. Guide early visually directed reaching along a surface. In those cases when the child *can* bring his arms up against gravity it is advisable to have him in supine. A side-lying board is helpful for those children who persist in keeping their arms in abnormal positions at their sides, out of their view (see Supine development, Figs. 8.68a–d).

(2) Once his hands are in front of him the child can be made aware of them by your touch and songs, shining a torch on them, putting sticky things such as jam on his hands, playing with his fingers, putting thimbles, rings, coloured ribbon, bracelets or bells on his wrist and fingers. Help him open his hands and rub his palms together, move his hands to stroke and touch his face and body and later clasp and unclasp hands, clutch materials and toys which are soft and easy to clutch. Commence guided reach along a surface.

Opening of hands

(1) Gradually desensitize a child's whole palm by rubbing it with rough textures, especially sand, during play activities.

(2) Rhythmical shake of a child's arm from his shoulder to relax his hand.

(3) Stroke the ulnar surface of his hand and little finger.

(4) You or the child press the heel of his hand on a firm surface especially combined with your giving pressure (joint compression) through a straight shoulder and extended elbow (Fig. 8.205).

(5) Hold the child's upper arms and rotate them outwards. Sometimes you only need to turn the elbow, so that the palm faces up. The child actively turns his elbow into supination as far as he can to hold a toy, ball or see a picture drawn on his hand. See other arm patterns of elevation in creep-

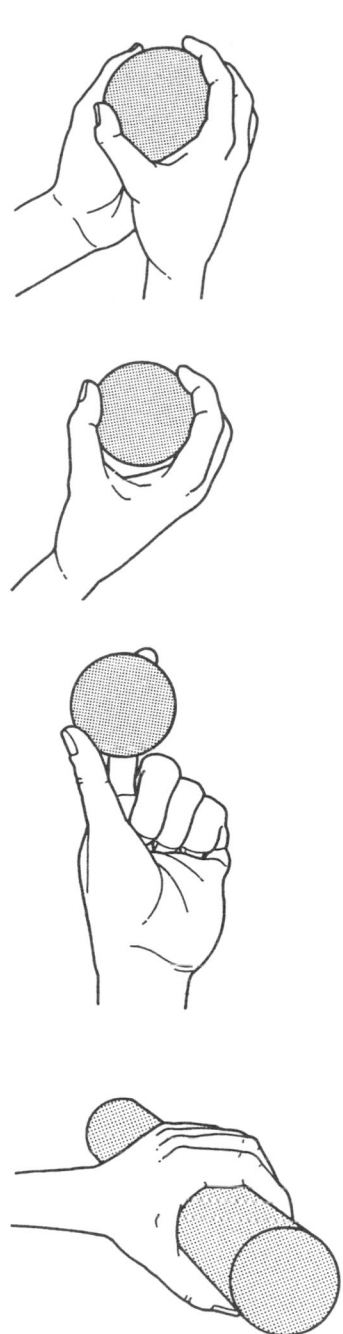

Fig. 8.206   Grasp patterns.

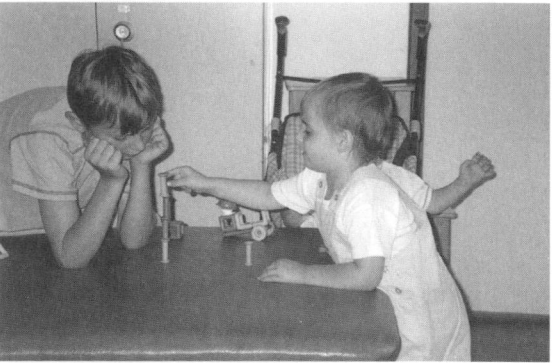

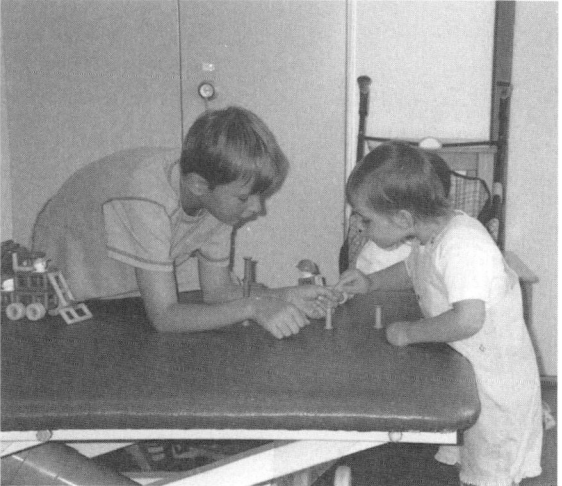

Fig. 8.207a,b   Brother playing with sister (with cerebral palsy) activating pincer grasp and fine release.

ing and rolling which include external rotation.

(6) Have the child's arms well away from his body. This avoids hand clenching in some children. Open the child's hand over a variety of large rubber, wooden or plastic objects. *Do not* give toys which stimulate clenching, such as squeezy toys. Have objects which are not too big for his small hands. Grasping a cone with the large end on the side of his little finger often helps to overcome hand clenching (Fig. 8.203).

(7) Open hands when child is prone leaning on elbows or hands, on hands and knees, sitting lean on hands, standing lean on hands. Open his hands by any of the above methods pressing the heel of the hand down. Pull the thumb or fingers out from the base and not from their tips.

Hand grasp

(1) See 'Abnormal hand grasps' above.
(2) Have a variety of objects that fit into the whole palm of his hand. Some children first learn to grasp soft objects more easily than hard ones or vice versa. Place different objects before him so that he chooses what he prefers.
(3) Light objects are often easier than heavy ones.
(4) Toys may be teething toys, hoops, teno-quoits, rattles, toy dumb bells, large rings, thick tubing with coloured liquid inside, cotton reels, sponge rubber toys. Avoid squeezy or tiny toys.
(5) Place his hands around large hand grips, handles, bars so that as a result he can sit up, kneel up or stand up or enjoy a ride on a tricycle, swing, rocking horse or see-saw.
(6) Thicken handles of spoons, pencils, toys with rubber, hardened clay, wood, a rubber ball or attach handles from, say, screwdrivers.
(7) See 'Practical points in training grasp' above.
(8) Encourage the child to hold rusks or spoon in feeding. Hold his hand on the spoon handle. Encourage him to hold a piece of his clothing as you help him undress; to hold his sponge in the bath, or hold his wet wash-cloth.

Besides placing objects of different shapes in his hand make sure to place other objects of different sensation into his hands, e.g. bean-bags, fur, velvet and suede objects, sandpaper, crinkling chocolate paper, shoe brushes, wooden, metal and natural objects. Use sand and water, dough, clay and modelling materials. Name these sensations for him as he feels them.

Help him to grasp and bring objects to his mouth to suck, lick, bite or chew, or to his nose to smell. Develop *grasp and press*, say a bath sponge, or large woollen pom-pom; *grasp and shake* a toy, rattle or maracas; *grasp and wave* a toy flag, ribbons, bells. *Grasp and drop* is present but it is not grasp and release which develops later (11 months). Grasp and push, grasp and pull, grasp and place and a variety of types of grasps usually develop later (Figs 8.206, 8.207).

5–7 MONTHS NORMAL DEVELOPMENTAL LEVEL

Common Problems

Delay in successful reaching in all or one direction, voluntary grip, palmar grasp, and manipulation of object in his hand, reach and grasp, taking weight on hands. Dropping of the object is normal but by 7 months a child usually holds a second block in the same hand and does not drop the first. Delay in hand to mouth activities to *mouth* everything; in bilateral then unilateral grasp of his feet, play with his toes. Delay in using both hands together.

Abnormal performance. As in 3–5 months level (see above). See 'Abnormal hand grasps' above.

Reflex reactions

(1) Saving reaction in arms down and forward is expected.
(2) Abnormal persistence of reflex reactions from earlier levels may be present.

Treatment Suggestions and Daily Care

(1) See above for 'Basic hand and arm patterns' and reach actions. See 3–5 months level for training grasp. See 'Abnormal hand grasps' above.
(2) Continue 0–5 months but combine reach *and* grasp. Practice of reach and grasp with a variety of objects begins to develop anticipatory grasp.
(3) Continue earlier treatment suggestions for reach and for grasp but now expecting the child to do more on his own. Expect him to

combine reach and grasp alone. See 6–9 months level in prone development, for taking weight on hands: used also in sitting and standing development. See also stimulation of saving and arm propping in prone and sitting development.

(4) See suggestions for *Inability to use both hands simultaneously* above.

7–9 MONTHS NORMAL DEVELOPMENT LEVEL

Common Problems

Delay in transfer from hand to hand, unilateral reach and grasp, grasp more than one block at a time, radial grasp, hand patting, banging, clutch, stroke, rake, scratch, bang two blocks together, release against a hard surface, use of hands in feeding and in holding on during sitting and standing. *Scissors* grasp (inferior pincer grasp) and use of fingertips may be delayed. Delay in anticipatory grasp in relation to size, shape, weight of object (9 months) (von Hofsten & Ronnqvist 1988).

Reflex reactions

(1) Saving and propping reactions expected.
(2) Abnormal persistence of reactions from previous levels may happen.

Treatment Suggestions and Daily Care

(1) See above for reach and grasp patterns and 'Abnormal release', 'Opening of hands'.
(2) Train child's active grasp in feeding, dressing, washing, toileting (Chapter 9). Begin training release by having the child release a block against a hard surface with the heel of his hand held down against the surface, or his other hand or his body. Release may be impossible if hand opening

has not yet been developed. See methods at 0–5 months level or training of hand opening.

(3) Ulnar grasp now develops into radial grasp.
(4) Transfer from hand to hand, banging blocks together and also holding on with one hand or leaning on one hand during unilateral reaching are particularly important for hemiplegia (Fig. 8.210a), and any child with asymmetrical function.
(5) Play with suitable toys, dough, sand, water can involve transfer from hand to hand, grasping more than one object at a time as well as patting, banging, clutching, stroking, raking, scratching and release against a hard surface.
(6) Patting with open hands may become a persistent pattern in some children with severe learning problems or visual disability. Activities involving grasp and manipulation at the child's developmental level counteract these and other *mannerisms*.

9–12 MONTHS NORMAL DEVELOPMENTAL LEVEL

Common Problems

Delay in finger/thumb opposition and development of crude and fine pincer grasp, no protrusion of index finger. Release of objects, casting haphazardly and delay of increasing control of release into containers of different sizes and building two-cube tower. Delay in a child's searching for a fallen object or hidden object perceived immediately before disappearance (permanence of objects). Supination may not develop. Delay in developing anticipatory grasp.

Abnormal performance See 'Basic arm and hand patterns, abnormal hand grasps, abnormal release' above. Abnormal arm patterns prevent increasing control of shoulder, elbow and hand. Abnormal grasp prevents pincer grasp, and index finger approach.

Reflex reactions

(1) Excessive avoiding reaction may prevent release becoming controlled as well as preventing maintained controlled grasp (casting toys is normal at this level of development but excessive hand extension is abnormal). See 'Abnormal release' above.

(2) Saving and propping backwards is expected at this level.

Treatment Suggestions and Daily Care

See training of reach and grasp, especially grasp in supination above and under 'Abnormal hand grasps' above.

Problems in anticipatory reach and grasp formation and for force regulation can be due to poor understanding of the properties of an object. Perceptual and cognitive problems need assessment and intervention by psychologist and occupational therapist.

Index finger approach to objects isolated finger pointing and pressing.

(1) Help the child to use toy telephones or ordinary telephones, using his index finger for dialling.

(2) Use index finger to press into dough, plasticine or sand. Later make lines and scribbles in sand.

(3) Put paint on finger tip and make dots and scribbles.

(4) Press-studs on clothes should be attempted. Press small button or knob which obtains interesting sound or visual appearance as, say, a jack-in-the-box or other pop-up toys. Help him switch on radios, TV and electric lights. Press Velcro straps on clothes or his own orthoses.

(5) Use finger puppets.

(6) Practise on the keys of a piano, computer keyboard, cash register or with an abacus.

Pincer grasp. Begin with larger objects then progress to smaller objects. Thumbs and all finger tips are used first before thumb and one finger, usually the index is used. (Crude and fine pincer grasp.) (Fig. 8.210b.)

(1) Pick up raisins, or small pieces of food and place in his mouth. The child may like to pick up buttons, wooden beads, marbles, under supervision as he may pop them into his mouth to swallow them.

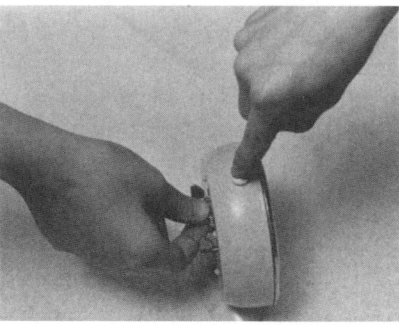

Fig. 8.208 Developing index finger pointing and pressing and a fine pincer grasp during action of pull, push and later to turn object, as in screwing movement.

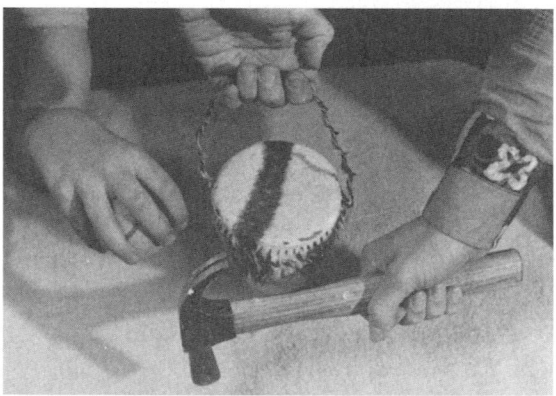

Fig. 8.209 Some hand grasps: to take hold of and to grip. Spherical with palm or fingertips only, hook grasp, cylindrical grasp. Others are lumbrical (Fig. 8.202), pincer (Figs 8.206, 8.207) with sides and with tips of fingers. *Remember* to train grasps in vertical, pronated, supinated and other hand positions.

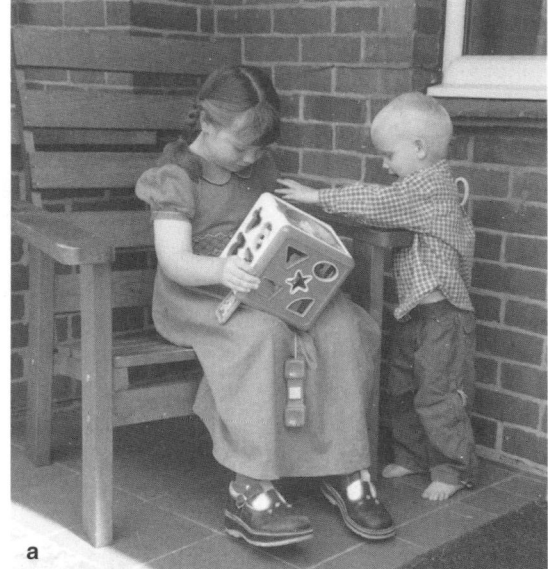

a

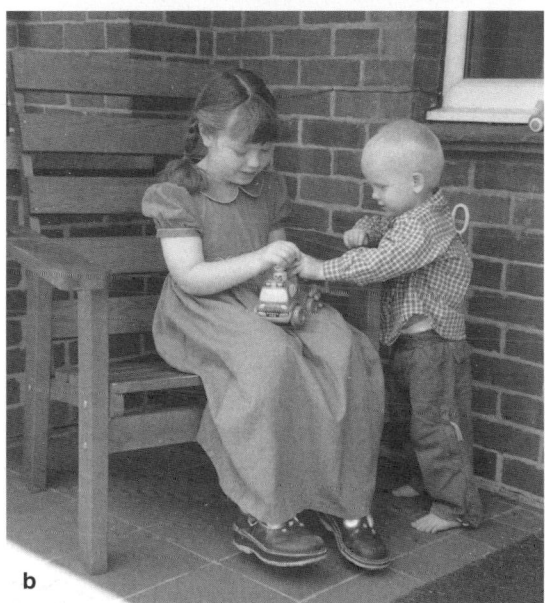

b

Fig. 8.210a,b   Girl with right hemiplegia using both her hands as she assists her able-bodied brother.

(2) Hold thick crayons and if possible pencils and thick chalk for making marks on paper or later writing (Fig. 8.205).
(3) Use toys with small knobs and of small size for fitting shapes.
(4) Hold small cup handles for drinking.

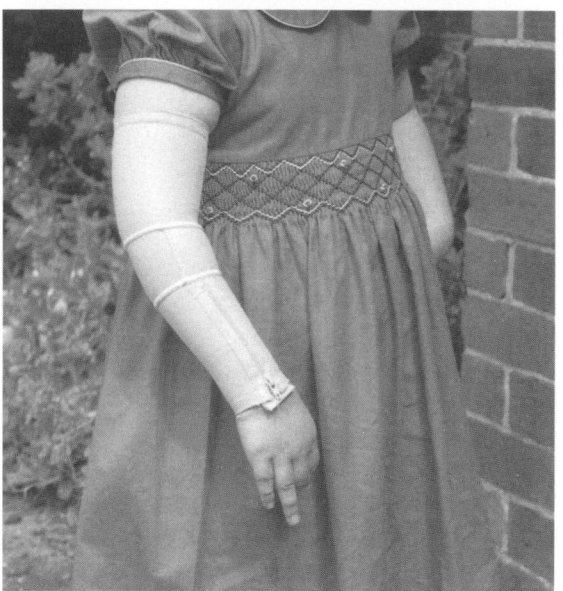

Fig. 8.211   Lycra arm splint.

(5) Wind clock and turn its knobs, press alarm bell to stop, press doorbells. Various toys have knobs and buttons to press and turn.
(6) Begin screwing action with large screw-toys, lids, etc. (Figs. 8.203, 8.208); progress to medium and fine screwing later.
(7) Pincer grasp includes thumb tip to finger tip, thumb to index-and-middle finger together and a ('key') lateral thumb to index pinch.

Allow the child to attempt the activities on his own. If he cannot manage to isolate his index finger, hold his little, ring and middle finger flexed for him until he can do this alone (Fig. 8.204). Use *finger plays* for index finger and for actively touching finger to thumb. For example hold finger-to-thumb to create 'eye spectacles'. Popping soap, bubbles with one finger and walking fingers on a table are among many ideas devised for playful therapy. Develop a greater variety of grasps (Fig. 8.209).

Continue training release. This involves dropping objects (beanbags) into container on the

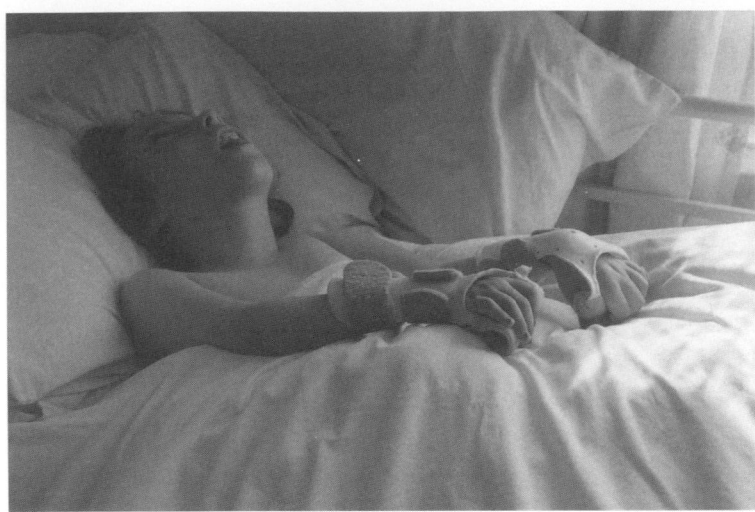

Fig. 8.212 Hand splints. Volar and dorsal splints for wrist and thumb with free finger motion.

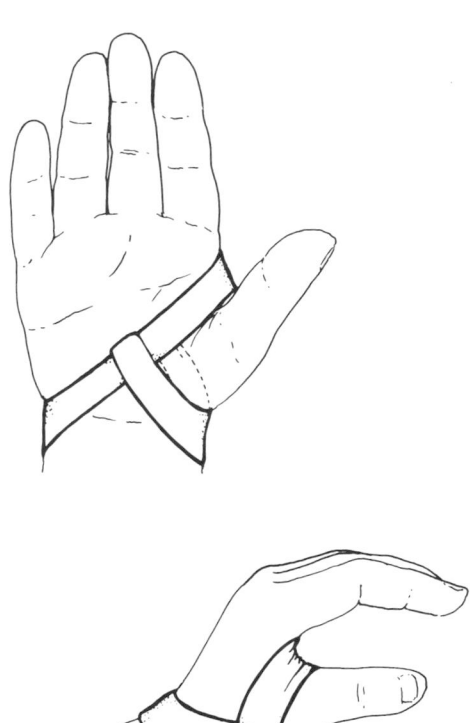

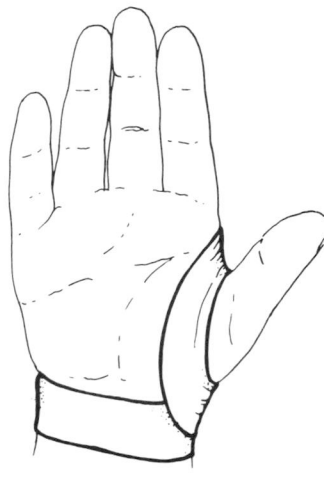

Fig. 8.213 Thumb splint to correct adducted-flexed thumb. A cock-up wrist splint to midline may be incorporated if palm flexion is excessive. Figure-of-eight thumb splint at base of thumb and over the wrist in soft pigskin or simply a handkerchief may be adequate for babies and young children.

ground below his chair, in front of his chair, at the side and behind his chair. Help him look and see 'where it dropped'. Later encourage him to place small objects in smaller containers until he learns to fit a peg in a formboard, and build one block on top of the other. Precise release is required for building a tower of blocks as well as for gaining perceptual and conceptual adequacy. Building blocks may be made of sponge rubber shapes, wood, plastic or be household objects, boxes, tins or pots, to develop hand function in this developmental period.

Manipulation and perception/conception

Manipulation is by now integrated with perceptual development of:

(1) Space and depth in, say, well coordinated reach and grasp activities.
(2) Form in placing a round peg in a round hole and similar matching.
(3) Size in placing objects into containers, according to size. Sorting objects of different sizes, shapes and textures.
(4) Colour and shape in use of matching toys (but not naming them), such as various posting boxes, mosaics and other sorting activities, jigsaws.
(5) Discrimination of soft, hard, scratchy, smooth sensations.
(6) Other cognitive and social activities such as wave bye-bye, point to visual stimulus, pat own face in mirror and smile at himself, and play pat-a-cake and similar games.

Perception, conception and fine motor manipulation continue to develop in such activities as threading large beads, smaller beads, other threading toys, scribbling, drawing, painting, pasting, using pegboards, draughts, jigsaws with knobs, using sewing cards, and a large variety of constructional toys, screwing toys, posting boxes and many more suggested in toy catalogues and by toy libraries and occupational therapists. Eye–hand coordination and rhythm, speed and precision of movement will need to be developed further after the basic arm and hand actions are trained. Occupational therapists and teachers need to be consulted for appropriate activities for individual children, adolescents and adults with cerebral palsy. *Consult* occupational therapists about hand splints, elbow back slab, lycra splintage.

9

Motor Function and the Child's Daily Life

Chapter 8 has presented ways in which the child may develop various postures, maintain these postures during movement, or disturbance of balance, get in and out of postures, obtain various forms of locomotion, and acquire the use of his hands. All these motor functions are used in the child's daily life and a few are summarized to demonstrate their use in self-care, perception, speech and language and socialization. The child's intellectual and emotional development are also involved as they interact with a child's achievement of motor control and learning.

It is also important to consider many recreational activities which can also be conducive to improved motor and sensory function, e.g. swimming, horse-riding, skiing and so on (see Leach 1993). (See Chapter 6.) There is a growing amount of research study on horse-riding and swimming showing their therapeutic value in cerebral palsy. See Appendix for addresses.

MOTOR FUNCTION AND FEEDING, DRESSING, TOILETING, WASHING, BATHING, PLAY AND COMMUNICATION

Those below are of particular significance although all motor functions are needed (see Levitt 1994).

Vertical head control in midline and slightly forward.
Obtained by: holding the child's shoulders forward with your arm when he sits on your lap when a baby; or next to you on his chair when older. Facing the child and holding his arms

stretched forward across the table between you or holding him in weight bearing on his forearms. Try using his own support with him either grasping a bar with straight arms, leaning against his table or onto his forearms.

This is especially needed for being fed, feeding himself, communication, visual exploration and other functions in his daily life.

Sitting on the floor and/or sitting on a chair of the correct size and design
Obtained by: sitting, leaning trunk against table, box or pouffe or other support, leaning on forearms and feeding, drinking, washing his face, playing, pulling off a jumper and so on (Fig. 9.1). Support is also possible by having the child grasp a rail or horizontal bar attached to the table, the wall, the bath, the toy shelves during daily activities (Fig. 9.2). Sitting astride his own chair and grasping its rungs may also be useful for communication, play, dressing and feeding. The child's one arm may be released for any activity, whilst his other controls his balance. Support may be needed for some children from behind by an adult sitting there and holding the child forward. She may only need to stabilize a child's pelvis with her knees, or with her feet and knees if she is sitting at a higher level to the child. A child can use his head and trunk control with or without his arm-hand support.

Sitting with support to the child's pelvis may be carried out with groin straps, diagonal strap across the hips or by firm pressure with an adult's hand in the lower area of the child's back, or holding his hips. The child can then carry out any particular activity using head,

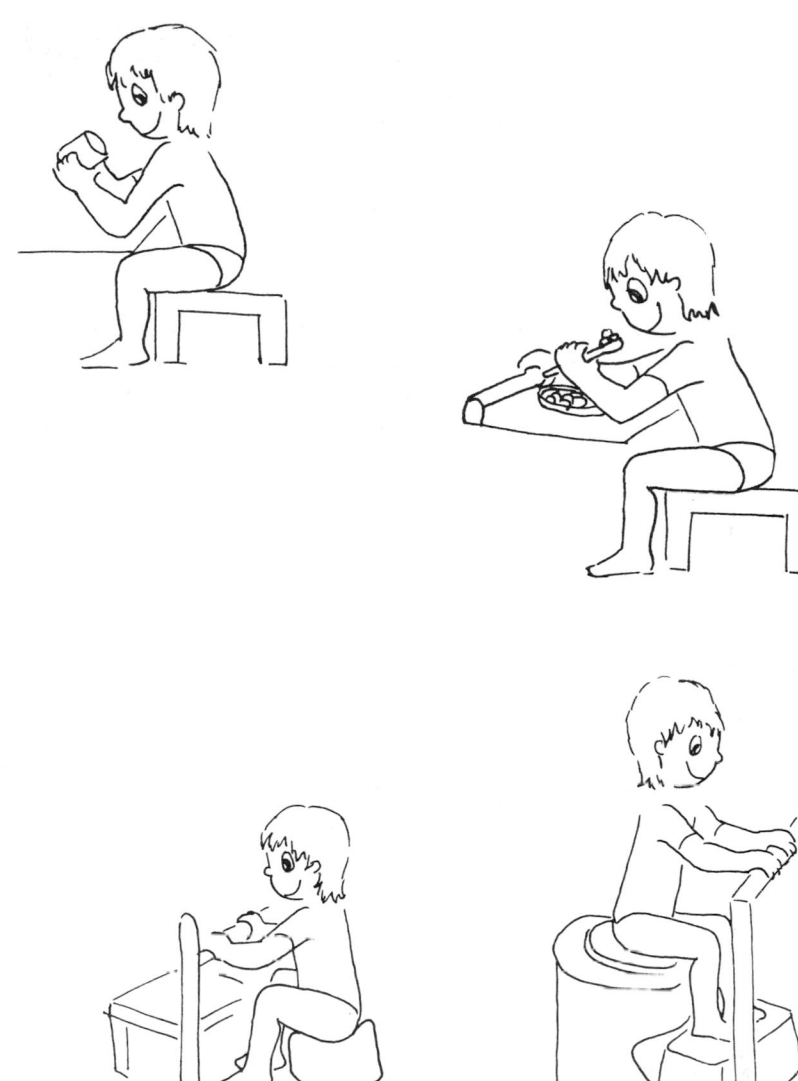

Fig. 9.1

Fig. 9.2

trunk and hand control. Sitting against a wall, in a room corner or on a variety of chairs may be used for particular children. Do not let the child slump or slide down during activities. Readjust his hips to be well back in a seat.

Correction of abnormal postures is needed so that the child can function (Fig. 9.3).

Prone and head control is used for play, communication, or when being washed and dressed,

on a wedge or lap. Some use this for chewing, sucking and swallowing to increase action of the muscles against gravity.

Obtained by: use of wedges, rolls, over your arms or lap, prone standers.

Standing or kneeling upright, holding on to tables, bars or rails for painting, drawing, washing, toilet for boys, dressing, communication and many other play activities.

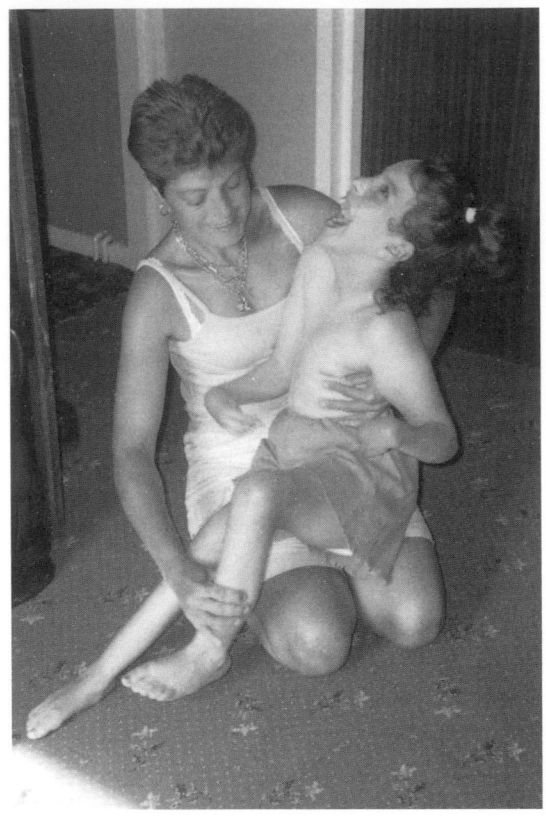

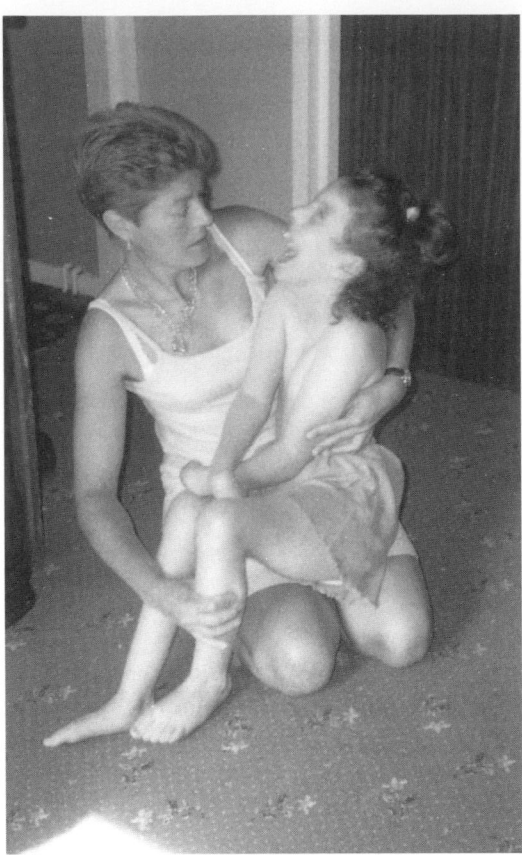

a

b

Fig. 9.3a,b   Positioning for communication with postural alignment. (See same child in Fig. 8.68.)

Obtained by: use of horizontal, sometimes vertical, rails on tables, walls, blackboards, easels, leaning against stable furniture, holding rungs of a chair or use of various standing frames.

On hands and knees may be needed for play with cars and trains, gardening, housekeeping activities, sandpits, painting.

Obtained by: cushions, wedge cut out to fit a child, over an adult's lap sitting on the floor, or have the child on a small roll which is stabilized. This position is *not* advisable for those children who sit back on their heels during the activity or who have tightly bent hips and knees.

Use of the hands is obviously required for all activities and cannot be condensed unless a particular activity is discussed in detail.

MOTOR FUNCTION AND PERCEPTION (Cratty 1970; Ayres 1979; Penso 1987)

All the training for motor function is also training perception. Thus during the motor developmental techniques the therapist needs to recognize and involve the following main features:

Tactile recognition and discrimination of textures, temperatures. Also feeling different shapes, sizes, weights, to develop stereognosis. Meanings of words are also associated with these experiences of say smooth, hard, scratchy, knobbly, rough, hot and cold. Later matching and discriminating of these sensations develops in specific learning activities.

Recognition of the child's own body by tactile recognition during motor training as when touching his mouth, face, grasping his foot or clasping his hands, as well as touching others and sitting close to others.

During motor training, communication and other activities a child can learn his body parts by having his nails painted, putting on rings, bells, bracelets, make-up moustaches, earrings, ribbons, bandages, thimbles or lighting up parts of his body with a torch. When handling the child in movement training rub, stroke, or use ice as well as words to draw attention to parts of his body. Use of vibrators is also valuable.

Drawing attention to the child's body parts leads to an awareness of his own spatial relationships or body scheme, i.e. where are his toes? – in front, below, and so on. This is also involved with his body planes (Cratty 1970) and which part of his body is moving and in which direction. Although this is experienced through sensation and proprioception, it need not be made conscious during motor training unless this conscious awareness is helpful to train movement itself or to train perception. This verbal, visual and proprioceptive linking is considered of importance by occupational therapists, psychologists, teachers and physical educators, for the child's future educational activities.

Intersensory development is encouraged by associating the movements trained with hearing and vision. During the training of hand function there is obviously linking between what the child grasps, feels, sees and even tastes and smells. Manipulation of objects with banging, throwing, squeezing, rolling, mouthing, break-

ing are linking many senses. This leads to another related perceptual experience, which is:

Appreciation of the qualities of objects and of their relations to one another. With gross motor activity and fine motor activity the child is offered learning experiences to recognize round, square, long, cylindrical shapes and discover which fits into which, which can be placed on top of which object and also which object is nearer, further away, or behind, in front of or next to the other. These perceptions and concepts are part of education and occupational therapy and need to be presented to children through various activities. Motor training overlaps into these areas.

Appreciation of the child's relationship to objects and space. These perceptual experiences also become involved with motor function. As the child learns to move through space he is also learning to appreciate how far he is from objects, how to get into and out of things, how to get on top of, under, around, behind and many other relationships to objects and space.

Thus the child finds out about his body parts, their relations to each other and also the relations of his body to objects and to space during gross motor development and fine motor development.

Development of praxia, motor planning or using the movements appropriate to a motor task such as dressing, writing, using a pair of scissors or other implements. Although this depends on perceptual experiences and on the training of the neuromuscular system and is helped in its development during motor developmental training, it could be defective on its own in brain damaged children. Specific teaching is therefore provided by occupational therapists and teachers.

Specialized perceptual and praxic training (including visuomotor training). This may be needed for many specific problems found amongst children with cerebral palsy with a primary motor impairment. These problems occur despite general perceptual experiences included in the motor developmental training. The specialized therapy and education needed is discussed elsewhere and advice must be sought from psychologists, teachers in special education and occupational therapists (Ayres 1979; Presland 1982; Fisher *et al.* 1991; Steel 1993).

Although special sessions of perceptual-motor training are needed it must be remembered that *perception is also being trained within the activities of feeding, dressing, washing, bathing, toileting and especially playing*, and is part of the whole therapy programme.

MOTOR FUNCTION AND SPEECH AND LANGUAGE

At first a child needs to pay attention to achieving motor control without the distraction of verbal instruction or he may not understand instructions. Nevertheless when a child is developmentally ready, language is linked with motor training. The motor training is then associated with words related to body parts, movements and the purpose of motor functions. Colours, shapes, sizes and all the other perceptual and conceptual experiences integrated with motor functions are greatly involved in development of speech and language.

Motor functions have already been summarized above for positions for communication, for feeding, for play, as well as other daily activities. All this promotes speech and language as well. The development of feeding develops the use of the oral musculature needed for speech. In addition, breathing exercises and stimulation of the facial muscles with neuromuscular techniques of touch, pressure, stretch, and resistance may be helpful. Short periods of ice application, or ice lollies reduce spasticity of tongues or mouths and promote speech. Quick ice stimulation of the mouth muscles may help

'flabby mouths' and make the child aware of his muscles of speech. This discourages dribbling by provoking mouth closure so facilitating swallowing. A large red handkerchief pinned to the child's clothes has motivated some children to remember to wipe their mouths and remember to swallow and keep lips closed. Unobtrusive pressure across the area between nose and upper lip or sometimes just below the lower lip provokes mouth closure and makes swallowing possible, instead of dribbling. Drooling is normal until about 15 months of age.

The development of speech and language requires special advice and treatment from speech therapists (Levitt & Miller 1973; Latham 1984; Stroh & Robinson 1991; Winstock 2003). See Chapter 5, Parent–child interaction.

Development of Communication – Brief Summary

(Hearing, speech, language and communication.)

0–3 months   Use of cry, facial expression. Stills to noise. Smiles at mother.

3–4 months   Sounds vary and beginning to babble.

4–6 months   Babbling, begins some intonations. Watches adult's lips.
    Turns to sounds; to mother's voice. Laughs, squeals, chuckles, annoyed screams. Excited limb motion as social responses.

6–8 months   Lip and tongue sounds. Syllables (baba a ba) begin.

8–12 months   Double syllables, first word. Turns to sounds that interest him instantaneously. Vocalizes to make personal contact. Associates sound with movement. Playful turn-taking.

12 months   Understands more than expresses. Follows adult's simple direction ('Give me', 'No'). Responds to his name. Single word. Real object labels.

12–20 months   Imitates adult speech. Echolalia. Two- or three-word phrases.

Responds and discriminates sounds, speech, simple commands.

24 months Loves listening to stories, jingles; verbal explosion.

3 years Simple sentences, many questions. Give own name. Nursery rhymes, talks to himself. Normal stutter. Unique dialogues.

Practical Suggestions

(1) Follow general guide of developmental levels and individual assessment by speech and language therapist and psychologist.

(2) Always try to communicate with the child with noises (at first not too loud and sudden), songs, smiles, gestures; talk near the child and with face-to-face contact.

(3) Speak slowly and distinctly but not with exaggerated articulation, as in 'baby talk'. Wait for any response by a child.

(4) Say names of familiar objects, colours, what they are used for, and demonstrate and name parts of the body, and talk about child's own experiences. Parents are expected to let therapists know about their child's interests and experiences.

(5) Child should be able to see your face in a good light during speech. Try to be at his eye level whenever possible.

(6) Play lip and tongue games, lick off jam, lollies, peanut butter and during feeding use babbling and speech and stimulate a child to do so.

(7) Encourage child to participate in songs, rhythms, body movements and hand/finger plays. However, do not pressurize a child to speak but create informal situations for conversation, especially in groups.

(8) Respond to a child's gestures, facial expressions, but wait for his voice, words if possible. Make it rewarding for him to use speech or have a need for speech by having to ask for things, indicate things, and so on.

(9) Praise but do not fuss about the child's attempts to speak and give him time to express himself. Do not finish sentences for him if he can do so in his own time. Avoid giving an answer for him if he can say something.

(10) Explore alternative forms of communication (symbolic), e.g. Bliss, Makaton, Paget-Gorman with experts. Respond to his use of electronic systems of communication and learn about them from experts.

Development of Feeding – Brief Summary

0–4 months Rooting reaction, sucking-and-swallowing reflex. Hypersensitive mouth or cardinal points reflexes, tongue thrust, open mouth and dribbling.

4–6 months Sucking dissociates from swallowing as child transfers liquids for swallowing. All reflexes disappeared. Bite reflex weak. Takes liquids from spoon. Recognizes bottle.

6–9 months Takes strained foods, solids, bites a biscuit. Holds a biscuit, may crumble in his hand. Up and down jaw motion in chewing, swallows with mouth closed.

9–12 months Finger feeds, chewing with lateral jaw motion, holds and drinks from bottle, from cup with help. Helps mother with spoon to mouth.

9–12 months Holds spoon alone but cannot bring to mouth with food.

12–15 months Uses spoon but turns it upside down before reaching mouth or within mouth. Holds and drinks from cup, often spills.

15–18 months Chewing established. Forward and rotary jaw motion. Feeds self clumsily.

2 years Uses spoon correctly, occasional spilling, holds glass and cup for drinking, plays with food. Understands what is edible and inedible. Begins straw drinking but bites edge.

2–3 years Feeds self completely with spoon, with fork. Pours liquids, obtains own drink from tap.

3–4 years   Serves self at table, spreads butter, cuts food.

Practical Suggestions (Fig. 9.4)

Unhurried feeding period, to try and give time for the child to actively participate. The speed of your feeding him should be slower and similar to the speed at which his own early attempts will start. Feeding himself and being fed should take place in as social and pleasant an atmosphere of an unhurried meal as you can make it. Speech and babbling in reply to your talk often occurs during such feeding periods. Sitting at meals with the family and other children at school also motivates feeding alone by imitation. Speech may then also occur for the social reasons as well as the fact that eating and drinking activates the speech muscles.

If the child cannot imitate due to impairments of intellect or vision, or because the others are eating too fast for him to feed himself at the same mealtime, it is essential to have private feeding therapy sessions. There is no distraction and he can concentrate on active achievements. Naturally he should join the others for the mealtimes, but be given something easy to do in the way of self-feeding or drinking.

Positioning for feeding should involve an upright position supported or if possible unsupported by special chairs or by the parent. Some feed more easily in a standing frame. See feeding positions in the section on motor function and feeding at the beginning of this chapter. The child's head should be held by you or preferably himself forward and upright whilst taking food, during eating and especially on swallowing. If he is allowed to swallow with his head back over the years, his growing oesophagus will trap food in its longer length and so prove dangerous. Swallowing with head upright also allows active participation in his training. Gently press his chest to help the head come forward and up and if his head drops give minimal support under his chin. Elbows on the table are recommended! Stability for head and hand to mouth action is promoted and babies and young children with visual disability are made aware of where they find the food and obtain security from the stable table.

Mouth actions in taking the food, keeping the mouth closed during eating, chewing actions and swallowing can be facilitated by your hands, supporting under his chin. Stroke under the chin and along his neck to stimulate a swallow whilst your other finger presses his lips closed. Fingers may have to be held above and below his lips to stimulate mouth closure. Simply achieving mouth closure may lead to his own swallow as the food or drink cannot spill out of his mouth. Stimulate chewing by massaging or manipulating the child's cheeks after he takes the small piece of food. Wait for him to bring his head forward and to take the food off the spoon offered below and in front of his mouth and do not scrape the food and spoon off the top of his teeth.

Weaning from liquids to tolerate various textures, tastes through semi-solids to solids is most important and may take longer in some children with disabilities. Children who are visually impaired, or severely intellectually impaired, may be conservative about any change or may use it as a means of controlling the overprotective adults around him. Change from liquids to semi-solids gradually by adding to his cup of favourite drink, yogurts, custards, apple sauce, stewed fruit, mashed banana, puddings, crushed fruit in dilution. Gradually transfer to a bowl. Spoon from cup of thickened liquid to spoon from bowl of food as a weaning process. Mashed semi-solids enjoyed by a child may have to be mixed with foods he does not like in semi-solids and solids. A meal of ice-cream and peas with mince and custard has been known to wean a difficult child to solids! Weaning to solids is not done only to socialize and improve nutrition but chewing solids

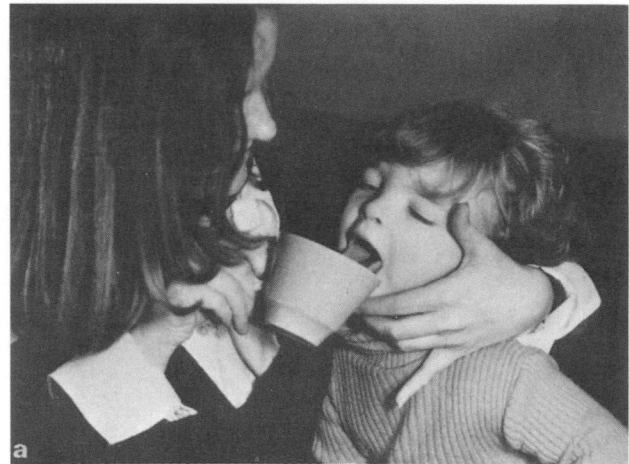

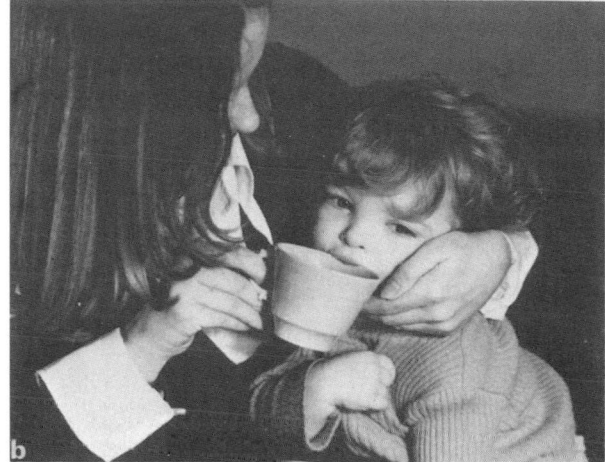

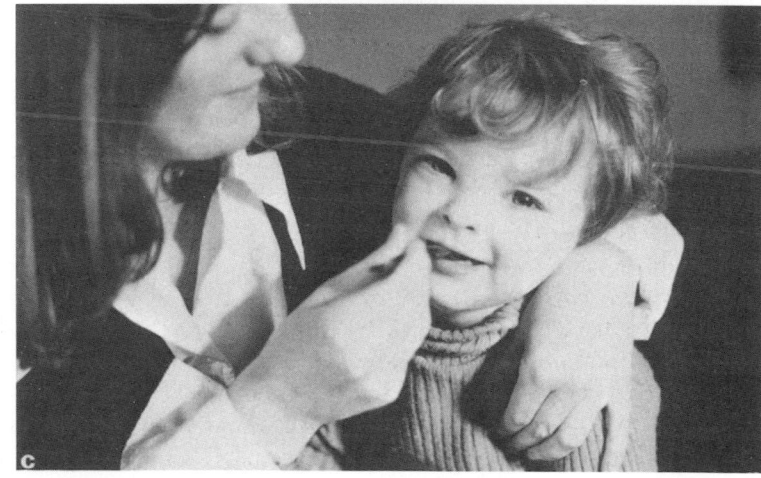

Fig. 9.4 a, Head extension and tongue thrust interfering with drinking and eating. b, Holding the child's head upright and forward, supporting her chin and stroking under her jaw trains drinking. c, Wait for the child to remove food from the spoon held below her mouth. Keep her head and shoulders well forward as she takes the food.

exercises the articulators for speech. Introduce a solid he can hold and likes in part of every meal from the beginning of training of feeding. Hold an apple slice, a sausage, rusk or cheese. You hold a sliver of meat and teach him to bite whilst you pull on the end of the meat. Always introduce lumps in food by a general 'lumpiness' rather than odd lumps in a smooth sauce, in the initial stages.

Gagging or choking. In severe cases, this may often be due to gastro-oesophageal reflux and is associated with aspiration into the lungs. In babies, drugs and positioning are used and many overcome this by 18 months. Medical opinion is essential, especially for older children. When gag and choking occur in other children without reflux, calmly and quickly tip the child forward and down. Avoid banging him on the back. An excessive gag reflex may be neurological and train its control by 'walking' the spoon gradually back on his tongue, give small amount and go slowly giving him time to take the food and swallow. The child may of course gag on foods he dislikes, to which he is allergic or if he has a behaviour problem. He may be reacting against a new person feeding him, an unfamiliar place, especially when in hospital, or he may be seeking the fuss and attention he gets from mother and others if he gags and vomits. Casualness in people's reactions and ignoring his 'performance' may stop this behaviour (see below). It also occurs in children with hypersensitive faces and mouths, which can be neurological or due to visual disability with fears, loss of body image, and unfamiliar situations.

Hypersensitivity of face and mouth can be treated by gradual *desensitization* methods used by speech therapists. Touch parts of the child's body in a game and gradually touch his face and then mouth. Stroke, use ice or ice lollies and tooth brushes, stroking his gums and other tactile games and gradually help the child accept handling of his face. Mouth actions described

above for lip closure, chew and swallow are all part of a total desensitization programme. Play with lipsticks and face paints and sticking on moustaches also helps.

Remember that desensitizing the child's face is best done with his own hands rather than those of the therapist. Many of us would dislike someone else handling our face and mouth for training techniques!

Gastrostomy and naso-gastric tube. Special feeding equipment is needed for children unable to feed orally because of the risk of aspiration. A naso-gastric tube either gives food to the stomach or drains gastric contents. It is used to administer medications.

A gastrostomy tube or button is used for feeding a child over time as a naso-gastric tube cannot be used over time. The gastrostomy is a surgical implant through the abdominal wall directly into the stomach. The catheter is secured. When not used a button for a feeding tube is less obtrusive and is usually preferred. Parent and nurse are responsible for feeding a child with gastrostomy and will advise therapists about handling and at appropriate times for the child. Nutrition is markedly improved so that a child has more energy for therapy.

Training self-feeding should begin with finger feeding so that the child feels his own fingers on his mouth, takes a small amount of food, learning how to manage that with his mouth and experiencing the texture, temperature and smell of the food and where he obtained it. Food coming at him from unseen places does not encourage a child with severe visual impairment to feed himself. Use sausage, biscuit pieces, raisins and other foods he can pick up himself. At first he will push it all into his mouth and in time release with a finer hand control. Train finger feeding one item at a time and so finish each item before putting the next piece of food into his mouth.

Feeding with a spoon follows, with the therapist guiding hand to mouth whilst controlling any extensor thrusts of the child. Do this from slightly behind and to the side of the child. Sit close to the child and hold him in his sitting posture with good head control as mentioned above. Guide his hand all the way from the bowl to his mouth at first. Feel at which point he seems to be actively moving hand to mouth himself and let go at that part. Usually the active control taken by the child is when he smells the food near his mouth. Later it is a few more inches away from his mouth, then more until he carries through the full hand to mouth action. Grasping the spoon may have to be trained separately or it may be all he can do at first. Perhaps a special handle or thickened handle with clay, rubber tubing strapped on which can be removed, or rubberzote removed as grasp improves, can be used. Occupational therapists supply many different spoons to help individual children and older persons.

Grasp, hand to mouth, taking food and eating is usually first achieved. Later, scooping up the food on the spoon is achieved. Use a bowl with sides to make this possible. Once again guide the child to scoop up food and select large, deep or small spoons to suit his ability. Use non-slip bowls, or have a non-slip mat on the table top.

Guidance is done by *hand over hand*, i.e. your hand over his hand on the spoon, or your hand alongside his hand on the handle, or by directing his elbow or his whole arm. Adducted arms may have to be held at right angles to release the hypertonus. There must be a semi or full abducted position of the upper arm to release flexed adducted tight arms. On taking the food to his mouth, the child must be taught to keep his head and trunk forwards, arm semi-abducted, or he may fall or extend backwards, with his mouth jerking open, gagging or choking, and perhaps hand losing grasp. At first, these basic movement and posture patterns will have to be taught without food and drink for easier learning.

Place a little on the spoon at a time, quietly approve of anything active that he does. Give some verbal praise but do not distract his attention as he will gain the reward of getting his food by himself.

Behaviour problems. The cause of inappropriate behaviour should be obtained using ideas from psychologists (Stroh *et al.* 1986). The child who refuses to eat *must* be checked for any medical, physical and psychological reasons first before behaviour methods are used. The training programme is checked to take account of his level of ability in understanding the relationships between him and objects, and between two objects such as spoon and food, spoon and bowl, as well as his physical ability (Kitzinger 1980). A child is never *forced* to eat when he refuses. Give a smaller helping and let him make the decision to take it. Calmly, and not as if he is being punished, take away his food so he does not eat at all if he still refuses to eat. Hungry children may be more willing to learn to eat. Sometimes a time for eating can be set with a kitchen timer and when that bell rings the food is removed calmly. He is taught that unless he eats in the *long period* set he gets no food. Many other ideas can be obtained from parents or from care staff and teachers to deal with behaviour problems other than accepting the child's decisions to make feeding a battleground in which all do exactly what he wants. His cooperation should be *expected* by you in a firm, matter of fact way, during training of feeding. It is of course essential to praise his smallest positive cooperation with the feeding programme. It should also be remembered that training feeding takes concentration on the child's part, so decrease distractions of having others present in the room, and check that a child with intellectual impairments, hyperactivity or a very young child has the attention span for the whole training session. Vomiting may be due to any pressure of tables or straps against his abdomen rather than his behaviour.

Special problems. Tongue thrusts, gag reflexes and hypersensitive mouths can be improved with use of a polythene (unbreakable) or bone spoon which is gently but firmly placed at the middle of the tongue. The child withdraws his tongue into his mouth as this is done so that he does not take food whilst pushing it out with his tongue thrust! Head in midline and firmly held in the upright and slightly forward is also essential. Bite reflexes are also best managed with non-metal spoons. Chewing development tends to decrease the primitive bite reflexes. Avoid the bite by slipping the spoon in at the side of the child's mouth between the teeth. Spastic tongues relax if ice lollies are used in some cases.

Floppy mouths associated with dribbling are helped by training of feeding, chewing and general stimulation of the mouth muscles with touch, pressure and quick icing. Speech therapists should be consulted with all these problems.

Aids. Occupational therapists should be approached about the correct selection of feeding aids. Assessment must be made as to whether they are necessary in the first place, and when they should be removed. The following may be used: non-slip bowls, table tops, high-sided bowls or suction bases for bowl or cup. Special feeding cups with weighted bases and with cut-out section at the lip so that the liquid can be seen, may be helpful. Feeder spouts may be used, but if the child sucks on it discard all such edges to a cup. Straws are discouraged as pouting rather than drinking actions of the lips may occur. Later straws are useful to activate mouths but not to train drinking actions. The holes on teats or feeder-cup nozzles may have to be widened in the weaning process from these aids to a regular cup. Two-handled cups are advisable for symmetrical use of hands and for children with visual disability who need to learn about both sides of a cup and to avoid spilling. An inclined lip on a cup may help to delay the flow of liquid and let the child see it

coming towards his lips. Thickening liquids may be easier to manage in some cases. Spoons of bone, unbreakable plastic, with special handles and inclined bent handles have to be selected for the individual child. Long-handled spoons, deep or shallow bowls of the spoon should be available to suit particular children. Unusual looking aids to feeding should be avoided until training is attempted for some years and the child's own ability assessed. The bent or curved spoon is used by older children if that becomes necessary.

Bibs which catch spills and are made of plastic are useful. Cover the floor with newspapers or a plastic cover to catch spills. Later forks and knives or a fork and knife on one implement or fork and pushers can be useful. A fork edge on a spade spoon may also be used by some children.

Training feeding involves patience, time and determination, but is worthwhile as independence in this area is something adult cerebral palsied people most appreciate having gained. Messing and spills are inevitable and adults who cannot bear this extended *normal* phase of learning to eat alone, should not be asked to take on the training of the children. If cleanliness is important one should in any event train the child to wipe his mouth, wipe the table and help to clear up.

Although speech therapists and occupational therapists are the experts on the training of feeding, physiotherapists are very much involved as well. Feeding and drinking methods are part of the training of head control, sitting, hand grasp and release and hand to mouth action without balance loss. It is motor function integrated with understanding, communication, body image and perceptual function. Mother–child relationships will be fostered by good physiotherapy methods used during feeding, as a child's difficulties can often create maternal anxiety. Support and approval of a mother's abilities is essential. Any emotional problems of a mother need to be appreciated. At some stages a mother may not feel able to take on the feeding training completely. A father can help and support his wife as soon as she is ready to learn to feed their child.

Development of Dressing – Brief Summary

6–12 months   Child is supported in sitting, during dressing.

10–12 months   Child may put out arm or leg for dressing and cooperate in other ways.

15 months   Take off shoes, hat.

18 months   Take off gloves, socks, unzip.

2 years   Take off pants. Put on shoes, hat, but unable to replace pants.

3 years   Take off all clothes. Confusion of back and front, right and left, two legs in one hole of trousers, etc.

4–5 years   Dresses self, becomes careless about details, such as tucking in shirt, etc. All buttons, laces, ties not possible until 6 years.

Practical Suggestions (Fig. 9.5)

(1) Development varies greatly and too much must not be expected of the child. Dressing, however, is important for training perception, balance, movements, and as a source for speech and language development.

(2) Begin any dressing activity for the child but let him finish it himself. If he can carry it all out himself, give him time and do not hurriedly do it for him if he is struggling on his own.

(3) Vary positions for dressing to discover the easiest one for the child. For example, side lying may enable a child to dress, take off socks and shoes. Lying and bridging allows him to remove the lower clothes.

(4) Dress and undress for bathing, swimming and other purposes but not as an exercise.

(5) Type of clothing: loose fitting garments, large sleeves and arm holes (raglan), elastic necks and waistbands, large buttons, zips with knobs, velcro fastenings are required.

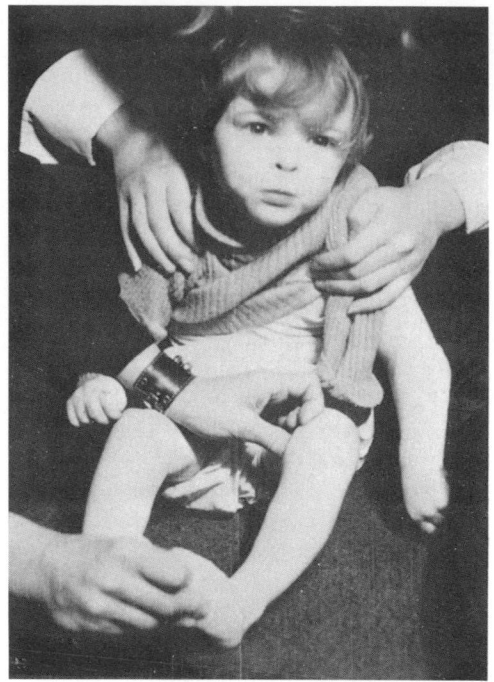

Fig. 9.5   The child is held flexed for dressing and play. Tailor-sitting is being obtained. Press beneath the big toe and bend hip and knee outward in order to overcome excessive leg extension-adduction for, say, a nappy change, sock removal and getting her into tailor-sitting.

Non-slippery materials are preferable. Tabs on front or top of shirts and dresses and back of boots are useful to guide the child. Avoid laces and small fastenings.

(6) Put the more affected arm in first. Try putting both arms in first then pull dress or jumper over the head.

Note. Occupational therapists will advise on dressing techniques and clothing ideas.

Development of Play – Brief Outline

This is the development of *learning through play*. This is closely correlated with the development of hand function and the development of intersensory relationships and perceptual-motor control.

0–6 months Visual fixation and pursuit, hand–eye coordination and bring hands to midline and grasp, drop, reach and grasp, touch, etc. Play with parts of body, mother's face, nearby materials. Amuses self for short intervals.

6–12 months Rolling, crawling, supported cruising and other gross motor activities to explore, strengthen body generally and enjoy moving. Hand function development using toys or objects. Investigates and experiments with increasing energy.

12 months–2 years Solitary play but imitates another child or adult. Uses large equipment, swings, balls, toys on wheels to push and pull. Sand and water play. Enjoys small objects such as shells, pebbles, buttons – often taken to mouth until 15 months of age.

2–3 years Rough and tumble play. As above only with more perceptual and conceptual ideas. Begins imaginative play ('Let's pretend'). Solitary and parallel play.

3–4 years Plays with other children. Imaginative play, dressing up. As above but not as energetic.

6 years Games with rules, arts and crafts. 'Tricks'.

Practical Suggestions

(1) Play differs at different ages, but it is impossible to have it strictly classified as the child's personality, opportunities and intelligence affect this. Social and cultural backgrounds also affect play.

(2) Play is usually a synonym for exploration and experimentation and is a serious affair for the child. Play can also be relaxing, working out emotions, imitating reality in order to understand it in imaginative play, and obtaining satisfaction and development of the child's personality. It is often messy, dirty, untidy and destructive as well as creative and constructive, in the adult sense.

(3) Show the child how to use a toy, but wherever possible see if he can find things out for himself.

(4) Do not interfere with any child who is concentrating on a play activity unless absolutely essential.

Techniques for Carrying the Child Correctly (Figs 9.6–9.11)

(1) To stimulate head control.
(2) To correct any abnormal postures.

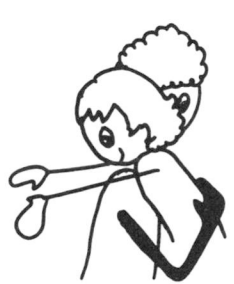

Fig. 9.6 Both the arms are over the adult's shoulder for symmetry, straighten back and raise head. Keep the legs apart, and hips flat if necessary in spasticity. Bring tight arms away from their habitual positions next to the child.

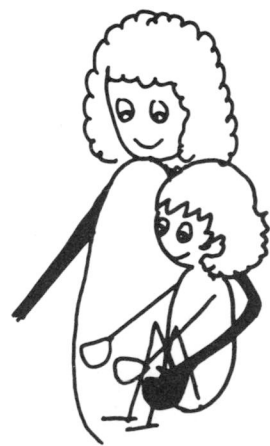

Fig. 9.7 For head control and correcting an excessively extended child, help bring hands down and together helps control an athetoid or floppy child.

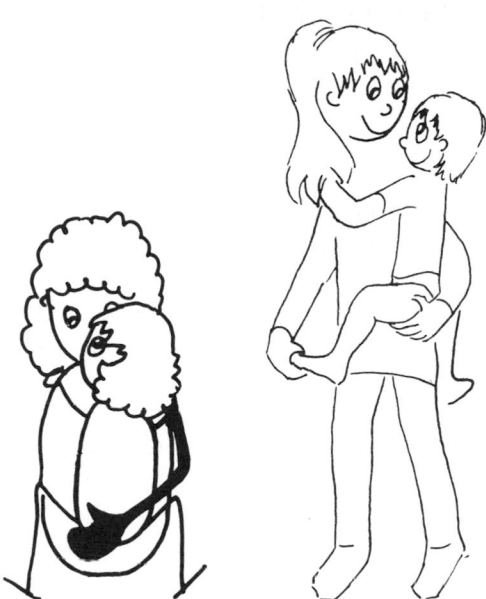

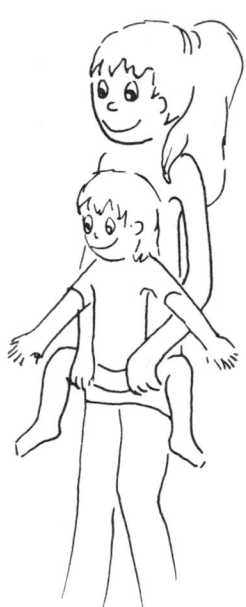

Fig. 9.8 and 9.9   Use of both arms, eye-to-eye contact, separate tightly adducted legs or very extended legs. Move the child to points around the adult's hips to find the most corrective posture of legs for him.

Fig. 9.10   Head and trunk control, if the child is moved slightly away from the adult's chest. Correct extended-adducted-internally rotated legs.

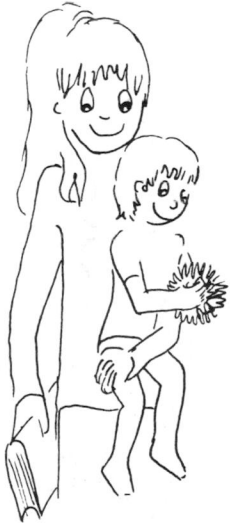

Fig. 9.11   Stimulates greater head and trunk control for floppy and other children. Hold child at chest and under his armpits and/or under his buttocks as well.

10 Problems of Deformity

Introduction

A deformity is an abnormal position of a joint. In cerebral palsied and other developmentally delayed children abnormal joint positions rarely appear or depend on only one joint and the total child must be examined.

The deformity may be mobile or dynamic, i.e. *unfixed*, which means that passive or active correction can take place. The deformity may have become *fixed* or a contracture when there is adaptive shortening of the soft tissues or bony changes. The therapist tries to prevent deformities developing as unfixed or fixed deformities. If unfixed deformities have already appeared they are treated, but little can be done for fixed deformities. Orthopaedic surgery is indicated for fixed deformities. However, in selected cases, orthopaedic surgery is also required for unfixed deformities (Bleck 1987).

Prevention and correction of deformities in therapy and daily care is particularly important as they can cause disability and discomfort. Therapists should consider the causes of the deformities. However, many different causes are suggested by various authorities. It is, however, possible for the therapist to combine many if not all viewpoints, as outlined in this chapter. The therapist may be able to classify the causes of deformity under the following headings. Some of these causes are interwoven and their relationships are discussed.

(1) Immobility – total or partial.
(2) Hypotonicity.
(3) Hypertonicity.
(4) Co-contraction and synergies (movement patterns).
(5) Weakness – general or specific.
(6) Abnormal reflex activity.
(7) Asymmetry.
(8) Involuntary movements in one repetitive pattern.
(9) Growth factors.
(10) Biomechanics.

CAUSES

Immobility – General

A general immobility of the child may be due to:

- *Physical impairment* of hypotonicity, hypertonicity, weakness, involuntary movements and severe spasms, abnormal reflex activity (see below). Severe deformities may have already developed and these prevent further movement. The deformities themselves may then become worse and also produce others.
- *Other causes* such as sensory loss (mainly blindness), severe perceptual-motor defects, especially those related to space and body image, emotional problems, especially if the child is fearful or withdrawn, severe intellectual impairment, social deprivation and malnutrition. Most of these reasons tend to create lethargic, unmotivated children, who prefer to be immobile.

When many of the above causes combine in the same child, deformities are likely to occur. Children who have severe multiple disabilities are usually more immobile and particularly prone to their deformities becoming contractures.

Immobility – Partial

Despite some or many of the above causes a child may acquire a few similar postures and a few stereotyped movements. This is well-known in children with cerebral palsy, especially with rigid muscles, (dystonia), short spastic muscles, overlengthened hypotonic muscles and intellectual problems. The few postures and movements children prefer are usually repeated in a few abnormal patterns which are seen in deformities.

Hypotonicity

The floppy baby or hypotonia may be due to many neurological causes affecting the muscles themselves, their spinal connections or the central nervous system. Hypotonic babies or children are immobile and may be left lying for long periods in one or two positions, which can create deformities. For example, the *frog position* of the legs in prone, supine or with the child propped up on pillows in the half-slumped sitting position may all lead to deformities in the legs, especially in the hips. Anterior subluxation or dislocation of hips need to be avoided in such cases.

A common characteristic of most floppy babies is the absence of all or some of the normal postural mechanisms. The neck, trunk, shoulder and pelvic girdle muscles are not being activated by these mechanisms, and appear weak and hypotonic. Hypotonia is not always associated with total weakness. Fair or even good voluntary movement may be present, but it is not enough to make the child mobile. Without the postural control of the postural mechanisms a child cannot get out of the few positions in which he is left during the day and night. Postural stability is absent or poor, preventing reliable function.

Some hypotonic children may develop some of the postural mechanisms and develop to sitting and standing. However, they carry out these levels of development in an abnormal way.

Common abnormal patterns of deformity are round backs, scoliosis, lordosis and hip flexion, hyperextended knees (*back-knees*), valgus knees (*knock-knees*) and valgus feet (*flat feet*). One or all of these postures may be present in the hypotonic child.

Hypertonicity

This is usually considered the most important cause of deformity. The creation of the deformities is, however, not dependent on the hypertonicity as such. There are other aspects that need consideration. Both neurological and orthopaedic (musculo-skeletal) views need to be combined, as well as the immobility already mentioned. Other factors such as abnormal coordinated movements, abnormal reflexes and growth are among those discussed below. The main aspects of hypertonicity, weakness and inefficient muscle work are related and will be outlined.

Hypertonicity. Hypertonic muscle groups tend to shorten and pull the joints into abnormal positions. In the baby and young child these abnormal positions can be anticipated by the tendency of the child to prefer certain postures and movements, and by the examination of the muscles using passive stretch. There is an abnormal reaction to sudden stretch, given by the examiner, called a *clasp-knife* spastic reaction. *A lead pipe* or *cogwheel* rigid reaction is felt throughout range, on stretching muscles. The tendency of spastic muscles is to shorten, which will cause *one aspect* of the deformity (Tardieu *et al.* 1982; Dietz & Berger 1983; Hufschmidt & Mauritz 1985). In the very young child this muscle shortening can be overcome, though threatening deformity, and in time become habitual and clearly observed. If left still longer such muscle transformations become fixed.

Shortening hypertonic ('hypoextensible') muscles pull the joints into abnormal motor patterns of the whole child or at least of the whole limb. However one joint may be more deformed than the others within the pattern. It is important to *check each joint* as well as observe the *pattern of abnormal posture* and movement.

Hypertonicity may pull the joints into abnormal positions at rest (Fulford & Brown 1976). Hypertonicity may be *absent at rest* but only elicited on passive stretch. When elicited on passive stretch, hypertonicity may still *not* produce abnormal positions in function. Hypertonicity may be absent at rest, minimal on passive stretch, and only obvious on *weight bearing* and during function. Finally, hypertonicity may create abnormal positions at rest, show very hyperactive or dystonic response on passive stretch and also the same abnormal, shortened positions in function. It depends on the age, severity and perhaps the history of treatment as to what is observed.

The therapist and especially those involved in daily care should treat the hypertonicity which appears *in function*, and in the developmental motor functions. See Abnormal postures in lying and sitting, Abnormal postures in standing, Abnormal hand function (Chapter 8) and some *gait patterns*.

The 'weak' antagonists to the spastic muscle groups. Sharrard (1971) states that spasticity alone does not create deformity. It is the muscle imbalance between the spastic muscles and their weak antagonists which leads to deformity. The antagonists of the spastic muscle groups are working at a mechanical disadvantage to the tight pull of spastic muscle groups. They cannot counter the pull of the spastic muscles and appear too weak to do so. In time they really become weak from disuse. It is necessary to treat this muscle imbalance by reducing the spasticity and strengthening the antagonists.

Although some orthopaedic surgeons talk of the muscle imbalance, they unfortunately say that the spastic muscles are *strong* and the antagonists are *weak*. This is rarely so in every case. It is the strong *pull* of the spastic muscle

that is strong, and not the spastic muscle work itself. Unless this is recognized, postoperative physiotherapy as well as therapy of children without operation will be inadequate.

Specific inefficiency of hypertonic especially spastic muscles. Spastic muscles are not paralysed muscles. They can contract. However, they are often *not* strong muscles. Spasm or spasticity must not be confused with strong and efficient muscle action.

Once spasticity is decreased, spastic muscles may reveal great weakness. Also spastic muscles may be able to act in only one part of their range and not in the rest of the range (Knott & Voss 1968). Cotton (1975a) emphasizes how children with, say, flexor spasticity of the hips cannot actively flex their hips in order to reach their feet. The limited range of motion in spastic muscles may be due to their inelasticity or weakness or both (Tabary *et al.* 1972, 1981). The electromyograph of the type of muscle contraction in spastic muscles has been shown as abnormal (Tardieu *et al.* 1982; Young & Wiegner 1987).

It may be that this inefficiency of action of the spastic muscles contributes to deformity. Their action as well as their tightness should not be ignored during the therapeutic regime for the prevention and correction of deformity. Motor activities should not only strengthen the apparently weak antagonists of abnormal motor patterns but also activate the spastic muscles themselves *in their full range* (Damiano & Abel 1998; Damiano *et al.* 1995, 2002; Wiley *et al.* 1998).

Abnormal Co-contraction and Abnormal Synergies

The abnormal postural mechanisms or their absence lead to abnormal postures against gravity. As discussed in Chapters 1, 3 and 8, compensations to maintain balance result in abnormal postures which if persistent become deformities. The abnormal co-contraction and abnormal synergies which include co-activation are not due to hypertonicity but caused by motor control problems (Shumway-Cook and Woollacott 2001). These incoordinated movements and postures need treatment within functional patterns. These patterns are normally seen in early development or early stages of learning a new motor skill.

Weakness – General and Specific

This heading is only given, as so many workers in cerebral palsy use this term. It should, however, be more clearly defined.

General weakness has already been discussed under hypotonicity and general immobility. The absence of the postural mechanisms creates general weakness.

Specific weakness has been discussed as the weakness of the antagonists in hypertonicity, the weakness of the spastic muscles themselves and, under asymmetry, the weakness due to inability of action on one side of the body. With any partial immobility, specific rather than general weakness will be the weakness usually observed.

Weakness may be present in a muscle test but be activated more effectively in a complex motor function.

On the other hand a specific muscle may act well on voluntary contraction but not transfer its action within a motor function (Damiano *et al.* 2002).

Abnormal Reflex Activity
(See Fig. 7.2 and Table 7.2)

These may be used by individuals with dyskinesia or spasticity. This may be persisting infantile reflex reactions or pathological reflex reactions. It is not the reflex *as such*, but the recurring stimulation of these patterns by those handling a person with cerebral palsy or by the child or older person in his own efforts to move, which may lead to deformity. However, not all children depend on a strategy of moving by

activating reflexes, or by an apparent domination by reflexes. Examples:

Asymmetrical tonic neck reactions or any other asymmetrical limb postures created by head turning may lead to deformities in the limbs, a scoliosis and/or a torticollis. Extensor postures are associated with asymmetrical tonic neck reactions. A 'windswept' hip, and later subluxating into flexion-adduction on the occipital side, may be associated with persistent reflex on one side.

Symmetrical tonic neck reflexes may occur in some very severe cases. Immobility and lack of treatment may lead to deformities within these patterns, or in remnants of them.

Reflex stepping may aggravate hypertonic plantarflexors, adductors and extensors if this reflex is used to 'walk' the child frequently.

Excessive supporting reaction or antigravity reflex may be overstimulated by, say, *baby bouncers* and increases the deformities of the legs, especially equinus and extensor-adductor postures.

Excessive suspension. If the child is lifted or suspended under the armpits and lowered to the ground, and there is an excessive plantarflexion.

Active use of total flexion reactions, withdrawal reflexes in kicking, during rolling, crawling, kneeling. The withdrawal reaction which combines hip-knee and ankle flexion rather than hip-flexion-knee *extension* and ankle flexion may be used in (heel strike) stepping. This hip and knee flexion is used in stepping instead of hip extension-knee flexion or other such synergia in swing-through or push-off in gait. The repeated use of flexion in all these movements or postures tends to flexion deformity.

Use of total extension reactions as in using the extensor thrust in active kicking, when bounced on the feet in standing, in order to achieve rolling and creeping along the floor, may lead to deformities into these patterns of extension.

Asymmetry

See abnormal postures and asymmetry in Development of standing, Development of sitting and Development in prone and supine (Chapter 8).

(1) Asymmetrical distribution of hypertonus.
(2) Asymmetrical development of tilt, saving and rising postural mechanisms.
(3) Asymmetrical use or uncontrolled persistence of abnormal reflex.
(4) Asymmetrical growth of legs.
(5) Hemianopia (of visual field), absent visual acuity or deafness in one ear augments asymmetry.
(6) Excessive weight bearing on one side of the body, arm or leg can lead to deformity. This is associated with asymmetry of postural stabilization and counterpoising. Using one hand only when the other is more impaired so that counterpoising develops more to one side increases asymmetry.

Involuntary Movement in One Repetitive Pattern

Any repeated flexor spasms or involuntary athetoid kicking with hip and/or knee flexion, or pawing an athetoid leg, may give rise to tightness in knees or hips and knee joints. Similarly and less commonly extensor spasms or rotary involuntary movement may create tightness. Dystonic athetosis is particularly worrying as a cause of deformity.

Growth Factors

There are four main factors which cause or aggravate the development of deformity.

(1) The difference in leg length, see asymmetry in abnormal postures in standing. (Difference in arm length is not related to the genesis of deformation).

(2) Spurts of growth in cerebral palsied children and adolescents are linked with deterioration and increase of deformities. The unequal growth of bone and muscle, increase in height and especially increase in weight seem to bring on deformities. Usually there would also be less mobility as older children need to spend longer hours at their studies.
(3) The mechanism of growth and spasticity have been studied by a number of workers. Sharrard (1971) believes it is the stronger spastic muscles imbalanced with their weaker antagonists, which pull unevenly on growing bones and create deformity. Tabary *et al.* (1972) showed that shortened muscles have a diminution of sarcomeres compared with normally mobile and extensible muscles. The weaker, inelastic, shortened spastic muscles grow abnormally in relation to bone and deformities increase with growth (Tardieu *et al.* 1982). Orthopaedic surgery is inevitable in their view (Sharrard 1971; Bleck 1987; Sussman 1992). Botulinum toxin injections aim to maintain muscle length during growth and delay surgery.
(4) The specific bony structure of the hip does not change as it normally would with growth, due to abnormal tone, abnormal posture and non-weight bearing. The neck of the femur remains in anteversion and the shaft/neck angle of valgus does not decrease. This is part of the reason for hip deformity, and dislocations.

Biomechanics

Every joint should be considered in the treatment of deformities, whether with or without orthopaedic surgery. This is due to the biomechanics of deformity. The biomechanics which create deformities are firstly dependent on the spastic muscle groups, each of which may flex one joint and extend another, e.g. hamstrings, rectus, gastrocnemius, and their relationship to weakness. Secondly, there are effects on the whole limb and the whole body in the biomechanics of spasticity. The more important clue is the presence or absence of the postural mechanisms of postural fixation, counterpoising and the locomotive reflexes which activate progression. When these are abnormal the child compensates by using abnormal postures in order to maintain balance in functions such as sitting, standing, crawling and walking. Green *et al.* (1995) have observed abnormal biomechanics in lying, sitting and standing. Butler and Major (1992), Farmer *et al.* (1999) have observed biomechanics in upright postures. Occasionally hip deformities or equinus deformity may disbalance the child, but it is usually the disbalance *of the child* which increases hip flexion in compensation for falling backward (see the Abnormal postures in standing and sitting section in Chapter 8). See Fig. 8.155e.

THERAPY AND DAILY CARE

Treatment aims based on the causes of deformity discussed are therefore:

(1) Motivation of movement throughout the day. However, movements must be varied and where possible of normal pattern.
(2) Frequent changes of the child's posture.
(3) Correct positioning of each part of a child's body in postures.
(4) Postures and movements must include:

   (a) Passive elongation of hypertonic muscles and soft tissues.
   (b) Active and full range of movement of antagonists to hypertonic muscles.
   (c) Active and full range of movement of hypertonic muscles including active work in their elongated position.

(5) Correct any asymmetries of posture, movement or balance and check postural alignments regularly.
(6) Train the normal postural mechanisms and locomotor reactions.

(7) Control recurring involuntary motion in one pattern.
(8) Counteract any use of relevant pathological reflexes. Train a variety of motor patterns if possible, so that reflexes need not be used.
(9) Treat the biomechanics of deformity and not just deformity in one joint.

As in the discussion of the causes, many of the aims interact with each other.

Techniques

Techniques for all the aims mentioned above are presented in the sections in Chapter 8 on Physiotherapy suggestions and suggestions for daily care throughout all developmental stages. There are, however, additional methods which may be required for individual children.

As malalignment of joints and spine by spasticity and weakness are common problems in children and older people, additional methods are needed for each individual. The association of muscle shortening with spasticity is treated with methods to reduce spasticity and elongate muscles. Examples are:

(1) *Ice treatments* to whole limb or on the spastic muscle groups to relax spasticity.
(2) *Prolonged stretch to spastic muscles* in correct positions in plasters (inhibitory casts), equipment and orthoses. Tardieu *et al.* (1988) found that stretch needs to be maintained for 6 hours daily to have an effect. This can be obtained in night splints or night positioning and/or by sessions in daily equipment. At least 30–60 minutes daily in different postures of lying, sitting and standing is advisable and selected according to age and daily activity. Using different postures avoids stretching only one group of spastic muscles; 30-minutes stretch maintains existing muscle length while 6 hours increases muscle length. Therefore a daily regime is worked out so that the more severely spastic muscle groups are stretched.

(3) *Gentle manual stretch* given together with ice treatments and especially with assisted active or active movement is more effective. Very young children as well as older individuals are easier to stretch in warm water at bathtime or in hydrotherapy. Manual stretching is not prolonged enough for changing muscle length but, after stretching, people with cerebral palsy report feeling looser and more able to carry out an activity. Stretching is also helpful before positioning a person in equipment and before the application of orthoses. Always give slow gentle stretch as forced stretches can tear muscles and soft tissues and quick stretches stimulate spasticity.

(4) *Passive ranges of movement* in as full a range as possible and with knowledge of normal ranges in infants and young children. Procedures to lengthen spastic muscles are not possible if joints are stiff from immobility or only moved in a limited range. Joint structures and soft tissues are kept flexible and in as full a range as possible. Passive ranges are not enough for overcoming problems of muscle length, but, if slow and rhythmic, do assist relaxation in children and adults in preparation for other procedures (Soames 2003).

(5) *Activation of antagonists* assists the correction of deformities. This lengthens the spastic muscles. However, some therapists suggest that activation of antagonists also reduces the spasticity of muscles by reciprocal inhibition (Stockmeyer 1967).

(6) *Holding a corrected position*. Lengthening muscles with orthoses, equipment or manual positioning and stretch needs to be more active for better effect. A child and an older person are trained to actively hold the correction once spasticity is reduced. A child who cannot understand can hold a position if he reaches out, stretches out his body in order to play with a person or toy.

(7) *Rotation and diagonal movements* have been observed to decrease spasticity and shortening observed in straight flexion and extension ranges.

(8) Vibration techniques (Rood 1962; Hagbarth & Eklund 1969; Eckersley 1990, 1993).

(9) Repeated contractions of spastic muscles to obtain autoinhibition (Rood 1962). An active contraction of the antagonists must follow immediately.

Botulinum toxin A

Botulinum toxin A injections are a relatively new treatment for spasticity (Corry *et al.* 1997; Cosgrove *et al.* 1994; a large multi-centre study by Baker *et al.* 2002). Botulinum toxin (BTX A) blocks the release of acetylcholine in the nerve endings at the neuromuscular junction. There is a reduction of spasticity of the individual muscle injected which commences between 24 and 72 hours. Muscle relaxation is most evident after 2 weeks following injection and disappears between 3–6 months and rarely lasts longer. Repeat injections are then indicated but may be limited as long-term damage is not yet known. Follow-up studies are still in progress, though the injections are currently found to be particularly safe with no serious side-effects (Forssberg & Tedroff 1997).

Parents and child need to know that the injection is given with a local anaesthetic with a mild sedative. Two hours post-injection is given for a child to overcome his sleepiness before he returns home. A few days of flu-like symptoms may occasionally happen in some children.

Selection of cases continues to be studied and the physiotherapist's view is expected by the team. Selection is based on ease of management or function as follows:

(1) Usually spastic hemiplegia and diplegia are preferred but tetraplegia is also selected for arm or leg muscle.

(2) The specific times for assessment for candidates for BTX A are:

- When a child pulls to stand and cruises, particularly with 'on-toes' pattern.
- When a walking (ambulant) child is at a plateau in walking skills, is losing balance, is continuing to have falls and a gait pattern is not improving.
- When a child wishes to progress to pedalling a bike (trike), climb stairs with less support, kick a ball and try other motor skills involving a better base for postural stability and counterpoising.
- When spastic adductors and plantar flexors limit transfers and base for sitting.
- When given injections for arms to counter asymmetry, which affects gait, and for function.
- When spasticity blocks nappy changes, hygiene of perineum or causes tight hands.

(3) High energy expenditure is causing poor endurance or decreasing skill such as reduction in distance walked in a specified time or decrease in motor repetitions.

(4) Anxieties of child, adolescent and families concerning appearance of gait.

(5) Difficulty applying orthoses and skin intolerance to them. Serial casting may precede the injection with BTX A.

(6) The candidate responds best when full joint ranges are present on static examination but dynamic shortening of spastic muscle takes place during activity.

(7) The reduction of spastic shortening of a muscle group shows the likely post-surgical biomechanics in the individual. In addition, surgical intervention can be delayed as muscle length is maintained during growth. The degree of surgery is also optimized following injections with continual physiotherapy.

Daily management following injections

Children having injections need priority for initial increased active physiotherapy and daily management consisting of:

(1) Daily range of motion with stretches and maintained stretch in day orthoses and night splints. Night splints immediately after injection worn for 6 hours or more (Tardieu *et al.* 1988). Orthoses may be increased initially and decreased from, say, ankle-foot orthosis to hinged ankle-foot orthosis to dynamic ankle-foot orthosis to supportive shoe with insole. Increased activity of leg muscles is enhanced with such progressive decrease of support.

(2) A sleeping system for postural correction depends on each child. See Appendix, Goldsmith *et al.* (1992).

(3) Strengthening injected muscles which appear weak after injection, their antagonists and postural control muscles.

(4) Re-educating gait pattern and gradually decreasing support that walking aids provide (see Fig. 8.155e).

(5) Checking that postural alignments in sitting, standing and lying are correct.

(6) Regular monitoring of parents and carers and school staff for daily stretching, use of postural management equipment and specific muscle strengthening. Their comments are especially important. Explain that a child will have an initial feeling of weakness of an injected limb or begin falling due to this and the change in his body image using a different base, say, plantigrade feet or more abducted thighs. The physiotherapy programme in which all participate improves all this. General weakness or other unexpected symptoms should be immediately conveyed to the consultant.

(7) Activities such as swimming, horse-riding and gym clubs become beneficial once specific treatment regimes are established.

Outcome measures. These include video analyses, Gross Motor Function Measure, goniometry for joint range, reports and diary by parents, carers, school assistant and child. Energy expenditure measures have also been used.

Measures are usually used at pre-injection, after 2 weeks, 6 weeks and 3–4 months after injection. It seems that long-term measures are not used once injections have worn off and spasticity has returned. Cosgrove *et al.* (1994) and others found improvement in gait. Studies continue to confirm that long-term improvements remain once injections are no longer used. Forssberg and Tedroff (1997) have queried the evaluation of the results of Botulinum injections.

Dumas *et al.* (2001) report a consensus of 41 paediatric physiotherapy experts in the USA and Canada which included a ranked importance of various direct interventions following Botulinum injection(s) for lower limb spasticity in cerebral palsy. Therapeutic exercise, functional training of self-care and function in the community and appropriate devices and equipment were most important in a list of seven components. However, precise descriptions of the procedures were not given. The report therefore suggests research of more detailed descriptions and their outcomes. The report also points out that as yet there are no studies of the influence of Botulinum toxin on the physical therapy plan of care. Most of the management procedures outlined by Harrison and Simpson (2001) are not particularly specific to post BTX A injections. However, more intense direct physiotherapy treatment and frequent monitoring of parents and school staff are emphasized. Stretching, strengthening and functional training are underlined, as they are in the American study by Dumas *et al.* (2001).

SPECIFIC DEFORMITIES

For a review of orthopaedic surgical procedures see Samilson (1975), Bleck (1987), Sussman (1992) and Cosgrove (2000).

Although a summary of each joint is given below, the whole child needs assessment. Multi-level surgery in one operation is preferred today for a whole view.

THE HIP DEFORMITIES
Hip Flexion-Adduction-Internal Rotation

One component may be greater than the others. The shape of the hip joint may be abnormal, e.g. the acetabulum is shallow, neck of femur anteverted; subdislocation and dislocation may occur, in time in bilateral cerebral palsy (Hiroshima & Ono 1979; Sussman 1992; Cosgrove 2000).

Hip subdislocation (subluxation) and dislocation increases deformity, causes pain, interferes with sitting and standing and daily care. Delayed weight bearing in standing is significant in causing dislocations. Scrutton and Baird (1997) and Scrutton *et al.* (2001) monitored hip migration and found that children who did not walk by 5 years had a 1 in 2 chance of hip dislocation. Late sitting or walking together with hypertonus, asymmetry and no weight-bearing in standing are risks for hip dislocation. Gudjonsdottir and Mercer (1997) clearly describe the development of hip and spine deformities for clinical work.

Therapy and Daily Care

Prevention of hip dislocation

Hypotonia or hypertonia and dystonia and/or marked asymmetry persisting beyond age 3 months need postural management, a variety of well aligned positions and later upright supported standing for weight bearing through hips, straight femurs and plantigrade feet. An hour of weight bearing 4–5 times a week is advised by Stuberg (1992) to improve joint and bone growth.

Positioning of a neonate and premature infant is needed to reduce the risk of subluxation/dislocation (Grenier 1988). This is part of general developmental care and are the positions of mid-range joints of shoulders and hips, well supported but not restrictive of movement. Excessive hip abduction-external rotation and flexion or hyperextension needs special attention in very young, unwell babies. The positioning is carried out by nurses and parents under supervision of physiotherapists in hospital and home. Positioning is essential from age 2 to 5 years.

Positioning in lying equipment needs to take account of sleeping problems and medical problems of sleep hypoxaemia, seizures or gastroesophageal reflux. Side-lying with correct abduction and body alignment is also used if supine or prone is not useful for any baby or child.

If there is any pain and decrease in a child's hip ranges of movement there should be referral to an orthopaedic surgeon immediately. Remember that range of motion and stretch of a child's hip flexors may rock the pelvis, increasing lordosis. Therefore in assessment and in exercises, stabilize the pelvis as shown in Figs 10.5–10.6.

Positioning. Prone lying, legs apart on conical-shaped pommel, in prone wedges, prone lying or supine positioning equipment, standing frames, standing tables, sitting with legs apart, externally rotated, tailor-sitting, sitting in chairs with pommels and corrective symmetrical hip-knee adaptations; stand or sit straddling equipment of rolls; carrying positions with legs apart and turned out pressing child's hip flat. Extension-abduction is most therapeutic (Goldsmith *et al.* 1992; Hankinson & Morton 2002; Pountney *et al.* 2002).

Splintage. Abduction padding/wedge used in all positions; abduction splint (Fig. 8.113) used in standing and walking; abduction in night splints or lying frames; rotation coil attached to pelvic band and shoe for external rotation (but check for any abnormal effect of tibial torsion), *twisters* (Fig. 8.167) for milder conditions of spasticity (see Fig. 8.155e).

Plaster of Paris. Long leg spicas or back slabs to incorporate hip extension-abduction rarely work. Excessive flexor spasms usually occur after removal. Use knee back slab only.

Ice treatment to reduce hypertonicity.

(1) Apply towels wrung out in chopped ice and water to adductor surface of leg for 3–4 minutes. In addition place the child in tailor-sitting or over a roll *while* the ice pack is tied on to his thighs. Repeat applications of ice packs. Carry out active abduction movements as well.

(2) Wring rough towels out in ice so that ice flakes cling to the towelling. Roll the whole leg from groin to feet in the towel for 3–4 minutes. Carry out leg patterns with rotation in the hip during and after ice application as well as positioning. Repeat.

Active exercise to antagonists

(1) See developmental training for active hip extension, hip abduction, hip external rotation in creeping, rolling from prone to supine, active extension in 'standing tall', in stand and reach overhead. Counterpoising techniques using leg extension, abduction, external rotation (Figs 8.37, 8.38, 8.163) in four-point kneeling and in standing, squatting with external rotation or sitting rise to standing, half-kneeling with front leg held in external rotation in rise to standing, and maintain abduction-external rotation-extension in lateral weight shifts.

(2) Other examples are given in Figs 10.1–10.10. Emphasize the movement of the antagonists to the deformity, e.g. the extensors in flexion deformities.

Active exercise to agonists and antagonists. See Developmental training of creeping (flexion and extension of legs), counterpoising techniques in crawling positions and standing position. Standing active bending down to floor/low table followed by stretch of hips in upright standing, see Figs 10.1–10.10.

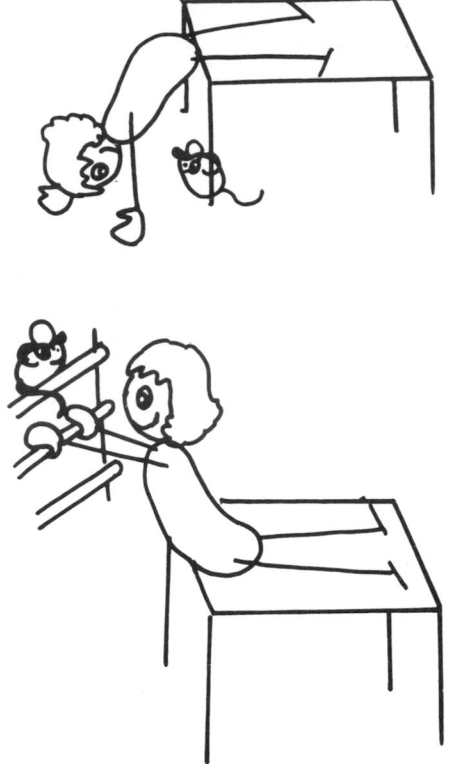

Orthopaedic surgery for hip deformities and dislocation. There are many different views and the surgeon involved will advise. Surgery may be soft-tissue surgery in younger children whose hips are not as severely migrating out of joint as others (Cosgrove 2000). Soft-tissue surgery includes muscle, tendon and connective tissue lengthening or releasing of adductors, flexors and hamstrings (Turker & Lee 2000). Bony surgery includes reconstruction of proximal femur and acetabulum, femoral and pelvic osteotomy, occasionally removal of the head of femur. Soft tissue releases with bone surgery may be used as well (Scrutton & Baird 1997; Cosgrove 2000; Bleck 1987). There are potential risks of surgery and it is best undertaken at a specialist centre where a surgeon is experienced in paediatric orthopaedics. Post-operative rehabilitation together with good postural management should be available (Turker & Lee 2000). For further reading on hip dislocation prevention and management contract Association of Paediatric Chartered Physiotherapists (Appendix).

Fig. 10.1 Bend over edge of mother's lap, large ball or couch, raise up and bend down again. Hold rungs and 'walk up' for level of hip extension. Keep legs apart and turned out if necessary. Child raises head and trunk up in association with hip extension. Initial support may be given by your hand on his chest. Avoid abnormal extensor thrust, excessive lordosis.

Hip Extension Deformity

Therapy and Daily Care

Positioning. Chairs to increase flexion and symmetry (see Seating in Chapter 8), Correct

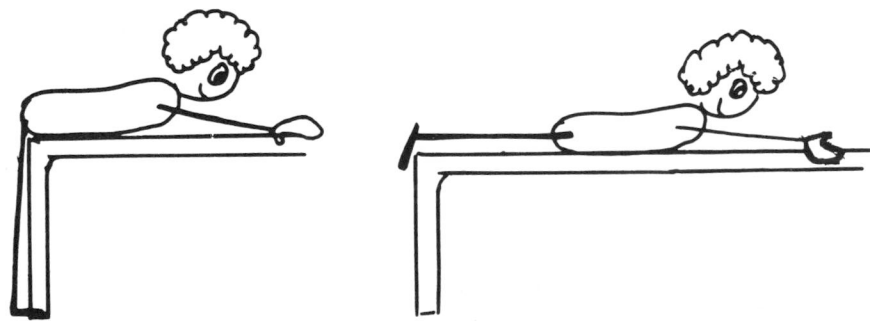

Fig. 10.2 Child's legs over mother's lap, edge of bed, large ball, or roll. Bring legs down to floor (hip flexion) into bed (hip extension). Hold knees and thighs apart in external rotation to encourage hip extension-abduction-external rotation if required. Raise *one* leg at a time to control lordosis (Fig. 10.6). Child may grasp side of table or both his arms are held elevated-abducted and externally rotated by adult if abnormal flexion in arm and trunk is present. Use these movements when getting up on to bed/plinth *or* getting out of bed.

carrying in flexion positions. Use some hip flexion in standing. Use heel-sitting, squatting and crook-sitting.

Splintage, plasters, ice not used as positioning seems to be simplest and more effective.

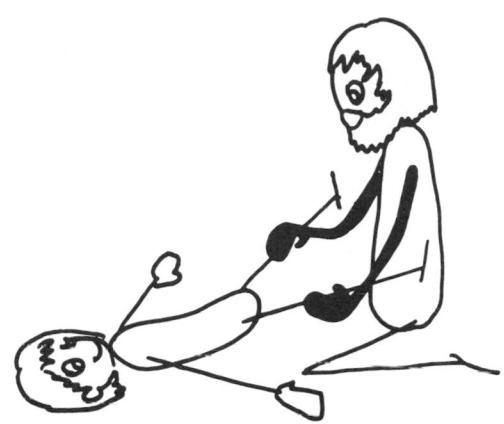

Fig. 10.3 Legs of child held in abduction-external rotation. Active raise of child's hips into extension. *Avoid* use of lordosis to do this. Legs may be on lap of therapist, on low stool or with his feet flat on the ground for 'bridging' the pelvis into extension. Manual resistance may be given to anterior superior iliac spines to augment extension. Obtain flexion by asking child to bend knees to chest then repeat hip extension activity. Use this action during play, dressing and washing.

Active movements of flexion and of flexion and extension, see developmental training of creeping, crawling and standing (see Fig. 8.168 on correcting hip extension in walking). See Figs 10.1–10.10.

Note. To overcome excessive extension of head, trunk, hips and knees, it is important to flex the child at his head and shoulders *and* at his hip joint. Hold his head and shoulders, hold under his knees and flex him 'into a ball'. His extensor spasm, thrust or constant extensor hypertonus decreases in this position. This may be easier in side-lying. Try different positions for flexion. *Orthopaedic surgery is used* (Bleck 1987; Sussman 1992). Drugs reduce hypertonus.

KNEE DEFORMITIES

Knee Flexion

Therapy and Daily Care

Positioning. Prone-lying with straight knees, sitting with straight knees on the floor, in floor seat or sit on a low chair if back rounds in sitting. Use knee gaiters in sitting (incline seat forward) and in standing.

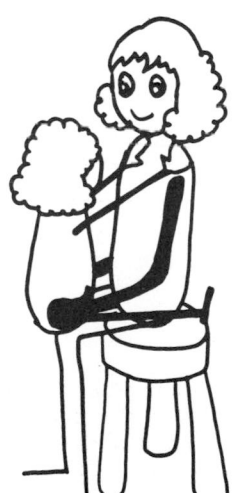

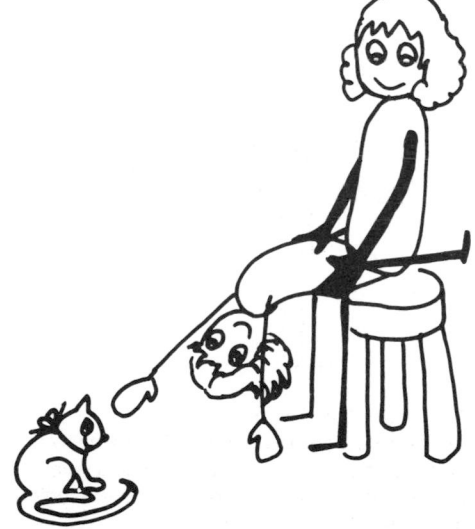

Fig. 10.4 The child actively stretches down and comes up to sitting with or without grasping your hands. For babies you may use the large ball, or roll. The child may also bend sideways to the floor for scoliosis correction.

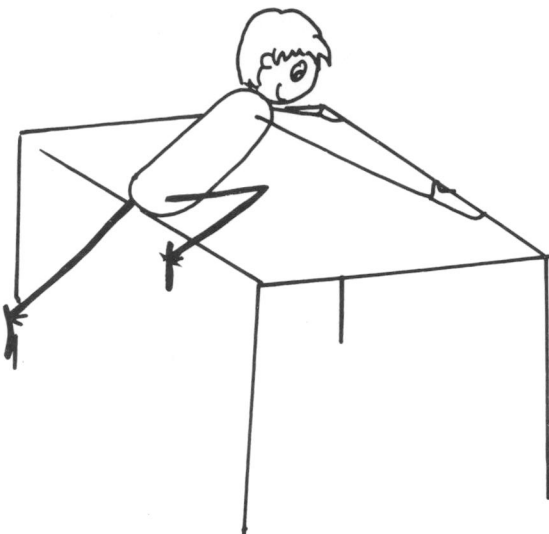

Fig. 10.5 One knee held bent to chest during hip extension of the other leg, to counteract lordosis. Carry this out in side-lying or in prone. Also flex-abduct-externally rotate extended leg for action of those agonists.

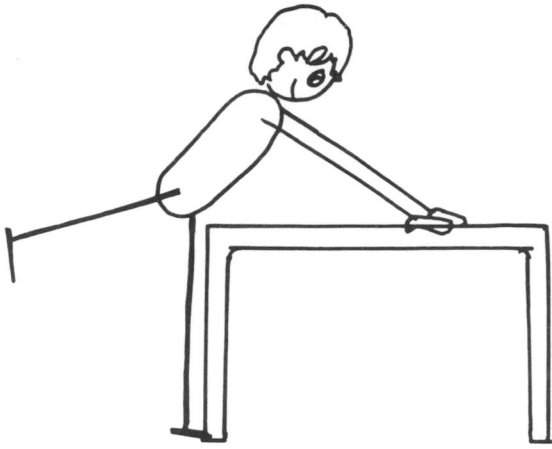

Fig. 10.6 Child leans forward onto ball, table, roll, during active hip extension of each leg. Lordosis is more easily controlled this way. Next, flex the leg so that foot reaches high bar or even table.

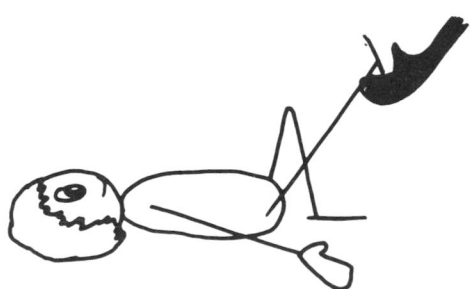

Fig. 10.7 One knee flexed to chest or flexed with foot flat. Press other leg into extension into adult's hand, sponge rubber surface, soft couch. Child's hips raise into extension with his weight on one foot. Full flexion of each hip should be carried out actively if required. Arms straight, and hands pressed flat or grasping edge of bed.

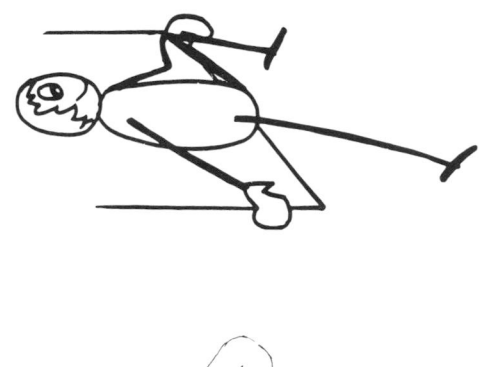

Fig. 10.8 *Activate agonists and antagonists* and full range of active hip and knee motion. Use of arm extension is incorporated in these exercises.

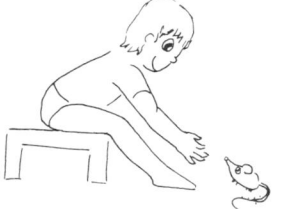

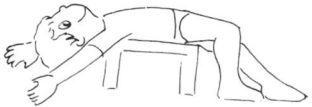

Fig. 10.9 *Activate agonists and antagonists* and full range of active hip and knee motion. Use of arm extension is incorporated in these exercises. Use hip flexion to manage socks and shoes.

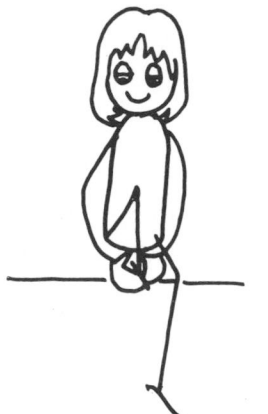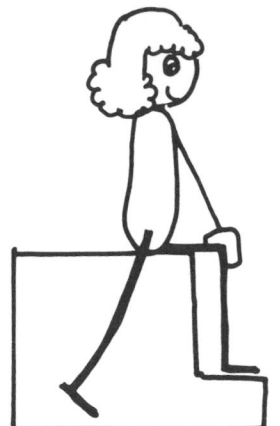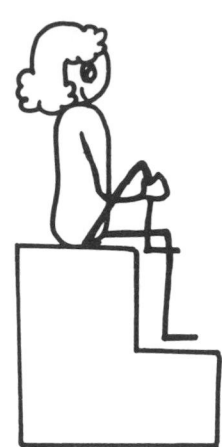

Fig. 10.10 *Activate agonists and antagonists* and full range of active hip and knee motion. Use of arm extension is incorporated in these exercises. Use these movements during dressing/washing.

Splintage. Knee gaiters, knee splints. Soft knee night-splints have been effective (Anderson *et al.* 1988).

Plasters from hip to ankle are useful (*stove pipe plasters*) or use back slabs.

Ice treatment to whole leg (see hip flexion above).

Active movements for knee extensors and for knee flexors and extensors. See developmental training for hip and Figs 10.1–10.10. Active sitting postural control may prevent a need for distal hamstring lengthening for round back.

Orthopaedic surgery. Various operations on the hamstrings to overcome crouch gait, improve sitting and knee flexion deformity 20–30°, such as partial hamstring tenotomy or hamstring slide, hamstring transplant, e.g. lengthen semitendinosus, transpose semimembranosus and detach gracilis, distal hamstring lengthening/release with rectus femoris transfer. Post-operative physiotherapy to strengthen hips, and knee extensors and flexors is important.

Knee Hyperextension
Therapy and Daily Care

Positioning. Delay standing development. A standing frame is better and needs to align knee posture and allow some flexion. Use sitting on chair, side-sit, tailor-sitting, upright kneeling avoiding excessive lordosis, crook-sitting. If child is standing already, stand with knee pieces preventing hyperextension; use shoes with higher heel to throw child's weight into knee flexion posture, *if* his plantarflexors are not shortened (see standing, Fig. 8.170).

Splintage. Knee pieces which lock with knee in midline, but allow knee flexion motion. Not necessary in many children.

Plasters and ice treatment for plantarflexors of the feet, if this is the cause of hyperextended knees, or for hamstrings.

Passive stretch and movement. Hyperextension may be due to tight plantarflexors. Maintain passive stretch of these muscles in orthoses or standing frames.

Active movement of knee flexors, but more important dorsiflexors of ankles if tight plantarflexors are present.

Active work for stabilization of pelvis, which is often the cause of hyperextended knees. See Crawling development, Standing development (see Fig. 8.170, and upright kneel) and use of *bear walk* in Prone development.

Orthopaedic surgery. If hyperextended knees are secondary to feet deformity or hip flexion deformity these joints may sometimes require surgery or be part of multi-level operations.

DEFORMITY OF THE FEET

Equinus and Equino-Varus

Therapy and Daily Care

Positioning. Prone lying with feet over edge of wedge or pillows, prone standers and upright frames with heels down; sitting in chairs with heels flat on ground; standing feet held flat on ground; standing in boots with raised soles; stand facing up on inclined platform; bear walk positions with heels down on ground.

Splintage and orthoses. Below-knee orthoses fixed; encouraging dorsiflexion or dynamic. Mild/moderate condition: correct with special boots having a raise on soles. Strap to keep the child's heel down in his boot. The strap should be wider and padded as it crosses the front of his ankle. Select ankle-foot orthosis to correct deformity more accurately. Orthoses usually worn post-operatively.

Plasters. Technique described below (Fig. 10.15). In close co-operation with orthotist and gait analysis. See Chapter 8, Development of Standing.

Ice treatment to whole leg or the ice pack to plantarflexors only. Quick ice stimulation to

dorsiflexors once relaxation and lengthening of plantar flexors is gained.

Passive stretch and movement. Hold the knee flexed with one hand, and grasp the heel and foot with your other hand. Gently dorsiflex foot as far as possible. Hold in dorsiflexion as you passively extend the child's knee.

Do not evert the child's foot as you push it up into dorsiflexion. Stretch must be slow and maintained. Ask child to hold foot up in dorsiflexion with you. Also stretch with inversion.

Suggestions for passive stretch, including active dorsiflexions:

(1) Child stands and leans forward to wall to stretch heel cords.
(2) With child's legs apart, turned out, push both his feet into dorsiflexion.
(3) Stand and lunge forward; half-kneeling lunge forward on front foot. (See Fig. 6.2)
(4) Sitting heels on small inclined foot board obtaining dorsiflexion; stand with heels down, child facing up on inclined board during classroom/play activity.
(5) Bear-walk with heels down (9–12 months developmental level).
(6) Standing on tipping board or rocker, slowly tipped back with child's heels held down (Fig. 8.181).
(7) Walk on heels if possible. Raise the soles of his shoes, or remove heels off his shoes.
(8) See Figs 10.2, 10.6, 10.7, 10.10.
(9) Child is reminded to sit in a chair with heels down. Squat with heels down. Slow rise from sit/squat to stand with weight forward. Slow stair ascent and descent.
(10) Stimulate creeping patterns for dorsiflexion. Other leg flexion patterns may do this (Fig. 8.37).
(11) Brushing, quick icing to dorsiflexors following passive stretch to plantarflexors, and during backward tilt in (6).

(12) *Bone pounding* or striking heel of foot on surface stimulates dorsiflexion. Use in context of gait training.

(13) Walk up inclined plane or ramps with heel down on surface.

(14) Draw faces on child's feet, and ask him to dorsiflex or raise his feet to look at the face, or to touch a toy and create similar games.

(15) Child to practise heel strike in walking. Attach flat squeezy toys to the heels of child's shoes. These create a sound on heel strike. This amuses a child and motivates the *heels down* action as a biofeedback during stance and step.

(16) Use pattern of hip flexion-adduction external rotation, knee extension, foot dorsiflexion, with child in sitting over edge of bed or in supported standing. Use stretch, touch, pressure and resistance if this method (PNF) is known (Fig. 8.163b).

Orthopaedic surgery. Surgeon may carry out lengthening of Achilles tendon (z-plasty) or often preferred gastrocnemius slide, e.g. Vulpius operation. Operation may need to be repeated with growth. Botulinum toxin delays this surgery so that young children need not have it until well after 6 years. Orthoses follow all these procedures.

Valgus Feet (Pronated)

Positioning. Have hips and knees turned out during sitting, round sit on the floor with feet in varus, hips externally rotated. Correct equinus if present as valgus is often overcompensation for this.

Splintage and bracing. Correct shoes or boots with inside raise, inside the shoe or outside on the sole or both; use moulded foot support to inner side of feet; below-knee orthosis; flare the heel or sole on the inner side so that it juts out slightly at the base.

Ice treatment. Occasionally may be used for reducing tone of spastic plantarflexion and for spastic peroneal muscles. Quick ice to dorsiflexors.

Plasters. See below.

Passive stretch as for equinus, but include some inversion.

Activity. As for equinus, but emphasize inversion. See Figs 10.11–10.14. Tap the bone at the heel and malleoli on one side to provoke inversion.

Orthopaedic surgery. If secondary to other deformities. Severely deformed feet may also be treated with Grice's operation to the joints (triple arthrodesis). There are a number of modified Grice operations, one with peroneus brevis lengthening.

Varus Feet

See equinus for treatment and Figs 10.12–10.14; tap bone at heel and malleoli all to

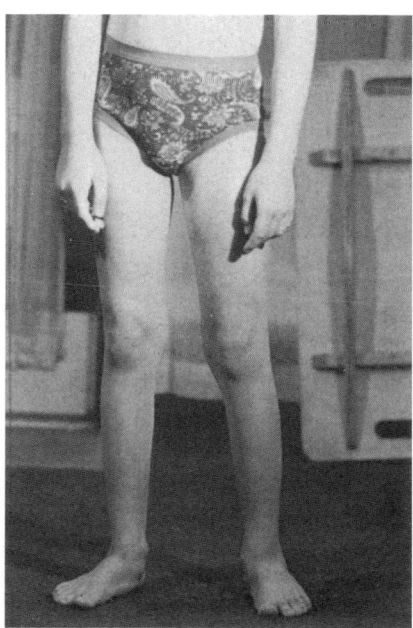

Fig. 10.11 Child with valgus feet.

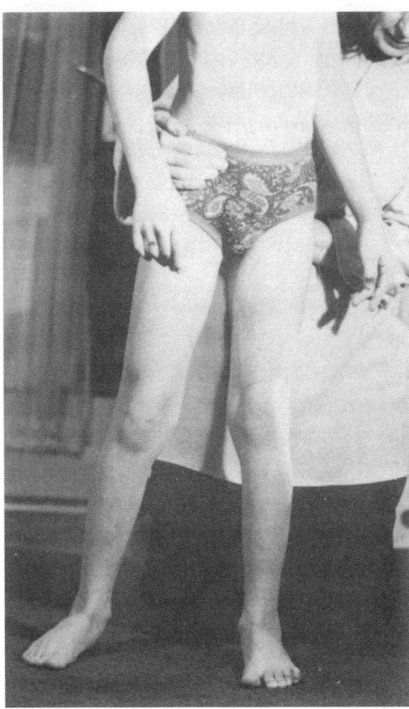

Fig. 10.12 Rotate pelvis to stimulate action of foot muscles to correct valgus. Rotate against your manual resistance at the hip in front and behind.

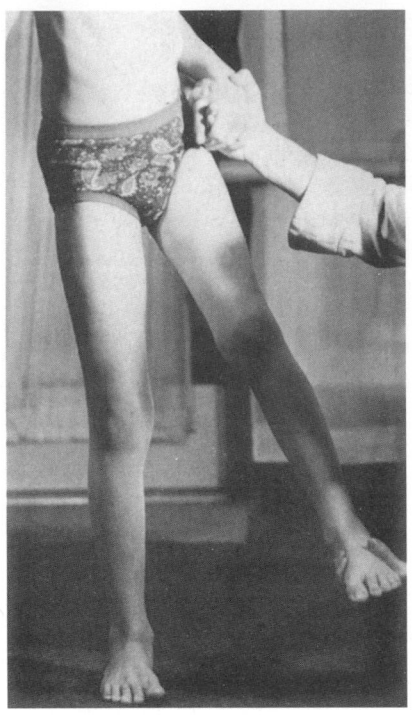

Fig. 10.13 Stand, tip the child on to outside of his foot to provoke action of foot muscles to correct valgus. Child may move his pelvis laterally against your hand to obtain inversion of feet, backwards for dorsiflexion, forwards for plantarflexion.

activate eversion. Plasters, splintage and orthoses are used with adjustment to the opposite side to that used for valgus.

This deformity is common as equinovarus.

Clenched Toes or Everted Toes

This disappears with correct weight-bearing and balance training. Heel must be on the ground and equinus treated. 'Flick' toes up as child takes weight. Use sponge or felt to hold toes corrected while balance develops. Excessive toe flexion occurs if standing is too early for the child. Incorporate toes into plaster or orthoses. This avoids clenching and inhibits spasticity.

ARM DEFORMITY

Orthopaedic surgery reviews are mainly on hemiplegia. Function of hands, cosmesis and hygiene (Bleck 1987; Cosgrove 2000) are main aims.

Shoulder Flexion-Adduction-Internal Rotation

Positioning. Elevation of arms on high table, over rolls. Hold the child's upper arms and turn them out (Figs 8.24, 8.106). Hold this position during play using his hands.

Splintage, plasters. These are not used. Occasionally a *figure 8 scarf* to hold his shoulders back is helpful. Lycra splints may help.

Ice treatment of the whole arm, together with active motion.

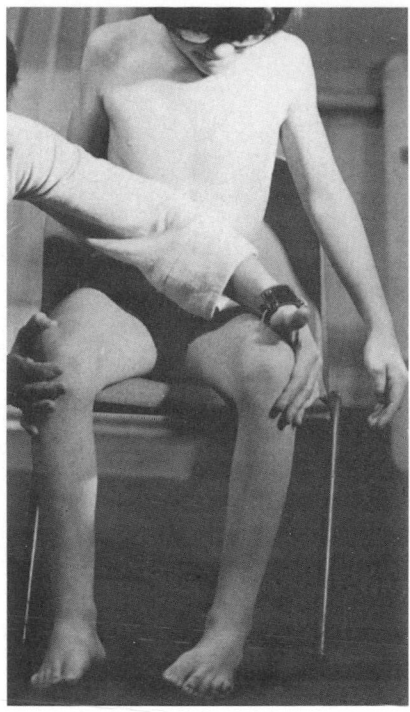

Fig. 10.14 Correction of abnormal adduction, internal rotation or valgus feet. Press his knees outward against your hands or the therapist turns his knees outwards for him. This may be done in sitting, in standing or in squatting positions.

Passive stretch and activity. In positioning and during activities. See Developmental training of creeping, crawling and counterpoising, sitting and counterpoising with arm elevation (Figs 8.185, 8.190), arms over large ball during training of standing, arm elevation in standing and counterpoising. Correct *shoulder retraction* in Developmental training and positioning equipment.

Elbow Flexion

Positioning. See section on shoulder and how to keep elbow straight in all Developmental training and Chapter 9 (Fig. 8.211).

Splintage. Elbow corsets (gaiters) and well padded in forearm area. Do not force into splint.

Passive stretch. None as this is dangerous. Slow range of motion to maintain existing mobility.

Active movements and correction of posture, see Sitting (Fig. 8.106), Arm patterns.

Ice treatment of the whole arm, together with active motion.

Wrist Flexion and Ulnar Deviation

See Developmental training and Hand function (see Abnormal hand grasps and treatment suggestions sections). See Figs 8.212 and 8.213 (hand splints).

Splintage. In midposition with thumb abduction. Hand-cone with a midposition splint. Wrist and hand splint for athetoid's grasp. Many new splints and materials appear and occupational therapists need to be consulted.

Orthopaedic surgery. Occasionally to wrist flexors, or stabilization of the wrist joint.

Hand and Thumb Deformities

Splintage. Thick thumb spacer (made of foam), figure 8 thumb splints and new splints appear on the market regularly. Consult occupational therapists about these and finger spreader, or opposition splints.

DEFORMITIES OF TRUNK AND HEAD

See Figs 8.28, 8.68a–c and 10.1–10.10. Position child in side-lying, observing correction with either a straightening of scoliosis when lying on side of convexity or on side of concavity. Raise hips and legs to stretch concavity. Use firm surface and keep legs apart (on padding) to avoid windswept positions. See also the prone stander (Fig. 8.156d). Windswept hips, asymmetrical weight bearing and scoliosis are seen together but which is the primary cause is unclear. See Fig. 8.155e.

See Developmental training, especially in Sitting and Standing. See chairs (see the section on Evaluating a chair for a child).

Orthopaedic surgeons recommend corsets or spinal orthoses for scoliosis and some operate as well, mainly in an older person. Surgery is considered when scoliosis and other joint contractures interfere with comfortable seating for older persons.

Passive stretch in side-lying with arm elevated. Rotate hips and shoulders in opposite directions in slow rhythm (Fig. 8.61).

GENERAL CONSIDERATIONS RELATED TO SURGERY

The physiotherapist should help the surgeon prepare the child and his family for surgery, if that has been recommended. *Their cooperation is most important.* The child and family and an older person with cerebral palsy need to have information and understanding of the following points:

(1) The surgery is not a cure, but an episode in the total rehabilitation programme. The degree of drive and *sometimes* intelligence of the child affects the results of surgery.
(2) There will be a setback before the ultimate progress is more obvious.
(3) How to look after the child in plaster.
(4) How to help with postoperative physiotherapy.
(5) How to apply any splintage or orthoses to maintain improvement by surgery.
(6) To try and maintain confidence and an encouraging atmosphere.

It is best if the child's own physiotherapist can be the one to treat him before the operation in the hospital and follow up in the home or centre. Otherwise she and the parents should at least introduce the child to the hospital environment, meet some of the staff and generally let the child know what is going to happen there. Possible psychological disturbance due to surgery and its associated hospitalization must not be ignored, as it has been known to affect children for years, and also hamper the physical advances gained by the surgery.

Surgeons have their own pre-/post-operative protocols and periods of immobilization and orthoses. Guidelines are presented for physiotherapy but may need modification according to the surgeon.

PRE-OPERATIVE PHYSIOTHERAPY

Hips, Knees and Feet

(1) Train all muscle groups *not only* the antagonists to the deformity.
(2) Train all *posture – balance reactions.* Results of surgery depend on activity of these mechanisms, or as many of them as possible.
(3) Measure child for any splints or orthoses ordered for the child's use postoperatively when indicated.

POST-OPERATIVE PHYSIOTHERAPY AND CARE

Hip and Knee Operations

In plaster. Spicas with broomstick to hold abduction or plaster from groins to feet, with the broomstick, may follow according to surgeon's plan. Some adductor tenotomies may not be followed by any plasters.

(1) Check that child's head and trunk are kept in alignment. Discourage sacral sitting, holding onto the broomstick (see positions in (3)).
(2) Carry young child over your shoulder keeping his hips flat with your hand.
(3) Change position from bed to sitting on chair with board for legs, or on foot supports. Use prone as on prone board in (4), and also in standing supported, in plaster. Weight bearing in plasters is important and

permission to do this must be obtained as soon as possible.

(4) Use prone board on wheels with wide board for legs. Keep hips flat with a band across them. Place ankles on roll of towels, pillow under chest.
(5) Plasters may be split at end of 3 weeks after knee operation.
(6) In plaster, carry out extension movement of head, arms and back. Sleep on pillows under his side and one leg whilst he lies slightly on his other side.

Out of plaster

(1) Use splintage for knees to control flexor spasms.
(2) Treat pain and swelling, dry skin as for all postoperative cases.
(3) Gentle movements in as much range as possible. Emphasize extension, abduction and improve motor patterns, which are new to the individual.
(4) Continue balance training whenever possible and preferably in standing. Therefore place the child on his feet as soon as possible with surgeon's permission. Stand and step in long leg plasters but return broomstick/abductor bar when child is at rest.
(5) Gently obtain hip and knee flexion by sitting on increasingly lower and lower chairs, over the edge of pillows and in exercises.
(6) No unrelieved sitting is to be resumed.

Harryman (1992) gives techniques following orthopaedic surgery.

Foot Operations

Foot operations may be followed by long leg plasters including the foot or below-knee plasters for 6 weeks.

(1) Train standing as soon as possible with surgeon's permission. Walking in plaster

must be emphasized. Correct pelvic-trunk alignments.
(2) Extension exercises for hips and knees in all positions are required, especially in sitting rise to standing.

Out of plaster

(1) Below-knee orthosis may be recommended by the surgeon.
(2) Active dorsiflexion encouraged (see above equinus – active motion; Figs 10.12–10.14).
(3) Continue training postural balance mechanism in pelvis and trunk in all positions, especially standing.
(4) Plantarflexion, walking on the toes and push off should be trained if possible.

USE OF WEIGHT BEARING PLASTERS (INHIBITORY CASTS)

Indications for below-knee plaster are:

(1) When child pulls up to stand on his toes only, or continues standing on toes.
(2) When child stands with heels down but walks on toes.
(3) When child is ready for standing and walking but cannot balance on deformed feet which are in either equinus, varus or equinovarus. When sitting balance is poor and feet are habitually in plantarflexion.
(4) To prevent any of the above becoming fixed deformities.
(5) To train a better walking pattern using the proprioceptive responses and body image of weight bearing with the heel down and the possibility of heel strike on stepping forward, made possible by the corrective plaster.

A number of research studies including those of Cusick and Sussman (1982), Bertoti (1986), Mosely (1997) show positive results from the use of below-knee casts. There is progress in foot position, postural alignment, balance and walking pattern.

Application of plaster. Based on work by H. de Rijke, Trengweath Centre, Plymouth, UK and Jones (1993). There are many casting materials available and those easily applied and removed, damp-proof and light are selected.

Position. Child lies prone with his knee bent so that dorsiflexion is easier to obtain, and to hold as the plaster is being applied.

Personnel. One person talks to the child and relaxes him and reads to him. One person applies the plaster and another person holds the foot in the corrected position. To shorten the time taken to apply the plaster an additional helper to cut and soak the plasters is needed.

Preparation of the foot and leg

(1) Clean skin, apply olive oil.
(2) Treat callouses, ingrown toenails and do not apply plaster if any skin abrasions have not yet healed.

Application of the plaster itself

(1) Apply stockinette, then thin cotton wool or orthopaedic bandage, allowing stockinette to hang over toes until plaster of Paris is completed.
(2) Apply compressed felt, with sides trimmed down, to ankle, heel and front of ankle. A shape may be cut so that a piece of felt covers the sole of the foot and the felt then wraps around from the heel to the front of the ankle. Do not overlap felt as this will act as a pressure area or the padding may shift under the plaster if it is too loose. Apply all materials evenly. The orthopaedic bandage may be over felt if this can be more even than under the felt.
(3) Wind wet plaster around ankle first. Do not use a figure 8. The *holder* keeps the foot at right angles or more whilst this plaster hardens slightly. It should be

applied with firm tension to hold the foot from slipping.
(4) Apply a plaster from toes to below the knee holding the foot at right angles or more. *Test* that the angle of dorsiflexion used in the plastering can be obtained passively with the child's knee straight. Gradually increase stretch into dorsiflexion in a series for very tight ankles.
(5) Slabs of plaster are put on along the back of the leg up to the toes. The holder keeps the toes *dorsiflexed* and spread out and presses into the centre of the metatarsal arch. The dorsiflexed toes hold the long arch firmly.
(6) Mould the plaster and dent it slightly on either side of the Achilles tendon. The holder must not let the calcaneus slip whilst this is being done. The calcaneus is being kept in the centre, with the Achilles tendon centre, only then is the forefoot corrected.
(7) Final plaster around foot, ankle and to below the knee (about 1 inch).
(8) Smooth and mould plasters to leg. Turn the top plasters back so that you can see all of the child's toes. Cut it at the sides to do this and also cut the stockinette and turn that backwards to reveal toes (Fig. 10.15).
(9) Reinforce the sole of the plaster or use a plaster boot for walking. A small flat heel may be set into the plaster. The plaster must cover the toes underneath and hold them in dorsiflexion to avoid toe clenching the edge of the plaster. Jones (1993) covers the whole cast in crêpe bandages for 4 minutes to aid bonding of layers. A raised sole to keep dorsiflexion is used.
(10) Plasters are said to dry in 30 minutes, according to the manufacturer. Keep child non-weight bearing for 24 hours. Check circulation by pressure on toes and observing immediate return of colour. Blue toes indicate the need to have the plaster removed immediately.

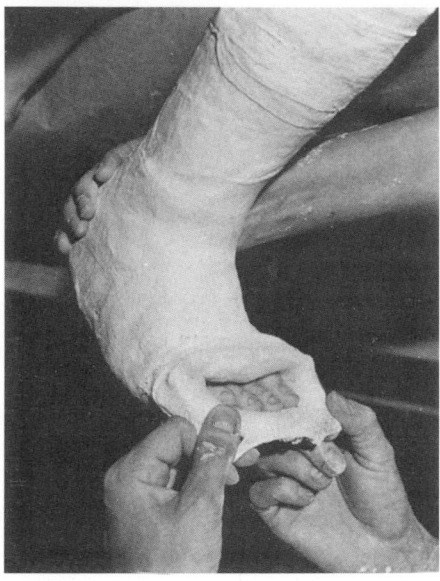

Fig. 10.15

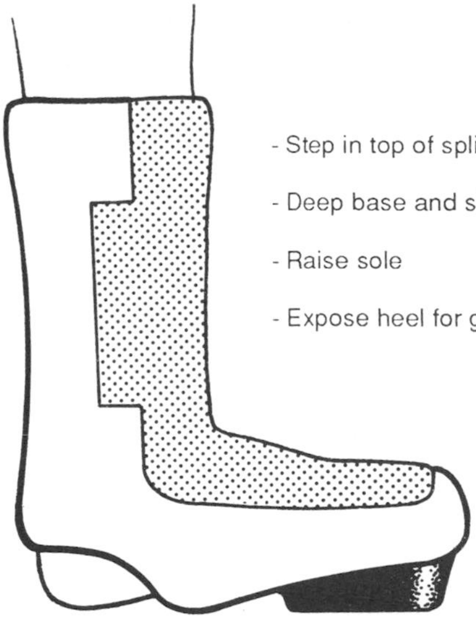

- Step in top of splint

- Deep base and shallow lid

- Raise sole

- Expose heel for ground contact

Fig. 10.16   Post plaster splint (removable) (day or night splint).

(11) Valium or other sedative may be needed for the first night in plaster. The strong pull of the child's hypertonic muscles may make him restless.

(12) Lift blankets off the child's feet by use of a cradle. Keep the child *off* his feet overnight. Plasters are damp-proof, but avoid wetting them as discomfort can be caused by this. Check that discomfort does not occur.

(13) Occasionally spasms of flexion appear in his knees or hips. Use knee gaiters and prone position for the first few days.

(14) Keep plasters on for 1 week in young children; 2–3 weeks in older children and 4 weeks in older and very stiff children. Check skin before application of next plaster.

Exercises in plaster. Emphasize extension movements of the knee and hip, and back (see Figs 10.1–10.10), e.g. straight leg lift backwards, knee stretching in sitting, side-lying extension. Weight bearing exercises after 3 days. Standing weight shift from leg to leg sideways and forward and back. Shift the pelvis forward over the weight-bearing foot, counteracting hip retraction. Sitting stretch up and stand up 'tall'. Stand walk as much as possible, with weight distributed on to both sides equally. Tilt reactions in standing on rocker board or sponge to increase weight bearing through the leg in plaster.

Exercises out of plaster must be continued with the same aims. A bivalved plaster cut down the side and stiffened with plastic material or fibreglass reinforcement may be used for walking. The plaster *shell* holds the foot and toes in dorsiflexion over the right angle if possible. Orthoses are worn as a follow-up of correction (see Fig. 8.155a–d).

Use a series of plasters for children who do not maintain correction. Have a short period of exercises and weight bearing before the next plaster is applied. The period between plasters has been from 2 years to a few weeks in different cases. Athetoids should only wear a plaster for a week at a time in case of involuntary movements within the plaster. Bot-ox for dystonia.

Foot and knee plasters have been applied simultaneously but others prefer below-knee plasters and knee plasters to be separated. After removal of plasters from hip and knee the child often needs exercises, particularly in water, bandaging of knees and treatment of knee swelling as well as long leg back slabs.

Cooperation of the parents is essential for good results, thus:

(1) Explain the purpose of the plaster and the importance of their help and encouragement to the child to wear the plaster for short periods.
(2) They should check the circulation often, be warned about possible restlessness and have a sedative for the child.
(3) Parents should protect the plaster and allow drying for $1^1/_2$ days. Child may sit with his leg or legs on cushions protected by waterproof material. An old sock, plaster boot or plastic covering may be used to cover plaster.
(4) Parents carry out home exercises and later as much standing and walking as possible.
(5) Discuss with parents which times are convenient for the periods of casting.
(6) Tell parents when the plaster comes off and they should know when their child is coming home with a plaster beforehand, or they may think he has broken a leg!
(7) If child's toes go blue, or if there is extreme pain and upset, the plaster *must* be removed by soaking it off in a bucket of warm water immediately. If there is discomfort some plasters can be removed with strong scissors.

11 Therapeutic Group Work

Children's need for group activities has long been recognized in the habilitation of children with disabilities. Such children are often isolated from their peers. Owing to motor disability, they may not be able to run up and join a group of children, put an arm round a friend or even push away an annoying child. Parents find it difficult to bring their child into contact with other children whether able-bodied or disabled. Children need group treatment for contact with other children, sharing an activity with others, feeling part of a group and responding to competition and cooperation. Group work in special or inclusive education as well as in therapy offers opportunities for the child's social and emotional development.

Groups have been used in a variety of ways:

- *In speech therapy* for stimulation of communication and development of speech and language.
- *In occupational therapy* for perceptual training, for play involving perceptual motor function, for recreation, social interaction and learning to play a game involving rules and taking turns, and so on.
- *In physiotherapy* for training children with a specific diagnosis to carry out a set of exercises, for games involving gross motor activity, for swimming and activities in water, and various sports for disabled people.

As the aims of these different therapy groups overlap it is possible to carry out *interdisciplinary groups* of two kinds:

Playgroups including toy libraries, adventure playgrounds, special or ordinary nursery schools, opportunity groups or nurseries, are orientated to each child's developmental levels and special problems. The therapists may advise or themselves work in the group setting, stimulating a few or occasionally all the children with play activities which involve gross motor, fine motor, perceptual and speech and language activities. The therapist may be in the playroom or nursery, relating to one child with specific problems and may or may not also bring in other children in the same activity. Classroom assistants are trained to position and handle children appropriately.

The children may all be in the same room and may or may not feel themselves to belong to the same group in all activities.

Songs, storytime, percussion band, games and music may be the only sessions when all the children carry out the same activity. Therapists are therefore working closely with teachers, psychologists, child care staff, nursery nurses, nurses and parents in the therapeutic play groups and classrooms.

The structured group works to treat or train a specific area of function. These groups integrate the gross motor, fine motor, perceptual, speech and language activities, but with more focus on any one of these areas. This focus may be on the major disability of the children in the group, say motor problems in cerebral palsied children. The focus may be on a specific area of function in one group session, whereas the focus will be on another area for that same group in other group sessions.

These structured interdisciplinary groups in Britain have been influenced by the ideas of

Petö, Hari, and the work of physiotherapists Ester Cotton (1965, 1970, 1974, 1975b), Dorothy Seglow (1984), Titchener (1983) and others who introduced these ideas in Britain. Many more Petö groups based on conductive education have developed in various parts of Britain (Hari & Tillemans 1984; Cottam & Sutton 1988; Hari & Akos 1990). Information can be obtained from SCOPE (The Spastics Society), London.

These groups may not follow the full system of the Petö approach, which involves very much more than a group session or group sessions. From studies with the staff of The Cheyne Centre for Children with Cerebral Palsy these structured interdisciplinary group sessions for multiply disabled children were invaluable and often essential for such children (1969–1979).

Some of the main observations are:

(1) Individual sessions sometimes create too much pressure on an older child and aggravate the normal or abnormal rebelliousness in a child. In the group such children often cooperate because all the other children present are doing what is expected of them.

(2) The one-to-one relationship in individual treatment may be too similar to the one-to-one relationship in the mother–child situation. This is normal in children under 3-year developmental level. Children with physical disabilities, however, are often over this age and need to relate to their peers *even though* their physical function may still be under a 3-year developmental level.

Although a child may need some private tuition in his school life and some disadvantaged children and children with very severe learning disabilities may still need this one-to-one relationship, many more need to 'grow out' of it emotionally and socially. Perhaps some of those who refuse to cooperate may be protesting at the dependency felt on being handled by the therapists all the time in this one-to-one situation.

(3) In the group, children follow a programme and imitate the other children. Imitation helps the children with partial hearing loss or learning disability to understand what is required of them. In addition, the children in groups are observed to instruct and help each other carry out the programme of work.

(4) Speech is stimulated as the adult's concentration on all the children seems to take off the *pressure* on one child to speak.

(5) Concentration of the children who are working at their own pace is great. The attention span is far longer than in individual sessions; children work hard in groups lasting one and a half hours whilst in individual treatment for only 20–40 minutes.

(6) The programme consists of integrating essential aspects of physiotherapy, occupational therapy, speech therapy together with group work. It is planned by the team but carried out by one therapist and one or two aides or assistants. In this way a number of children are helped at the same time with economy on staff and on time spent getting children to and from each therapy department, as well as on time required to establish rapport with each different professional.

(7) Physiotherapists, occupational therapists, speech therapists, teachers, and nursery nurses welcome interdisciplinary groups as they can then see the total child and the relationship of their specialty to those of the others in his total function. On planning and using the structured group session the different disciplines are enabled to share their knowledge with one another so that practical integrated group activities can be created. Different disciplines have then to clarify their main aims with each child and make certain they are understood by everyone in the planning of the programme and

in its execution. It is not possible for each professional to convey all her expertise to the other different disciplines, but rather to learn how to discover the overlap of her particular discipline with others. In this way the overlap becomes a practical achievement and enriches the teamwork.

GENERAL MANAGEMENT OF GROUPS

Number of children. This varies according to the numbers of children in each centre, school or unit, from whom selections may be made. No matter how many children are in a group, they must be *involved* and preferably participating.

Staff. One staff member leads the group with another assisting her. The assistant should be from another discipline. If the children are all severely disabled, more help may be indicated. However, the adults present must be kept to a minimum, or their one-to-child relationship rather than a child-to-child relationship may occur. The leader may alternate with her assistant each week or alternate days in conducting the group.

All assistants need to work according to the leader's action and not divert the child's attention away from the group by private conversation with them or with each other.

Venue. The group is best done in the child's own classroom or where there are no unfamiliar distractions and a coming and going of adults or other children.

Arrange children during the group session so that they can see the leader of the group at all times, and also so that the children see each other. Semi-circles or L-shaped seating arrangements are best, but the positions will change in a class with particular motor activities and walking exercises.

Length of sessions should be planned for 1 to 2 hours depending on the children's ability to continue participating, and the programme of work.

Frequency. Group sessions are best done daily or three times a week depending on the aims of the group programme. Some aims only require twice a week. The main object is that the children work together for not less than two or three times a week so that they know each other and develop a group dynamic.

Behaviour. If a child refuses to join in, make sure that the programme is not too difficult for him. If it is not, let him watch for a while, ignoring him. The other children may be given a particularly pleasant activity or they may occasionally be told 'let's do that again for so-and-so to try as well'. Other ideas may be offered by the parent or team members who know the child. However, if non-participation continues or if the child seems oblivious to other children and cannot imitate others, the group cannot 'carry' him indefinitely. He may not be ready or not suitable for group treatments, and this is not always obvious in the beginning.

Children with behaviour problems may become disruptive to the group. Hyperkinetic children may be particularly difficult. However, try a trial period of partial sessions with the group, increase to full sessions and the techniques above. Restless children may settle down and join in with the others. Finally, good selection of children and programme planning makes organized management easier.

SELECTION OF CHILDREN

The basis for selection varies and ideas are still developing. The early days of group treatment both for staff and children seem to be easier if the disparity between the children is not great. A group with children who have hemiplegia and are at the walking level and at approximately the same chronological age and have intelligence form a group which works well. Such a group is best for inexperienced staff and for those professionals beginning group work. The hemiplegic group might enlarge itself to encompass other diagnostic types of cerebral palsy who have asymmetry. Mental levels of children may be varied. A variety of developmental levels among motor developmentally delayed children may be contained in one group. The following points influencing selection may be helpful.

PROBLEMS OF CHILDREN

Motor Problems

Selection of children according to diagnosis is not usually helpful. Select the children according to their problems. Although it is difficult to generalize them, motor problems are usually some or all of the following:

(1) Head control – postural stability, particularly in the upright position.
(2) Head and trunk in midline, symmetrical arm and leg postures.
(3) Head and trunk counterpoising so that arms and legs can move into various asymmetrical postures or movements.
(4) Grasp to hold on, and grasp and release.
(5) Corrective movements and postures for any recurring abnormal positions of any joints; e.g. in spastic or athetoid conditions, elbow flexion, shoulder retraction, hip extension or semiflexion, adduction, knee flexion, equinus feet.
(6) Form of locomotion.
(7) Ability to sit or stand.
(8) Ability to rise from the floor or from a chair.

It is possible, say, to have a *pre-sitting group* with a selection of motor activity building up to sitting, prone to hands and knees and weight bearing on feet with trunk support (see developmental channels in Appendix, 0–6 months level). It is possible to have a group on *sitting and prewalking* with activities taken from the channels of development of 6–12 months (Appendix) or an ambulant group, 12 months and over (Appendix). The motor abilities selected for training will depend on the children with these problems. It is obviously essential to have individual assessments to plan for the problems. The other impairments and disabilities in the child should be considered, although motor problems are primary.

Age of Child

Children should be around the same chronological age, as their developmental levels alone will offer a range of children. It is sometimes an unhappy situation if a large boy aged 11 with a developmental level of, say, sitting equal to about 6–9 months normal level is in a group with 3-year-olds also at this developmental level.

Cognitive Level

The cognitive level should not cross too wide a spectrum. Some prefer keeping intelligent children in one group whilst others find it useful to mix as the cognitively impaired child will imitate the intelligent child in carrying out the motor activity or other activities which do not demand high intelligence. Intellectually disabled children may also be better at movement than, say, children with severe physical disabilities, and intelligence as, say, in dyskinesia. The programme therefore allows each child to demonstrate his assets and abilities.

Personality and Behaviour

Personality of the children is rarely a consideration unless a child is excessively disruptive and management ideas for behaviour fail (see above). A child's emotional and social stages of development influence whether he or she is suitable for a particular group.

Other Disabilities

Deaf, partially sighted or children with severe visual impairment may find it more difficult to join a group if the focus is on the motor disability. However, again some children with partial hearing loss and some children with partial sight have responded well to groups through imitation, lip reading or augmented visual clues, as well as the fact that a good group session focused on problems other than specific hearing and severe visual problems. Children with profound intellectual impairment may be too oblivious of the group dynamics being used and remain in their own world, and be unsuitable for such group work.

It must be remembered that factors for selection are still being explored by those working with groups in therapy and education.

Whatever the basis for selection the 'answer' to the best way to select children finally rests on whether group programmes of work can be created by the staff and on the ability of the leader of the group to weld her group of children together, so that they work together and there is a group spirit.

THE PROGRAMME

(1) It is essential to have this prepared before the group commences.

(2) It can be modified once used and *must* be changed as the children change and progress.

(3) The group leader needs to have the programme in front of her so that she does not delay and lose any group impetus and collaboration gained. She must know 'what comes next', to maintain group concentration.

(4) The programme should not be too long, but it is better to spend more time on each item. The items are after all only chosen because they are to be trained and repetition is needed. Time is given so each child can be active.

(5) Occasionally, have an easy item already achieved, as well as items *just beyond* the capacity of the children. If the children experience a successful achievement this motivates them further.

(6) Use action songs to carry out motor activities for the children; as they use the same songs each time, their familiarity is often appreciated. For many children, the programme should contain familiar elements, either songs, the same assistant and leader, the room, the time of day or days of the week and the general outline. However, the activities must gradually develop and change and not remain so predictable that the children do not progress or become bored!

Items of the Programme

The programme and its further modifications needs to be assessed and reassessed, not only by the group leader, but also together with the other professional workers in the centre. Ongoing consultations are necessary to make sure that the items selected for the children motivate *all* the children and that any child is not 'carried' as a non-participant for too long.

Select items from the treatment suggestions in the chapters on developmental training and the problems of deformity. Give preference to those items which do not depend on holding or handling the child or there may be too many adults required. The presence of many adults disrupts the growing child–child relationships in the group. Select items which are at first easy and become more difficult as the children develop in the group programme. In addition, such selected items may be used in groups to allow some children to function better than the others. This motivates the others to work towards these more advanced levels, which they can observe in their peers. In this way the therapist can have children at different levels of motor development in one group. She must have components selected so that they *build up* a particular motor function.

For example

All the children sit around a large table. Children at 3–6 months developmental level of sitting will have to lean their trunks against the table and grasp a horizontal bar attached to the table or grasp a slatted table. The children from 6–9 months level do not lean against the table, but only grasp the support, and the children from 9–12 months level who can sit alone, do so with their hands at their sides or on their laps. All children may sing or use language and visual activities while practising sitting.

Similarly, standing may be modified from standing leaning on arms or against the table with grasp support, stand and grasp, and stand alone.

Also prone lying raise head, prone lying raise head and rise on to elbows, and prone lying raise head and rise on to hands can be included simultaneously. With careful planning and assessment of the children many more examples will be found.

All motor activities must be associated with perceptual experience of direction, spatial relationships, colour, body awareness, various

matching activities in relating shapes, sizes, textures as well as speech and language, social awareness and of course the fun of children working and playing together (Fig. 11.1).

Music and movement, songs, action songs, fingerplays and any other children's songs and music are enjoyed in group work. However, as with the other activities, these are modified to relate to the children's levels of development and interest. Imaginative activities such as 'pretend you are a tree in the wind' or 'let's wave our arms like birds' which are used for children's groups are not advisable unless the children understand them and are at the 'let's pretend' level of play development. This is about the level of understanding of normally developing 2 to 3-year-olds.

Children's group games and party games may also be adapted and used in group work. Whatever items are selected they *must not* be random, but selected according to aims of therapy with each child. There will be aims of therapy which cannot fully be realized in the group sessions, or not at all. *Individual sessions* will be necessary for the children. However, if a child has the items well chosen for him in the group, individual sessions may not be essential for him, for a period.

It is not possible to give programmes for groups as these must be composed around the

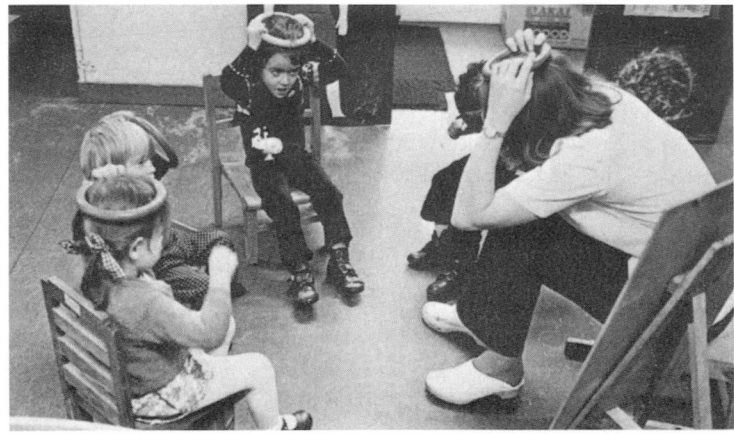

Fig. 11.1

children themselves. However, the following are necessary for groups:

(1) Start and end with a dressing activity, e.g. taking shoes and socks off, or taking a cardigan off.
(2) Fetch and put away any equipment for the group.
(3) Use gross motor activities for one session, integrating this with perception and language activities.
(4) Use hand classes for a session, integrating this with perception and language activities.
(5) Have a meal or tea for the group in order to include feeding training and washing hands.
(6) Suggested group games for walkers and non-walkers. These may include crawling hand ball, passing ball or objects in sitting, throwing beanbags into large containers, obstacle course, croquet, ring toss, deck quoits, carpet bowls, shuffle board, rolling balls on the table or floor, ping-pong with the ball attached to a high horizontal wire for ball retrieval and other play activities. Board games need to have large counters

or handles on the draught pieces or holes for the pieces and other adaptations. (Catalogues of adapted playthings are available from organizations for children with disabilities.)

SUMMARY

Interdisciplinary group work is valuable in the treatment of cerebral palsied and motor delayed children. They require consultations between staff:

(1) To assess children's functions in all areas before and *during* group sessions.
(2) To plan, monitor and progress the items of the group programmes.

It is best for one person to carry out the programme with perhaps other professionals occasionally assisting but *not* interrupting during the group session itself. Adjustments of the programme can be discussed after the session is over.

Teachers and therapists depend on each other to create dynamic group sessions and therefore need to work closely together.

Appendix 1

Developmental Levels

Function	0–3 months		3–6 months	
PRONE				
SUPINE				
SITTING				
STANDING WALKING				

6–9 *months*   9–12 *months*

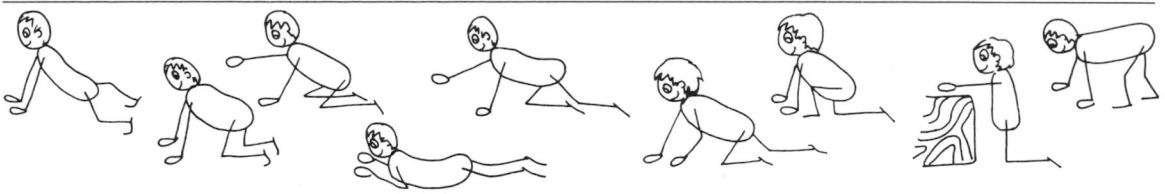

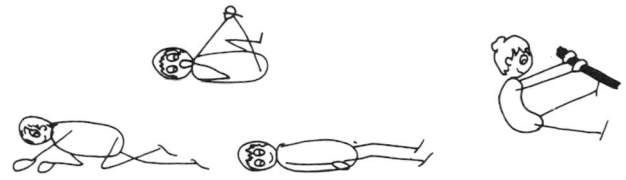

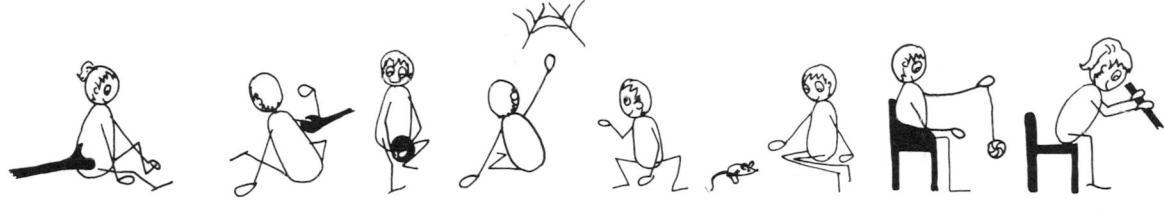

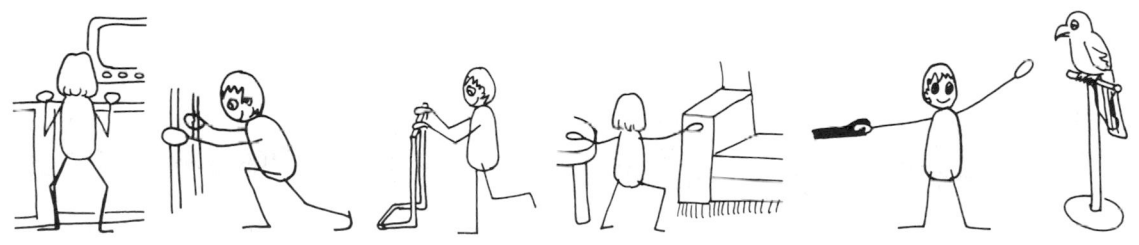

Physical ability assessment guide

SCORING KEY

0 – No ability, no initiation
1 – Initiates alone
2 – Partial, laboured, unreliable or infrequent
3 – Completes alone reliably but very abnormal
  performance
4 – Completes reliably with near normal/
  normal performance

Maintains posture – 10 seconds
Locomotion – 10 steps
Stairs – 4 steps

PRONE

0–3 months	Can be placed, head turns
	Raises head up
	Maintains head up
	On forearms, head, chest up
	Rises on to knees and forearms
3–6 months	Reaches forward with right arm (extended)
	Reaches forward with left arm (extended)
	Rolls over to right
	Rolls over to left
6–9 months	Creeps on abdomen
	Maintains on hands, elbows straight
	Rises on to hands and knees
	Maintains hands and knees
	Reaches forward with one hand, on hands posture
9–12 months	On hands and knees, lifts arm and opposite leg
	Pivots body using limbs to right
	Pivots body using limbs to left
	Crawls reciprocally
	Achieves sit from hands and knees

	Half-kneels with hand supports
	Rises to upright kneeling with hand supports
	Walks on hands and feet
12–24 months	Creeps on to table/couch
	Crawls upstairs
	Crawls downstairs backwards
	Kneels upright, hips straight, no support
	Half-kneels upright, no support
	Knee walks forwards
	Rises to stand, no support

SUPINE

0–3 months	Can be placed, head turns
	Head lag overcome slightly
	Reaches out along floor, to side
3–6 months	Head maintained in midline, symmetrical weight bears
	Hands together, symmetry
	Head raises, head lag overcome
	Reaches up, across body
	Bridges hips into extension, feet flat
6–9 months	Rolls over to right
	Rolls over to left
	Reaches, grasps foot
	Lying straight, arms down, head midline, turns
9–12 months	Rises to sitting through right side-lying, alone
	Rises to sitting through left side-lying, alone
	Pulls self to sitting

SITTING

0–3 months	Can be placed, head, trunk supported, flexes, hips
	Vertical head control, trunk supported
	Leans on forearms or hands, trunk supported

3–6 months	Sits leaning on hands, no support to upper then lower trunk
	Sits in chair with back, sides or chest support
6–9 months	Sits with one hand support, uses other hand
	Saves self on hands forwards
	Sits arms free, alone
	Saves self to right side
	Saves self to left side
	Sits leaning forwards, re-erects alone
9–12 months	Sits, reaches across, to side, above head
	Sits and turns, reaches to right
	Sits and turns, reaches to left
	Side-sits on right hip
	Side-sits on left hip
	Changes to hands and knees
	Sits alone on regular chair
	Sits on chair, reaches in all directions
	Rises from sit to standing, holding on
	Sits and pivots on floor
	Sits and pivots on chair
	Bottom shuffles along floor
	Tilt reactions anterior-posterior
	Tilt reactions laterally
12–18 months	Seats self on low stool
	Rises from sit to stand, no holding
	Sits on high stool, legs dangling
	Squats at play
	Squat rises to stand and returns to squat
	Saves self if tipped backwards

STAND AND WALK

0–6 months	Weight bears, plantigrade feet, full then lower trunk support
	Steps, trunk supported

6–9 months	Stands, forearm leaning or holding on, pelvis supported
	Stands, holds on alone, hips may flex, feet flat
9–12 months	Pulls self to standing, holds on
	Stands, holds on, lifts right leg
	Stands, holds on, lifts left leg
	Cruises using two hands
	Stands, holds one hand, reaches in all directions
12–18 months	Stands alone
	Stands stoop and recover
	Walks, two hands held or grasps walker
	Walks, one hand help
	Walks alone
	Walks, carrying object
	Rises to stand from all positions, no support
	Walks backwards
	Walks upstairs, holds both sides, two feet per step
	Protective stagger reaction if pushed sideways
	Protective stagger reaction if pushed forward
	Protective stagger reaction if pushed backward
18–24 months	Stands, kicks ball
	Throws ball overhead
	Runs
	Walks, stops and turns (pivot)
	Walks upstairs, holding one rail, two feet per step
	Walks downstairs, both rails, two feet per step
2–3 years	Jumps in place
	Jumps off 6-inch step
	Pedals tricycle
	Broad jump (8 inches)
	Walks downstairs, on rail, alternate feet
	Walks upstairs, no hold, alternate feet
	Walks downstairs, no hold, alternate feet

3–4 years	Stands on preferred leg (5–10 seconds)
	Hops on preferred leg
	Heel-to-toe walk
	Catches bounced ball
	Uses large bat
4–5 years	Balances on one leg, 10 seconds
	Walks on narrow, straight line
	Walks between 8-inch parallels
	Walks on narrow plank/bench
	Steps over knee-high stick with right
	Steps over knee-high stick with left
	Backward, heel-to-toe walk

Note:

- Ages are in approximate sequence.
- Select items in each section (prone, supine, sit, stand) as aims/objectives in a developmental therapy plan.
- Record items achieved with dates; use scoring key for outcomes/evaluations.
- All gross motor items from the Denver developmental screening test are included and based on those ages (Frankenberg *et al.* 1970).
- This guide is similar to the gross motor function measure which was validated as responsive to changes in child's function with inter-rater and intra-rater reliability (see Russell *et al.* 1989).

Wheelchair use

Development of abilities – assessment outline:

Sits upright in wheelchair
Finds and grasps wheel on right side
Finds and grasps wheel on left side
Grasps both wheels simultaneously
Moves right wheel forward slightly (2 inches)
Moves left wheel forward slightly (2 inches)
Moves right wheel forward over 1 foot
Moves left wheel forward over 1 foot
Moves both wheels forward over 1 foot
Moves right wheel backward
Moves left wheel backward
Moves both wheels backward
Travels forward, brings wheelchair to a halt
Travels backward, brings wheelchair to a halt
Starts from stationary, turns wheelchair to right, 180°
Starts from stationary, turns wheelchair to left, 180°
Propels wheelchair round obstacles
Propels wheelchair between two objects forward
Propels wheelchair between two objects backward

- Increase distances and speed
- Explore child's own strategies

Transfers

Sitting, uses brake to halt wheelchair
Sitting, lifts leg rests out of way
Sit slides forward in seat pushing on arm rests
Sit slides forward in seat using semipivot pelvis
Sit rises to stand on plantigrade feet, uses arm rests or
Sit rises to stand, uses arms forward to grasp support
Sit transfers laterally to bed, to toilet, to chair
Sit slides along transfer board to new seat, uses hand
Sit transfers out of seat downward, to kneel or sit
Sit rises to stand using arm rests or grasping support
Sit to stand, changes to new seat
Repeats any of the above in safe return to wheelchair

- Modify this list according to each child's own strategy and condition
- Therapist uses physical guidance and support to teach
- Demonstrate transfers to parents *and* carers so that they bend hips and knees correctly, and protect their own backs (see Fig. 8.179, rising)

Appendix 2

Equipment

Equipment lists and related information may be obtained from various voluntary organizations, other parents of disabled children, Departments of Health, Social Services and Education in local authorities or other Government departments and equipment lists from various Medical Equipment firms, Toy manufacturers and Education suppliers.

Consult organizations such as*:

Association of Paediatric Chartered Physiotherapists, c/o Chartered Society of Physiotherapy, 14 Bedford Row, London WC1R 4ED.

Association for Spina Bifida and Hydrocephalus, Tavistock House North, Tavistock Square, London WC1H 9HJ.

Association of Swimming Therapy (Halliwick) c/o ADKC Centre Whitstable House, Silchester Road, London W10 6SB.

British Sports Association for the Disabled, 13 Brunswick Place, London N1 6DX.

Capability Scotland (Scottish Council for the Welfare of Spastics), 22 Corstophine Road, Edinburgh EH12 6HP.

College of Speech and Language Therapists, 2 White Hart Yard, London SE1 1NX. (Enquire for centres offering communication aids and advice.)

Disabled Living Foundation, 380/384 Harrow Road, London W9 2HU.

Down's Syndrome Association, 153 Mitchum Road, London SW17 9PG.

Headway (National Head Injuries Association), 4 King Edward Court, King Edward Street, Nottingham NG1 1EW.

Kidsactive (Adventure Play for Children with Disabilities and Special Needs), Pryor's Bank, Bishop's Park, London SW6 3LA.

Mencap, Royal Society for Mentally Handicapped Children and Adults, 117/123 Golden Lane, London EC1Y 0RT.

Muscular Dystrophy Group of Great Britain, 7–11 Prescott Place, London SW4 6BS.

*addresses correct at time of going to press

National Association of Paediatric Occupational Therapists, c/o British Association of Occupational Therapists, 106–114 Borough High Street, London SE1 1LB.

National Association of Swimming Clubs for the Handicapped person, The Willows, Mayles Lane, Wickham, Hants PO17 5ND.

National Association for Toy and Leisure Libraries, 68 Churchway, London NW1 1LT.

Riding for the Disabled Association, Avenue R, National Agricultural Centre, Kenilworth, Warwickshire CV8 2LY.

Royal National Institute for Deaf people, 19–23 Featherstone Street, London EC1Y 8SL.

Royal National Institute of the Blind, 224 Great Portland Street, London W1N 6AA.

SCOPE (for people with cerebral palsy), 6 Market Road, London N7 9PW.

SENSE (National Deaf, Blind and Rubella Association), 11 Clifton Terrace, London N4 3SR.

SPOD (Sexual and Personal relationships of the Disabled), 286 Camden Road London, N7 0BJ.

Basic equipment

Imaginative parents and therapists require a mat, chairs of different sizes, tables of different sizes and everyday objects in the home, especially in the kitchen, and also use of grass, sand, water, leaves and so on outside the house.

Additional equipment is selected *according to the children* and a therapist's assessment of them.

Postural management for day and night. Equipment includes lying, seating for chairs and wheelchairs, prone standers and upright standing frames. Wedges and other sponge rubber shapes are also used for correct positioning throughout the 24 hours.

Note. A Manual Handling Assessment by an expert trainer is important for lifting patients, placing them in equipment and taking them out of equipment. There are also increasing numbers of designs on the market for safe manual handling such as electrical lifting appa-ratus, electric lifting mechanisms on standing frames, hoists, bathroom apparatus, electric wheelchairs and other equipment. *Contact should be made with each therapist's profes-sional association for further information.* See booklet *Paediatric Manual Handling – Guide-lines for Paediatric Physiotherapists*, Associa-tion of Paediatric Chartered Physiotherapists, UK.

Lying equipment currently developed are the Chailey lying frame for supine or prone, the Goldsmith Symmetrical Body Support 'Sym-metrisleep' for rest and night positioning, and the Dreama modular mattress designed by Jenx Ltd, Sheffield. This night-positioning mattress allows for support pads to be placed and locked almost anywhere for correcting individual pos-tures of a child or older person in supine, prone or side lying. Side-lying boards/equipment used during the day with positioning of body and abducted legs and both arms forward are avail-able from various manufacturers.

Wedges, other sponge rubber shapes or firm cushions.

Sponge rubber rolls of different diameters. Cover wedges, shapes, rolls with waterproof and washable material. Diameters of rolls are small for prone lying, chest support, to take weight on elbows or hands; take weight on knees, or sit astride. Large diameters for tilt reactions, arm saving reactions; lower to stand-ing; standing arm support on roll, stepping push roll along.

Large inflatable balls including beach balls may be used instead of rolls. Therapy balls of large diameter such as 44 inches (1100 mm) and 32 inches (800 mm). Small beachballs of various sizes.

Seating. See the development of sitting in Chapter 8. This includes special chairs or adap-tive seating; adjustable corner seat or floor seat with tray fitment and simple chairs with non-slip seats, backs and sides (removable) of dif-ferent sizes to fit children. The slatted chair (Petö) is also useful for training various motor tasks as well as sitting. There are a variety of toilet seats, potties, hoist seats, car seats, bath seats, portable shower seats on wheels on the market. Variable height tables should be obtained whenever possible. Cut-out tables should also be adjustable. Tables which tilt to different angles are available.

Crawlers. A canvas sling, under the child's abdomen and supports on casters, is essentially the basic principle used in crawlers when indi-cated. Many adjustments may be required to prevent *shooting* into abnormal extension or arms pushing into the area beneath the child's abdomen. Prone scooter boards or platforms on wheels, wedges on wheels (casters) or toy creations such as the dolphin on casters are also used by some children for crawling on hands only, on knees only, or on hands and knees.

Apparatus for supported standing. Various standing frames are available. The child can also show ability to stand and hold parallel or vertical bars; backs of chairs or stationary walking aids (see Chapter 8).

Note. Standing aids do not train standing unless the aid is vertical with the line of gravity going from the child's head (ear) down to just behind his ankle. Adjust the foot pieces or straps to obtain the correct alignment, with symmetry and feet held at right angles.

Prone standing frame attached at a forward angle to a table for schoolwork or hand activi-ties corrects abnormal postures of the legs, keeps the trunk straight and stimulates head control and arm function. Periods of passive stretching of tight (spastic) muscles and joints are given to prevent deformities. Some prone standers are adjustable to become upright standers. Prone 20–30° incline is advisable.

Walking aids. There are a great variety and they should be carefully selected (see Chapter 8).

- *With trunk support* given by a padded support to chest or by chest slings attached overhead.
- *Without trunk support.* A four-point walker which can be pushed with grasp on the sides of the child or grasp in front of the child. Toy walkers or doll's prams are very popular. Large soft toys on wheels, large trucks, large toy boxes on casters and similar normal toys should be stable, weighted and checked for size according to the child. Pushing stable children's or adult's chairs which slide easily but not too quickly as well as boxes on skis and other simple aids also train walking. The slatted back walker is also useful.

Note. Check that wheels on walkers are correct for the child. If they 'run away', preventing correct postures and establishment of the child's own control of his balance, use the walkers with crutch tips at each of the four points, ski sliders or other modifications. Crutches, elbow crutches, quadripods, tripods and thick based sticks are used for *selected* children (Fig. A2.1). Frequently progress is made from crutches to sticks. Check length, hand grasps and stability.

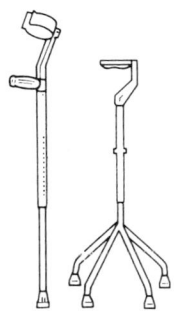

Fig. A2.1 Walking aids.

Some sticks may be linked together with a centre piece for initial stability.

Note. All walking aids should be checked for height so that the child does not grasp them with abnormal shoulder hunching, excessive flexion of the elbows and radial deviation of wrists. If grasp is not possible without these abnormalities try a walking aid which requires pushing with flat hands and straight elbows, or use a chair.

Parallel bars. These should be adjustable in height, sometimes in width. Hand slides are used if the child cannot grasp and release to use the parallel bars. A chair at the end of the bars may be used for training standing up from sitting. Eversion boards, foot prints and abduction boards have been placed between the bars when needed.

Appliances for correct posture in standing, weight bearing, trunk control; and to *weight* the boots of unstable athetoids or ataxics' shoes:

- *Knee gaiters* or polythene knee moulds, plaster back-slabs to keep knees straight (Fig. A2.2).
- *Elbow gaiters* which keep elbows straight for correct arm push and grasp of walkers and other poles in other functions (Fig. A2.3).

Boots may:

(1) Be padded at the tongue to fit well around the ankle.
(2) Have a strap to cross the front of the ankle to press heel well down.
(3) Have an inside mould at the inside arch to control valgus.
(4) Have an external heel extension on the inner side of the sole to prevent pronation (valgus) of the foot: on the outer side of the sole to prevent supination (varus).
(5) Have a raise on the heel, with a flare on the inner side for valgus; outer side for varus.
(6) Boots may be worn with special orthoses.

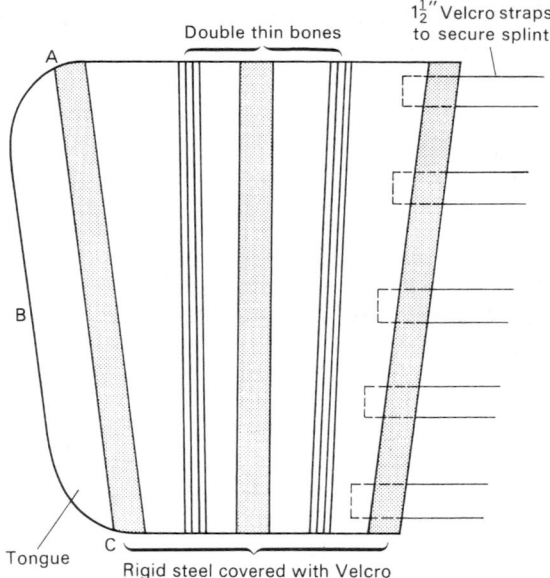

Fig. A2.2 Leg gaiter made of white coutil. It is wrapped around the leg bringing Velcro straps over the front side of 'B'. (1″ ≈ 25 mm)

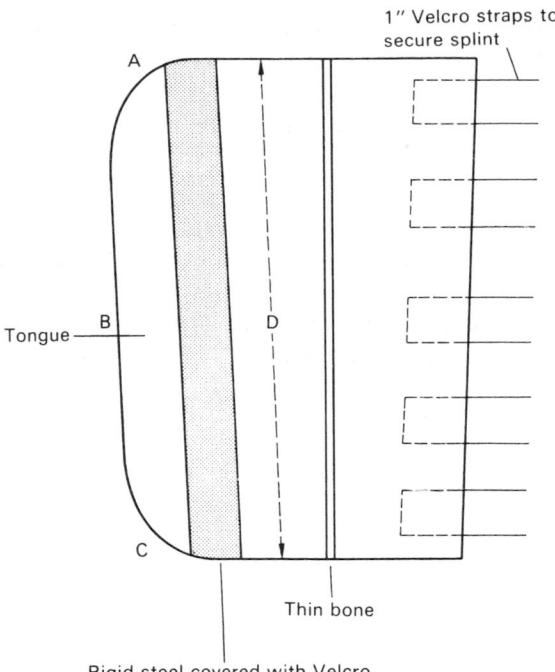

Fig. A2.3 Arm splint made of white coutil. Wrap splint around arm bringing Velcro straps over side B.

(7) Boot may have a sole raised to provoke forward weight shift to step, or to stretch heel cords. Sometimes just removal of the heels and thick soles stops toe walking in a mild spastic child.

(8) Boots or shoes may have a weighted base to add stability for, say, ataxic children.

(9) Stiffening on the boot leather may be given on the inside or outside to stop the foot rolling over into either pronation or supination, respectively. Heel cups on their own or with moulded extension to correct all foot arches may be needed.

(10) Toes of boots often have to be protected with thick rubbers, plastic coatings or metal to avoid the frequent wearing of the leather in *toe walkers* or *crawlers* who are just beginning to walk.

(11) Crawling children or non-walkers have boots and shoes to keep their feet warm, without any modifications. Booties or *trainers* stay on their feet better. Crawling is not possible in below-knee orthoses.

Note. Putting on and off shoes and boots is facilitated by the use of laces down to the toes as in Piedro shoes. Toes can then be held flat during application of boots. Velcro instead of laces makes it possible for some children to put their own shoes on and off. A tab on the back of the boot helps the child to pull on his boot.

Stairs with bannisters can be part of the physiotherapy department. Stairs should vary in height.

Ramps, uneven ground, various floor surfaces should be available for training walking.

Mirrors to floor level may be a help in training sitting, standing and walking.

Aids to activities of daily living
Consult occupational therapists.

Feeding

Dycem mat, long-handled spoons, spoons of different sizes, metal and unbreakable polythene/bone spoons, rubberzote and other handles, dishes with and without sides. Suction rubbers to hold bowl on table. Bibs. Cups; non-slip, weighted, cup-and-straw, baby mugs with non-spill aids and training lids with small opening. Mugs with two handles or one handle which are easy to grasp.

Dressing

Velcro. Zips and special designs. Detachable fronts for children who drool or mess. Large buttons, hooks or other fastenings.

Bathing

Non-slip mat in bath, small bath within large bath. Special bath seats, and safety neck supports. Liquid bath cleansers to avoid soaping when there are difficulties.

Toilet

See sections on chairs and sitting in Chapter 8. Many more are available.

Sleeping Bags, Cots, Baby Toys, etc.

As for normal babies.

Prams, Pushchairs and Baby Buggies

As for normal children but check postures more carefully. Special inserts for pushchairs and buggies which correct posture are available on the market.

Wheelchairs

A variety are available. References should be made to manufacturers of medical equipment, departments of health and voluntary organizations as lists of wheelchairs and their designs change and improve (see list of organizations and local seating clinics). The principles of correct seating discussed in Chapter 8 on the development of sitting is applied to the child in wheelchairs with the added considerations:

(1) Can he propel the chair himself or must it be pushed? Can he transfer?
(2) Facilities of the child's home for containing a wheelchair – stairs, doorways, sizes of rooms, use of table heights available, etc.
(3) Is the wheelchair useful indoors, outdoors or both?
(4) Can the wheelchair 'grow' with the child. What modifications?
(5) Can the wheelchair be transported, stored, put on public transport?

Special Aids in the Classroom

Typewriters; electronic aids to communication (augmented communication aids and also called communication systems). Advice and professional skills can be obtained from communication advice centres. Contact: ISAAC (International Society for Augmentative and Alternative Communication), Centre for Human Communication, Oak Tree Lane, Selly Oak, Birmingham B29 6SA. Various aids such as page-turners, pencil holders, page and book holders, various clips for drawing/writing paper and special low vision aids are among many classroom aids offered by manufacturers of medical and educational equipment in their lists. Occupational therapists and speech and language therapists should be consulted (see addresses in list above).

Aids to Mobility

Aids other than walkers, crawlers and wheelchairs such as go-karts, powered chariots; tricycles with adaptations. Hand-propelled tricycles and other special tricycles. Corner seat on casters. A variety of mobility toys is in development by engineers, research workers, parents, therapists and toy manufacturers. See Adventure Playground organizations, e.g. Kidsactive, and the Disabled Living Foundation, in address list above.

Many toys and mobility aids are now operated by a variety of switches for severely impaired people. Enquire to Occupational Therapy Association and voluntary organizations about these electronic devices.

General

Helmets to protect the child's head if he falls frequently. Toy catalogues. Toy libraries' catalogues for appropriate toys. Gym apparatus (balls, hoops, ropes, climbing apparatus). Playground apparatus, playthings and equipment. Rocking boards, rocking toys, swings with supports and straps, slides, climbing frames.

Note. Treatment tables in physiotherapy should be high for some physiotherapy techniques and low for training the child to get off the treatment table into standing.

References

Albright, A.L. & Neville, B. (2000) Pharmacological management of spasticity. In *The Management of Spasticity Associated with the Cerebral Palsies in Children and Adolescents* (eds A.L. Albright & B. Neville), pp. 121–133. Churchill Communications, Secaucus.

Almeida, G.L., Campbell, S.K., Girolami, G.L. *et al.* (1997) Multi-dimensional assessment of motor function in a child with cerebral palsy following intrathecal administration of baclofen. *Phys. Ther.*, 77, 751.

Amiel-Tison, C. & Grenier, A. (1986) *Neurological Assessment during the First Year of Life.* Oxford University Press, New York.

Andre-Thomas, C.S., St Anne Dargassies, S. & Chesni, Y. (1960) *Neurological Examination of the Infant.* Heinemann – Spastics International Medical Publications, London.

APCP (2002) *Paediatric Physiotherapy Guidance for Good Practice.* Available from Association of Paediatric Chartered Physiotherapists, c/o CSP, 14 Bedford Row, London WC1R 4ED.

Ayres, A.J. (1979) *Sensory Integration and the Child.* Western Psychological Services, Los Angeles.

Bailey, D.B. & Simeonsson, R.J. (1988) *Family Assessment in Early Intervention.* Merrill, Columbus, Ohio.

Bailey, D.B., Simeonsson, R.J., Buysse, V. & Smith, T. (1993) Reliability of an index of child characteristics. *Dev. Med. Child Neurol.*, 35, 806.

Bairstow, P., Cochrane, R. & Hur, J. (1993) Shortened version: *Evaluation of Conductive Education for Children with Cerebral Palsy (Final Report).* HMSO, London.

Bairstow, P., Cochrane, R. & Rusk, I. (1991) Selection of children with cerebral palsy for conductive education. *Dev. Med. Child Neurol.*, 33, 984.

Baker, R., Jasinski, M. *et al.* (2002) Botulinum toxin treatment of spasticity in diplegic cerebral palsy: a randomized, double-blind, placebo-controlled, dose-ranging study. *Dev. Med. Child Neurol.*, 44, 666–675.

Bardsley, D.G.I. (1993) Seating. In *Elements of Paediatric Physiotherapy* (ed. P. Eckersley). Churchill Livingstone, Edinburgh.

Barnes, M., Crutchfield, C. & Heriza, C. (1978) *The Neurophysiological Basis of Patient Treatment. Reflexes in Motor Development.* Stokeville, Morgantown.

Bayley, N.A. (1993) *The Bayley Scales of Infant Development.* The Psychological Corporation, San Antonio.

Beach, R.C. (1988) Conductive education for motor disorders: new hope or false hope. *Arch. Dis. Child.*, 63, 211.

Belenkii, V.Y., Gurfinkel, V.S. & Paltsev, Y.I. (1967) Elements of control of voluntary movements. *Biophysics*, 12, 135.

Bertoti, D.B. (1986) Effect of short leg casting on ambulation in children with cerebral palsy. *Phys. Ther.*, 66, 1522–1529.

Bidabe, L. & Lollar, J.M. (1990) *MOVE/Mobility Opportunities Via Education.* MOVE International, Bakersfield.

Blair, E., Ballantyne, J., Horsman, S. & Chauvel, P. (1995) A study of a dynamic proximal stability splint in the management of children with cerebral palsy. *Dev. Med. Child Neurol.*, 37, 544–554.

Bleck, E.E. (1987) *Orthopaedic Management in Cerebral Palsy. Clin. Dev. Med.* No. 99/100, MacKeith Press, Blackwell Scientific Publications, Oxford.

Bobath, B. (1965) *Abnormal Postural Reflex Activity Caused by Brain Lesions.* Heinemann, London.

Bobath, B. (1971) Motor development, its effect on general development and application to the treatment of cerebral palsy. *Physiotherapy*, 57, 526.

Bobath, B. & Bobath, K. (1975) *Motor Development in the Different Types of Cerebral Palsy.* Heinemann, London.

Bobath, K. (1971) The normal postural reflex mechanism and its deviation in children with cerebral palsy. *Physiotherapy*, 57, 515.

Bobath, K. (1980) *A Neurophysiological Basis for the Treatment of Cerebral Palsy. Clin. Dev. Med.* No. 75, SIMP, Heinemann Medical, London.

Bobath, K. & Bobath, B. (1972) Cerebral palsy, part 1, and the neurodevelopmental approach to treatment, part 2. In *Physical Therapy Services in the Developmental Disabilities* (eds P.H. Pearson & C.E. Williams). C.C. Thomas, Springfield, Illinois.

Bobath, K. & Bobath, B. (1984) The neurodevelopmental treatment. In *Management of the Motor Disorders of Children with Cerebral Palsy* (ed. D. Scrutton), p. 6. SIMP, Blackwell Scientific Publications, Oxford.

Bohannon, R.W. & Smith, M.B. (1987) Interrater reliability of a modified Ashworth scale of muscle spasticity. *Phys. Ther.*, **67**, 206–207.

Bower, E. & Ashburn, A. (1998) Principles of physiotherapy assessment and outcome measures. In *Neurological Physiotherapy* (ed. M. Stokes), pp. 43–55. Mosby, London.

Bower, E. & McLellan, D.L. (1992) Effect of increased exposure to physiotherapy on skill acquisition of children with cerebral palsy. *Dev. Med. Child Neurol.*, **34**, 25.

Bower, E., McLellan, D.L., Arney, J. & Campbell, M.J. (1996) A randomised controlled trial of different intensities of physiotherapy and different goal-setting procedures in 44 children with cerebral palsy. *Dev. Med. Child Neurol.*, **38**, 226–237.

Bower, E., Michell, D., Burnett, M., Campbell, M.J. & McLellan, D.L. (2001) Randomized controlled trial of physiotherapy in 56 children with cerebral palsy followed for 18 months. *Dev. Med. Child Neurol.*, **43**, 4–15.

Boyce, C., Gowland, C., Rosenbaum, P.L. *et al.* (1995) The Gross Motor Performance Measure: Validity and responsivity of a measure of quality of movement. *Phys. Ther.*, **75**, 603.

Brazelton, T. (1976) Case finding, screening, diagnosis and tracking. Discussants' comments. In *Intervention Strategies for High Risk Infants and Children* (ed. T.D. Tjossem). University Park Press, Baltimore.

Brunnstrom, S. (1970) *Movement Therapy in Hemiplegia – A Neurophysiological Approach.* Harper & Row, New York.

Burns, Y.R. & MacDonald, J. (eds) (1996) *Physiotherapy and the Growing Child.* Saunders, London.

Butler, C. & Darrah, J. (2001) Effects of neurodevelopmental treatment (NDT) for cerebral palsy: an AACPDM evidence report. *Dev. Med. Child Neurol.* **43**, 778–790.

Butler, P.B. & Major, R.E. (1992) The learning of motor control: biomechanical considerations. *Physiotherapy*, **78**, 1–6.

Butler, P.B. & Nene, A.V. (1991) The biomechanics of fixed ankle-foot orthoses and their potential in the management of cerebral palsied children. *Physiotherapy*, **77**, 81.

Butler, P.B., Thompson, N. & Major, R.E. (1992) Improvement in walking performance of children with cerebral palsy (preliminary results). *Dev. Med. Child Neurol.*, **34**, 567.

Campbell, S.K. (1999) The infant at risk for developmental disability. In *Decision Making in Pediatric Neurologic Physical Therapy* (ed. S.K. Campbell), pp. 260–332. Churchill Livingstone, New York.

Campbell, S.K., Vander Linden, D.W. & Palisano, R. (2000) *Physical Therapy for Children.* 2nd edn. Saunders, London.

Cantrell, E.G. (1997) Adult cerebral palsy. In *Rehabilitation of the Physically Disabled Adult*, 2nd edn. (ed. C.J. Goodwill, M.A. Chamberlain & C. Evans), pp. 295–313. Stanley Thornes, Cheltenham.

Capute, A.J., Accordo, P.J., Vining, E.P.G., Rubenstein, J.E. & Harryman, S. (1978) Primitive reflex profile. *Monographs in Developmental Pediatrics*, Vol. 1. University Park Press, Baltimore.

Capute, A.J., Palmer, F.B., Shapiro, B.K., Wachtel, R.C., Ross, A. & Accordo, P.J. (1984) Primitive reflex profile: a quantitation of primitive reflexes in infancy. *Dev. Med. Child Neurol.*, **26**, 375.

Carlsen, P.N. (1975) Comparison of two occupational therapy approaches for treating the young cerebral-palsied child. *Am. J. Occup. Ther.*, **29**, 267.

Carmick, J. (1993) Clinical use of neuromuscular electrical stimulation for children with cerebral palsy. Part I: Lower extremity & Part II: Upper extremity. *Phys. Ther.*, **73**, 505 & 514.

Carr, J.H., Shepherd, R.B. (1987) A motor learning model for rehabilitation. In *Movement Science: Foundations for Physical Therapy in Rehabilitation* (eds J.H. Carr & R.B. Shepherd), p. 31. Aspen, Rockville, Maryland.

Chappell, F. & Williams, B. (2002) Rates and reasons for non-adherence to home physiotherapy in paediatrics: pilot study. *Physiotherapy*, **88**, 138–147.

Chiou, I.L. & Burnett, C.N. (1985) Values of activities of daily living. *Phys. Ther.*, **65**, 901.

Cioni, G., Ferrari, F. & Prechtl, H.F.R. (1989) Posture and spontaneous motility in fullterm infants. *Early Human Dev.*, **18**, 247.

Cioni, G., Ferrari, F. & Prechtl, H.F.R. (1992) Early motor assessment in brain-damaged preterm infants. In *Movement Disorders in Children* (eds H. Forssberg & H. Hirschfeld), p. 72. Karger, Basel.

Collins, J. & Brinkworth, R. (1973) *Improving Babies with Down's Syndrome*, 5th edn. N.I. Region, National Society for Mentally Handicapped Children, Annadale Ave., Belfast.

Collis, E. (1947) *A Way of Life for the Handicapped Child*. Faber & Faber, London.

Collis, E., Collis, R., Dunham, W., Hilliard, L.T. & Lawson, D. (1956) *The Infantile Cerebral Palsies*. Heinemann, London.

Cooper, J., Moodley, M. & Reynell, J. (1978) *Helping Language Development*. Edward Arnold, London.

Cordo, P.J. & Nashner, L.M. (1982) Properties of postural adjustments associated with rapid arm movements. *J. Neurophysiol.*, **47**, 287.

Corry, I.S., Cosgrove, A.P., Walsh, E.G., McClean, D. & Graham, H.K. (1997) Botulinum toxin A in the hemiplegic upper limb: A double-blind trial. *Dev. Med. Child Neurol.*, **39**, 185–193.

Cosgrove, A. (2000) Orthopaedic surgery in spastic cerebral palsy. In: *The Management of Spasticity Associated with the Cerebral Palsies in Children and Adolescents*. (ed. A.L. Albright & B. Neville), pp. 75–92. Churchill Communications, Secaucus.

Cosgrove, A.P., Corry, I.S. & Graham, H.K. (1994) Botulinum toxin in the management of the lower limb in cerebral palsy. *Dev. Med. Child Neurol.*, **36**, 386–396.

Cottam, P. & Sutton, A. (1988) *Conductive Education: a System for Overcoming Motor Disorder*. Croom Helm, London.

Cotton, E. (1965) The Institute for Movement Therapy and School for Conductors, Budapest, Hungary. *Dev. Med. Child Neurol.*, **17**, 437.

Cotton, E. (1970) Integration of treatment and education in cerebral palsy. *Physiotherapy*, **56**(4), 143.

Cotton, E. (1974) Improvement in Motor Function with the use of Conductive Education. *Dev. Med. Child Neurol.*, **16**, 637.

Cotton, E. (1975a) *The Basic Motor Pattern*. The Spastics Society, London.

Cotton, E. (1975b) *Conductive Education and Cerebral Palsy*. The Spastics Society, London.

Cratty, B.J. (1970) *Perceptual and Motor Development in Infants and Children*. Macmillan, London.

Cummins, R.A. (1988) *The Neurologically Impaired Child: Doman-Delacato Techniques Reappraised*. Croom Helm, London.

Cusick, B. & Sussman, M. (1982) Short leg casts. Their role in the management of cerebral palsy. *Phys. Occup. Ther. Pediatr.*, **2**, 93.

Damiano, D.L. & Abel, M.F. (1998) Functional outcomes of strength training in spastic cerebral palsy. *Arch. Phys. Med. Rehabil.*, **79**, 119–125.

Damiano, D.L., Vaughan, C.L. & Abel, M.F. (1995) Muscle response to heavy resistance exercise in children with spastic cerebral palsy. *Dev. Med. Child Neurol.*, **37**, 731–739.

Damiano, D.L., Dodd, K. & Taylor, N.F. (2002) Should we be testing and training muscle strength in cerebral palsy? *Dev. Med. Child Neurol.*, **44**, 68–72.

Dietz, V. (1992) Spasticity: exaggerated reflexes or movement disorder? In *Movement Disorders in Children* (eds H. Forssberg & H. Hirschfeld), p. 225. Karger, Basel.

Dietz, V. & Berger, W. (1983) Normal and impaired regulation of muscle stiffness in gait: a new hypothesis about muscle hypertonia. *Exp. Neurol.*, **79**, 680.

Doman, G., Doman, R. *et al.* (1960) Children with severe brain injuries. Neurological organisation in terms of mobility. *JAMA*, **174**, 257.

Drillien, C.M. & Drummond, M.B. (eds) (1977) *Neurodevelopmental Problems in Early Childhood: Assessment and Management*. Blackwell Scientific, Oxford.

Drillien, C.M. & Drummond, M.B. (1983) *Developmental Screening and the Child with Special Needs*. Heinemann, London.

Dumas, H.M., O'Neil, M.E. & Fragala, M.A. (2001) Expert consensus on physical therapist intervention after botulinum toxin A injection for children with cerebral palsy. *Pediatr. Phys. Ther.*, **13**, 122–132.

Dunn, C., Willams, V. & Young, C. (1990) *Guidelines for Good Practice*. Association of Paediatric Chartered Physiotherapists, c/o CSP, 14 Bedford Row, London WCIR 4ED.

Eckersley, P.M. (1990) Cerebral palsy and profound retardation. In *Profound Retardation and Multiple Impairment* (eds J. Hogg *et al.*). Chapman & Hall, London.

Eckersley, P.M. (ed.) (1993) *Elements of Paediatric Physiotherapy*. Churchill Livingstone, Edinburgh.

Edwards, S., Partridge, C.J. & Mee, R. (1990) Treatment schedules for research: a model for physiotherapy. *Physiotherapy*, **76**, 605.

Egan, D.F. (1990) Developmental examination of gross motor skills. In *Developmental Examination of Infants and Preschool Children*, p. 71. Clinics in Developmental Medicine, No. 112, Mac Keith Press, London.

Ellenberg, J.H. & Nelson, K.B. (1981) Early recognition of infants at high risk for cerebral palsy: examination at age four months. *Dev. Med. Child Neurol.*, 23, 705.

Farber, S.D. (1982) A multisensory approach to neurorehabilitation. In *Neurorehabilitation: A Multisensory Approach* (ed. S.D. Farber). Saunders, Philadelphia.

Farmer, S.E., Butler, P.B. & Major, R.E. (1999) Targeted training for crouch posture in cerebral palsy. *Physiotherapy*, 85, 242–247.

Fay, T. (1954a) Rehabilitation of patients with spastic paralysis. *J. Intern. Coll. Surgeons*, 22, 200.

Fay, T. (1954b) Use of pathological and unlocking reflexes in the rehabilitation of spastics. *Am. J. Phys. Med.*, 33(6), 347.

Featherstone, H. (1981) *A Difference in the Family*. Basic Books, New York.

Feldenkrais, M. (1980) *Awareness Through Movement*. Penguin Books, London.

Finnie, N. (1997) *Handling the Young Cerebral Palsied Child at Home*, 3rd edn. Butterworth-Heinemann, Oxford.

Fisher, A.G., Murray, E. & Bundy, A. (1991) *Sensory Integration: Theory and practice*. Davis, Philadelphia.

Foley, J. (1977a) Cerebral palsy – physical aspects. In *Neurodevelopmental Problems in Early Childhood: Assessment and Management* (eds C.M. Drillien & M.B. Drummond), p. 269. Blackwell Scientific Publications, Oxford.

Foley, J. (1977b) Cerebral palsy – associated disorders. In *Neurodevelopmental Problems in Early Childhood: Assessment and Management* (eds C.M. Drillien & M.B. Drummond), p. 282. Blackwell Scientific Publications, Oxford.

Foley, J. (1983) The athetoid syndrome. *J. Neurol. Neurosurg. Psychiatry*, 46, 289.

Foley, J. (1998) *Human Postural Reactions*. Available from Association of Paediatric Chartered Physiotherapists, c/o CSP, 14 Bedford Row, London WC1R 4ED.

Folio, R., Fewell, R. & DuBose, R.F. (1983) *Peabody Developmental Motor Scales and Activity Cards*. Teaching Resources Corp, Hingham.

Forssberg, H. (1985) Ontogeny of human locomotor control I. Infant stepping, supported locomotion and transition to independent locomotion. *Exp. Brain Res.*, 57, 480.

Forssberg, H. & Hirschfeld, H. (eds) (1992) *Movement Disorders in Children*. Karger, Basel.

Forssberg, H. & Tedroff, K.B. (1997) Botulinum toxin treatment in cerebral palsy: intervention with poor evaluation? *Dev. Med. Child Neurol.*, 39, 635–640.

Fox, A.M. (1975) *They Get This Training But They Don't Really Know How You Feel: Transcripts of Interviews with Parents of Handicapped Children*. Institute of Child Health, London.

Fraiberg, S. (1977) *Insights from the Blind*. Human Horizon Series. Souvenir Press (Educational and Academic), London.

Frankenburg, W.K., Dodds, J.B. & Fandel, A.W. (1970) *Denver Developmental Screening Test*. University of Colorado Medical Center, Denver.

French, J. & Patterson, M. (1992) Psychological development of the child: its implications for physiotherapy practice. In *Physiotherapy: A Psychosocial Approach* (ed. S. French). Butterworth-Heinemann, London.

Fulford, G.E. & Brown, J.K. (1976) Position as a cause of deformity in children with cerebral palsy. *Dev. Med. Child Neurol.*, 18, 305.

Gentile, A.M. (1987) Skill acquisition: action, movement and neuromotor processes. In *Movement Science: Foundations for Physical Therapy in Rehabilitation* (eds J.H. Carr & R.B. Shepherd), p. 93. Aspen, Rockville, Maryland.

Gesell, A. (1971) *The First Five Years of Life*. Harper & Row, New York.

Girolami, G.L. & Campbell, S.K. (1994) The efficacy of a neurodevelopmental treatment program for improving motor control in preterm infants. *Pediatr. Phys. Ther.*, 6, 175.

Giuliani, C.A. (1992) Dorsal rhizotomy as a treatment for improving function in children with cerebral palsy. In *Movement Disorders in Children* (eds H. Forssberg & H. Hirschfeld), p. 247. Karger, Basel.

Goff, B. (1969) Appropriate afferent stimulation. *Physiotherapy*, 55, 9.

Goff, B. (1972) The application of recent advances in neurophysiology to Miss M. Rood's concept of neuromuscular facilitation. *Physiotherapy*, 58, 409.

Goldkamp, O. (1984) Treatment effectiveness in cerebral palsy. *Arch. Phys. Med. Rehab.*, 65, 232.

Goldschmied, E. (1975) Playing with babies. In *Creative Therapy* (ed. S. Jennings). Pitman, London.

Goldsmith, E., Golding, R.M., Garstang, R. & MacRae, A. (1992) A technique to measure windswept deformity. *Physiotherapy*, 78, 235–242.

Goodman, M., Rothberg, A.D. & Jacklin, L.A. (1991) 6 year follow up of early physiotherapy intervention in very low birthweight infants. In *Proceedings of the World Confederation of Physical Therapy Congress*, p. 1211. WCPT, London.

Gordon, J. (1987) Assumptions underlying physical therapy intervention: Theoretical and historical perspectives. In *Movement Science: Foundations for Physical Therapy in Rehabilitation* (eds J.H. Carr & R.B. Shepherd), p. 1. Aspen, Rockville, Maryland.

Gordon, N.S. & McKinlay, I.A. (eds) (1986) *Neurologically Handicapped Children: Treatment and Management*. Blackwell Scientific Publications, Oxford.

Granger, C.V., Hamilton, B.B. & Keith, R.A. (1986) Advances in functional assessment for medical rehabilitation. *Topic. Geriat. Rehabil.*, 1, 59–74.

Green, E.M., Mulcahy, C.M. & Pountney, T.E. (1995) An investigation into the development of early postural control. *Dev. Med. Child Neurol.*, 37, 437–448.

Greer, J.G. & Wethered, C.E. (1984) Learned helplessness: a piece of the burnout puzzle. *Exceptional Children*, 50, 524.

Grenier, A. (1988) Prevention of early deformations of the hip in brain damaged neonates. *Annales Pediatrica*, 35, 423–427.

Griffiths, M. & Clegg, M. (1988) *Cerebral Palsy: Problems and Practice*, Chapter 3. Souvenir Press, London.

Griffiths, R. (1967) *The Abilities of Babies*, 4th edn. University of London Press, London.

de Groot, L. (1993) *Posture and Motility in Preterm Infants: A clinical approach*. VU University Press, Amsterdam.

Gudjonsdottir, B. & Mercer, V.S. (1997) Hip and spine in children with cerebral palsy: Musculoskeletal development and clinical implications. *Pediatr. Phys. Ther.*, 9, 179–185.

Hagbarth, K.-E. & Eklund, G. (1969) The muscle vibrator – a useful tool in neurological therapeutic work. *Scan. J. Rehab. Med.*, 1, 26.

Hagberg, B., Hagberg, G., Olow, I. & von Wendt, L. (1996) The changing panorama of cerebral palsy in Sweden. The birth year period 1987–90. *Acta Paediatr. Scand.*, 85, 954–960.

Haley, S.M., Coster, W.J., Ludlow, L.H., Haltiwanger, J. & Andrellos, P. (1992) *The Pediatric Evaluation of Disability Inventory: Development Standardization and Administration Manual*. New England Medical Center, Boston.

Hall, D.M.B. (1984) *The Child with a Handicap*. Blackwell Scientific Publications, Oxford.

Hankinson, J. & Morton, R.E. (2002) Use of a lying hip abduction system in children with bilateral cerebral palsy. *Dev. Med. Child Neurol.*, 44, 177–180.

Hanzlik, J. (1990) Nonverbal interaction patterns of mothers and their infants with cerebral palsy. *Educ. Train. Mental Retard.*, 25, 333.

Hari, M. & Akos, K. (1990) *Conductive Education*. Routledge, London.

Hari, M. & Tillemans, T. (1984) Conductive education. In *Management of the Motor Disorders of Children with Cerebral Palsy* (ed. D. Scrutton), p. 19. SIMP, Blackwell Scientific Publications, Oxford.

Harryman, S.E. (1992) Lower extremity surgery for children with cerebral palsy: physical therapy management. *Phys. Ther.*, 72, 16–24.

Hartveld, A. & Hegarty, J. (1996) Frequent weight-shift practice with computerised feedback by cerebral palsied children – four single-case experiments. *Physiotherapy*, 82, 573–580.

Hazlewood, M.E., Brown, J.K., Rowe, P.J. & Salter, P.M. (1994) The use of therapeutic electrical stimulation in the treatment of hemiplegic cerebral palsy. *Dev. Med. Child Neurol.*, 36, 661–673.

Held, R. (1965) Plasticity in sensory motor systems. *Sci. Am.*, 213(5), 84.

Hicks, C.M. (1995) *Research for Physiotherapists*. Churchill Livingstone, Edinburgh.

Hinojosa, J. (1990) How mothers of pre-school children with cerebral palsy perceive occupational and physical therapists and their influence on family life. *Occup. Ther. J. Res.*, 10, 144.

Hiroshima, K. & Ono, K. (1979) Correlation between muscle shortening and derangement of the hip joint with spastic cerebral palsy. *Clin. Orthopaed. Rel. Res.*, 144, 186–193.

Hirschfeld, H. (1992) Postural control: acquisition and integration during development. In *Movement Disorders in Children* (eds H. Forssberg & H. Hirschfeld), p. 199. Karger, Basel.

von Hofsten, C. (1992) Development of manual actions from a perceptual perspective. In *Movement Disorders in Children* (eds H. Forssberg & H. Hirschfeld), p. 113. Karger, Basel.

von Hofsten, C. & Ronnqvist, L. (1988) Preparation for grasping an object: a developmental study. *J. Exp. Psychol.*, **4**, 610.

von Hofsten, C. & Rosblad, B. (1988) The integration of sensory information in the development of precise manual pointing. *Neuropsychologia*, **20**, 461.

Holt, K.S. (1966) Facts and fallacies about neuromuscular function in cerebral palsy as revealed by electromyography. *Dev. Med. Child Neurol.*, **8**, 255.

Holt, K.S. (1973) Discussion of Equinus in *CDI Cahiers*, English edition, No. 1. Masson et Cie, Paris.

Holt, K.S. (ed.) (1975) *Movement and Child Development*, chapters by Holt; Rosenbloom; Wyke; Brand & Rosenbaum; Rosenbaum, Barnitt & Brand; Rosenbloom & Horton. Heinemann – Spastics International Medical Publications, London.

Holt, K.S., Jones, R.B. & Wilson, R. (1974) Gait analysis by means of a multiple sequential camera. *Dev. Med. Child Neurol.*, **16**, 742.

Horak, F.B. (1992) Motor control models underlying neurologic rehabilitation of posture in children. In *Movement Disorders in Children* (eds H. Forssberg & H. Hirschfeld), pp. 21–30. Karger, Basel.

Horn, E.M., Warren, S.F. & Jones, H.A. (1995) An experimental analysis of a neurobehavioral motor intervention. *Dev. Med. Child Neurol.*, **37**, 697–714.

Hufschmidt, A. & Mauritz, K-H. (1985) Chronic transformation of muscle in spasticity: a peripheral contribution to increased tone. *J. Neurol. Neurosurg. Psychiatry*, **48**, 676–685.

Hurvitz, E.A., Leonard, C., Ayyangar, R. & Nelson, V.S. (2003) Complementary and alternative medicine use in families of children with cerebral palsy. *Dev. Med. Child Neurol.*, **45**, 364–370.

Hylton, N. (1989) Postural and functional impact of dynamic AFOs and FOs in a paediatric population. *J. Prosthet. Orthot.*, **2**, 40–53.

Hylton, N. & Allen, C. (1997) The development and use of SPIO Lycra compression bracing in children with neuromotor deficits. *Pediatr. Rehabil.*, **1**, 109–116.

Illingworth, R.S. (1975) *Basic Developmental Screening 0–2 years*. Blackwell Scientific Publications, Oxford.

Illingworth, R.S. (1983) *The Development of the Infant and Young Child, Normal and Abnormal*, 8th edn. Churchill Livingstone, Edinburgh.

Jan, J.E., Freeman, R.D. & Scott, E.P. (1977) *Visual Impairment in Children and Adolescents*. Grune & Stratton, New York.

Jones, M. (1993) Serial splinting in hemiplegic cerebral palsy. In *Elements of Paediatric Physiotherapy* (ed. P.M. Eckersley), p. 364. Churchill Livingstone, Edinburgh.

Jones, R.B. (1975) The Vojta method of treatment of cerebral palsy. *Physiotherapy*, **61**, 112.

Jonsdottir, J., Fetters, L. & Kluzik, J. (1997) Effects of physical therapy on postural control in children with cerebral palsy. *Pediatr. Phys. Ther.*, **9**, 68–75.

Kabat, H. (1961) Proprioceptive facilitation in therapeutic exercise. In *Therapeutic Exercise* (ed. S. Licht), 2nd edn, Chapter 13. Licht, New Haven, Connecticut.

Kabat, H., McLeod, M. & Holt, C. (1959) The practical application of Proprioceptive Neuromuscular Facilitation. *Physiotherapy*, **45**, 87.

Kanda, T., Yuge, M., Yamori, Y., Suzuki, J. & Fukase, H. (1984) Early physiotherapy in the treatment of spastic diplegia. *Dev. Med. Child Neurol.*, **26**, 438–444.

Katz, R.T., Campagnolo, D.I., Goldberg, G., Parker, J.C., Pine, Z.M. & Whyte, J. (1995) Critical evaluation of clinical research. *Arch. Phys. Med. Rehabil.*, **76**, 82–93.

Kazdin, E. (1982) *Single-case Research Designs*. Oxford University Press, London.

Kerr, G. (1992) Book review. *Physiotherapy Theory & Practice*, **8**, 127.

Kinsman, R., Verity, R. & Walker, J.A. (1988) A conductive education approach for adults with neurological dysfunction. *Physiotherapy*, **74**, 277–280.

Kitzinger, M. (1980) Planning management of feeding in the visually handicapped child. *Child: Care, Health and Development*, **6**, 291.

Knott, M. & Voss, D.E. (1968) *Proprioceptive Neuromuscular Facilitation. Patterns and Techniques*, 2nd edn. Harper & Row, New York.

Knox, V. (2002) Evaluation of the Sitting Assessment Test for Children with Neuromotor Dysfunction as a measurement tool in cerebral palsy: Case study. *Physiotherapy*, **88**, 534–541.

Knowles, M. (1984) *The Adult Learner: A Neglected Species* (3rd edn). Gulf, Houston.

Kogan, K., Tyler, N. & Turner, P. (1974) The process of interpersonal adaptation between mothers and their cerebral palsied children. *Dev. Med. Child Neurol.*, **16**, 518.

Kong, E. (1987) The importance of early treatment. In *Early Detection and Management of Cerebral*

Palsy (eds H. Galjaard, H.F.R. Prechtl & M. Velickovic), p. 107. Martinus Nijhoff, Dordrecht.

Kraus de Camargo, O., Storck, M. & Bode, H. (1998) Video-based documentation and rating system of the motor behaviour of handicapped children treated with physiotherapy – a new outcome measure. *Pediatr. Rehabil.*, **2**, 21–26.

Latham, C. (1984) Communicating with children. In *Paediatric Developmental Therapy* (ed. S. Levitt). Blackwell Scientific Publications, Oxford.

Leach, M. (1993) *Activities for People with a Multiple Disability.* The Spastics Society, London.

Lee, D.N. & Aronson, E. (1974) Visual proprioceptive control of standing in human infants. *Percept. Psychophysiol.*, **15**, 529.

Leonard, C.T., Hirschfeld, H. & Forssberg, H. (1988) Gait acquisition and reflex abnormalities in normal children and children with cerebral palsy. In *Posture and Gait: Development, Adaptation and Modulation* (eds B. Amblard, A. Berthoz & F. Clarac), p. 33. Elsevier, Amsterdam.

Leonard, C.T., Hirschfeld, H. & Forssberg, H. (1991) The development of independent walking in children with cerebral palsy. *Dev. Med. Child Neurol.*, **33**, 567.

Lesney, I. (1993) Sensory disorders in cerebral palsy: two point discrimination. *Dev. Med. Child Neurol.*, **35**, 402–405.

Levitt, S. (1962) *Physiotherapy in Cerebral Palsy.* Thomas, Springfield, Illinois.

Levitt, S. (1966) Proprioceptive Neuromuscular Facilitation techniques in cerebral palsy. *Physiotherapy*, **52**, 46.

Levitt, S. (1969) The treatment of cerebral palsy and proprioceptive neuromuscular facilitation techniques. In *On the Treatment of Spastic Pareses.* Institute Neurology, Stockholm. *Sjukgymnasten*, **27**, 3.

Levitt, S. (1970a) Principles of treatment in cerebral palsy. *Fysioterapeuten*, **10**.

Levitt, S. (1970b) Adaptation of PNF for cerebral palsy. In *Proceedings of the World Confederation of Physical Therapy Congress, Amsterdam.* WCPT, London.

Levitt, S. (1974) Common factors in the different systems of treatment in cerebral palsy. *CDI Cahiers*, No. 59, Masson et Cie, Paris.

Levitt, S. (1976) Stimulation of movement: A review of therapeutic techniques. In *Early Management of Handicapping Disorders* (eds T.E. Oppé & F.P. Woodford). IRMMH. Associated Scientific Publishers, Amsterdam, reprinted from *Movement and Child Development* (ed. K.S. Holt), Heinemann – Spastics International Medical Publications, London.

Levitt, S. (1982) Movement training. In *Profound Mental Handicap* (ed. D. Norris). Costello, Tunbridge Wells.

Levitt, S. (ed.) (1984) *Paediatric Developmental Therapy.* Blackwell Scientific Publications, Oxford.

Levitt, S. (1986) Handling the child with paediatric developmental disability. *Physiotherapy*, **72**, 161.

Levitt, S. (1987) Therapy for the motor disorders. In *Early Detection and Management of Cerebral Palsy* (eds H. Galjaard, H.F.R. Prechtl & M. Velickovic), p. 113. Martinus Nijhoff, Dordrecht.

Levitt, S. (1991a) International therapy workshops. In *Proceedings of the 11th International Congress of the WCPT*, p. 283. WCPT, London.

Levitt, S. (1991b) Family-centred physiotherapy. In *Proceedings of the 11th International Congress of the WCPT*, pp. 1236–1238. WCPT, London.

Levitt, S. (1994) *Basic Abilities – A Whole Approach.* Souvenir Press, London.

Levitt, S. (1999) The collaborative learning approach in community based rehabilitation. In *Cross-cultural Rehabilitation.* (ed. R.L. Leavitt), pp. 151–161. Saunders, London.

Levitt, S. & Goldschmied, E. (1990) As we teach, so we treat. *Physiotherapy Theory & Practice*, **6**, 227.

Levitt, S. & Miller, C. (1973) The interrelationships of speech therapy and physiotherapy in children with neurodevelopmental disorders. *Dev. Med. Child Neurol.*, **15**, 2.

Lin, J-P. (2000) The pathophysiology of spasticity and dystonia. In *The Management of Spasticity Associated with the Cerebral Palsies in Children and Adolescents* (eds A.L. Albright & B. Neville), pp. 11–38. Churchill Communications, Secaucus.

Logan, L., Byers-Hinley, K. & Ciccone, C. (1990) Anterior vs posterior walkers for children with cerebral palsy: A gait analysis study. *Dev. Med. Child Neurol.*, **32**, 1044.

Long, T. & Toscano, K. (2002) *Handbook of Pediatric Physical Therapy.* 2nd edn. pp. 162–164. Lippincott Williams & Wilkins, Philadelphia.

McCarthy, G.T. (ed.) (1992) *The Physically Handicapped Child*, 2nd edn. Faber & Faber, London.

McClenaghan, B.A., Thombs, L. & Milner, M. (1992) Effects of seat surface inclination on postural stability and function of the upper extremity of children with cerebral palsy. *Dev. Med. Child Neurol.*, **34**, 40.

McConachie, H. (1986) Parents' contribution to the education of their child. In *The Education of Children with Severe Learning Difficulties: Bridging the Gap between Theory and Practice* (eds J. Coupe & J. Porter), p. 253. Croom Helm, London.

McGraw, M. (1989) *The Neuromuscular Maturation of the Human Infant*. Clinics in Dev. Med. Mackeith Press, London.

McKinlay, I.A. (1989) Therapy for cerebral palsy. *Seminars Orthopaed.*, 4, 220.

McKinlay, I.A., Hyde, E. & Gordon, N.S. (1980) Baclofen: a team approach to drug evaluation of spasticity in childhood. In *Baclofen: A Broader Spectrum of Activity*, p. 26. A supplement to *Scott. Med. J.*

McLaughlin, J.F., Bjornson, K.F., Astley, S.J., Graubert, C., Hays, R.M., Roberts, T.S., Price, R. & Temkin, N. (1998) Selective dorsal rhizotomy: efficacy and safety in an investigator-masked randomized clinical trial. *Dev. Med. Child Neurol.*, 40, 220–232.

McLellan, L. (1984) Therapeutic possibilities in cerebral palsy: a neurologist's view. In *Management of the Motor Disorders of Children with Cerebral Palsy* (ed. D. Scrutton), p. 96. SIMP, Blackwell Scientific Publications, Oxford.

Marsden, C.D., Merton, P.A. & Merton, H.B. (1981) Human postural responses. *Brain*, 104, 513.

Martin, J.P. (1965) Tilting reactions and disorders of the basal ganglia. *Brain*, 88, 855.

Martin, J.P. (1967) *The Basal Ganglia and Posture*. Pitman Medical Publications, London.

Mayston, M.J. (1992) The Bobath concept – Evolution and application. In *Movement Disorders in Children* (eds H. Forssberg & H. Hirschfeld), pp. 1–6. Karger, Basel.

Miedaner, J. (1990) An evaluation of weight-bearing forces at various angles for children with cerebral palsy. *Pediatr. Phys. Ther.*, 2, 215.

Milani-Comparetti, A. & Gidoni, E.A. (1967) Routine developmental examination in normal and retarded children. *Dev. Med. Child Neurol.*, 9, 625.

Miller, C.J. (1972) The speech therapist and the group treatment of young cerebral palsied children. *Br. J. Disord. Commun.*, 7, No. 2.

Mitchell, R.G. (1977) The nature and causes of disability in childhood. In *Neurodevelopmental Problems in Early Childhood: Assessment and Management* (eds C.M. Drillien & M.B. Drummond), Chapter 1. Blackwell Scientific Publications, Oxford.

Montgomery, P.C. (1998) Predicting potential for ambulation in children with cerebral palsy. *Pediatr. Phys. Ther.*, 10, 148–155.

Morris, K. (1996) Physiotherapy management of the neonate and infant – developmental problems. In *Physiotherapy and the Growing Child*. (eds Y.R. Burns & J. MacDonald), pp. 343–357. Saunders, London.

Morris, C. (2002) A review of the efficacy of lower-limb orthoses used for cerebral palsy. *Dev. Med. Child Neurol.*, 44, 205–211.

Mosely, A.M. (1997) The effect of casting combined with stretching on passive ankle dorsiflexion in adults with traumatic brain injuries. *Phys. Ther.*, 77, 240.

Mossberg, K., Linton, K. & Friske, K. (1990) Ankle-foot orthoses: Effects on energy expenditure of gait in spastic diplegic children. *Arch. Phys. Med. Rehabil.*, 71, 494.

M.O.V.E. Europe (2001) *Mobility Opportunities Via Education*. Available from The Disability Partnership, Wooden Spoon House, 5 Dugard Way, London SE11 4TH.

Msall, M.E., DiGaudio, K., Rogers, B.T., Laforest, S., Catanzaro, N., Campbell, J., Wilczenski, F. & Duffy, L.C. (1994) The Functional Independence Measure for Children (WeeFIM): conceptual basis and pilot use in children with developmental disabilities. *Clin. Pediatr.*, 33, 421–430.

Mulcahy, C.M., Pountney, T.E., Nelham, R.L., Green, E.M. & Billington, G.D. (1988) Adaptive seating for motor handicap: problems, a solution, assessment and prescription. *Br. J. Occup. Ther.*, 51, 347.

Mulder, T. (1985) *The Learning of Motor Control Following Brain Damage: Experimental and Clinical Studies*. Swets & Zeitlinger, Lisse.

Mulder, T. (1991) A process oriented model of human motor behavior: implications for rehabilitation medicine. *Phy. Ther.*, 71, 157.

Mulder, T. & Hulstijn, W. (1988) From movement to action: The learning of motor control following brain damage. In *Complex Human Movement Behavior* (eds O.G. Meijer & K. Roth), p. 247. Elsevier, Amsterdam.

Myhr, U. & von Wendt, L. (1990) Reducing spasticity and enhancing postural control for the creation of a functional sitting position in children with cerebral palsy: A pilot study. *Physiotherapy Theory & Practice*, 6, 65.

Nashner, L.M., Shumway-Cook, A. & Marin, O. (1983) Stance posture in select groups of children with cerebral palsy: deficits in sensory organisation and muscular condition. *Exp. Brain Res.*, **49**, 393.

Nathan, P. (1969) Annotation: treatment of spasticity with peri-neural injections of phenol. *Dev. Med. Child Neurol.*, **11**, 384.

Neistadt, M.E. (1994) Perceptual retraining for adults with diffuse brain injury. *Am. J. Occup. Ther.*, **48**, 877.

Nelson, K.B. & Ellenberg, J.H. (1982) Children who 'outgrew' cerebral palsy. *Pediatrics*, **69**, 529.

Neville, B. (2000) Introduction. In *The Management of Spasticity Associated with the Cerebral Palsies in Children and Adolescents* (eds A.L. Albright & B. Neville), pp. 1–10. Churchill Communications, Secaucus.

Newson, E. (1976) Parents as a resource in diagnosis and assessment. In *Early Management of Handicapping Disorders* (eds T.E. Oppé & F.P. Woodford), p. 105. Associated Scientific Publishers, Amsterdam.

Nichols, D.S. & Case-Smith, J. (1996) Reliability and validity of the Pediatric Evaluation of Disability Inventory. *Pediatr. Phys. Ther.*, **8**, 15.

Norén, L. & Franzén, G. (1982) An evaluation of 7 postural reactions selected by Vojta in 25 healthy infants. *Neuropediatrics*, **12**, 308.

Nwaobi, O.M. (1987) Seating orientations and upper extremity function in children with cerebral palsy. *Phys. Ther.*, **67**, 1209.

Nwaobi, O.M., Brubaker, C., *et al.* (1983) Electromyographic investigation of extensor activity in cerebral palsy children in different seating positions. *Dev. Med. Child Neurol.*, **25**, 175.

Olow, I. (1986) Children with cerebral palsy. In *Neurologically Handicapped Children: Treatment and management* (eds N.S. Gordon & I.A. McKinlay), p. 60. Blackwell Scientific Publications, Oxford.

Oppenheim, R.W. (1981) Ontogenetic adaptations and retrogressive processes in the development of the nervous system and behavior: A neuroembryological perspective. In *Maturation and Development* (eds K.J. Connolly & H.F.R. Prechtl), p. 73. Heinemann, London.

Oppenheim, W.L., Staudt, L.A. & Peacock, J.W. (1992) The rationale for rhizotomy. In *The Diplegic Child* (ed. M.D. Sussman), p. 271. American Academy of Orthopedic Surgeons, Rosemont.

Ottenbacher, K.J. (1986) *Evaluating Clinical Change: Strategies for Occupational and Physical Therapists*. Williams & Wilkins, Baltimore.

Paine, R.S. (1962) On the treatment of cerebral palsy – The outcome of 177 patients, 74 totally untreated. *Pediatrics*, **29**, 605.

Paine, R.S. (1964) The evolution of infantile postural reflexes in the presence of chronic brain syndromes. *Dev. Med. Child Neurol.*, **6**, 345.

Paine, R.S. & Oppé, T.E. (1966) *Neurological Examination of Children*. Heinemann Books – Spastics International Medical Publications, London.

Palisano, R., Rosenbaum, P., Walter, S., Russell, D., Wood, E. & Galuppi, B. (1997) The development and reliability of a system to classify gross motor function in children with cerebral palsy. *Dev. Med. Child Neurol.*, **39**, 214–223.

Palmer, F.B., Shapiro, B.K., Wachtel, R.C., *et al.* (1988) The effects of physical therapy on cerebral palsy. *N. Engl. J. Med.*, **318**, 803.

Parette, H.P. & Hourcade, J.J. (1984) A review of therapeutic intervention research on gross and fine motor progress in young children with cerebral palsy. *Am. J. Occup. Ther.*, **38**, 462.

Parker, D.F., Carriere, L., Hebestreit, H., Salsberg, A. & Bar-Or, O. (1993) Muscle performance and gross motor function of children with spastic cerebral palsy. *Dev. Med. Child Neurol.*, **35**, 17–23.

Patton, M.Q. (1980) *Qualitative Evaluation Methods*. Sage, Beverly Hills.

Paus, T., Zijdenbos, A., Worsley, K., Collins, D.L., Blumenthal, J., Giedd, J.N., Rapoport, J.L. & Evans, A.C. (1999) Structural maturation of neural pathways in children and adolescents: in vivo study. *Science*, **283**, 1908–1911.

Peacock, W.J. & Staudt, L.A. (1991) Functional outcomes following selective posterior rhizotomy in children with cerebral palsy. *J. Neurosurg.*, **74**, 380–385.

Pearson, P.H. & Williams, C.E. (eds) (1972) *Physical Therapy Services in the Developmental Disabilities*. Thomas, Springfield, Illinois.

Pederson, E. (1969) *Spasticity, Mechanism, Measurement, Management*. Thomas, Springfield, Illinois.

Penso, D.E. (1987) *Occupational Therapy for Children with Disabilities*. Croom Helm, London.

Phelps, W.M. (1949) Description and differentiation of types of cerebral palsy. *Nerv. Child*, **8**, 107.

Phelps, W.M. (1952) The rôle of physical therapy in cerebral palsy and bracing in the cerebral palsies. In *Orthopaedic Appliances Atlas 1*, pp. 251–522. Edwards, Ann Arbor.

Piper, M.C. & Darrah, J. (1994) *Motor Assessment of the Developing Infant*. Saunders, Philadelphia.

Plum, P. & Molhave, A. (1956) Clinical analysis of static and dynamic patterns in cerebral palsy with a view to active correction. *Arch. Phys. Med.*, **37**, 8.

Pountney, T., Cheek, L., Green, E., Mulcahy, C. & Nelham, R. (1999) Content and criterion validation of the Chailey levels of ability. *Physiotherapy*, **85**, 410–416.

Pountney, T., Mandy, A., Green, E. & Gard, P. (2002) Management of hip dislocation with postural management. *Child: Care, Health Develop.*, **28**, 179–185.

Pountney, T.E., Mulcahy, C.M., *et al.* (2000) *Chailey Approach to Postural Management.* Active Design, Birmingham.

Prechtl, H.F.R. (1981) The study of neural development as prospective of clinical problems. In *Maturation and Development* (eds K.J. Connolly & H.F.R. Prechtl). Heinemann, London.

Prechtl, H.F.R. (2001) General movement assessment as a method of developmental neurology: new paradigms and consequences. *Dev. Med. Child Neurol.*, **43**, 836–842.

Prechtl, H.F.R., Einspieler, C., Cioni, G., *et al.* (1997) An early marker for neurological deficits after perinatal brain lesions. *Lancet*, **349**, 1361.

Presland, J.L. (1982) *Paths to Mobility in 'Special Care'*, pp. 19, 35–8. British Institute of Mental Handicap, Kidderminster.

Price, E., Thylefors, I. & von Wendt, L. (1991) The role of the physiotherapist in the Swedish paediatric rehabititation teams. In *Proceedings of the World Confederation of Physical Therapy Congress, London*, p. 1187. WCPT, London.

Radtka, S., Skinner, S.R., Dixon, D.M. & Johanson, M.E. (1997) A comparison of gait with solid, dynamic and no ankle foot orthoses in children with spastic cerebral palsy. *Phys. Ther.*, **77**, 395–409.

Reid, D.T. (1995) Development and preliminary validation of an instrument to assess quality of sitting of children with neuromotor dysfunction. *Phys. Occup. Ther. Pediatr.*, **15**, 53–81.

Reid, D.T. (1996) The effects of the saddle seat on seated postural control and upper extremity movement in children with cerebral palsy. *Dev. Med. Child Neurol.*, **38**, 805–815.

Reid, D.T. (1997) *The SACND: A standardised protocol for describing postural control.* Therapy Skill Builders, San Antonio.

Reiner, A.M., Steinbok, P. & Kestle, J.R. (1996) The relationship of baseline motor skills to functional outcome in a study of therapeutic electrical stimulation. Abstract. *Dev. Med. Child Neurol. suppl.*, **74** (38), 23.

Reynell, J. & Zinkin, P. (1975) New procedures for the developmental assessment of young children with severe visual handicaps. *Child: Care, Health and Development*, **1**, 61.

Riddoch, J. & Lennon, S. (1991) Evaluation of practice: The single case study approach. *Physiotherapy Theory & Practice*, **7**, 3.

Roberts, D.M. (1978) *Neurophysiology of Postural Mechanisms*, 2nd edn. Butterworth, London.

Robson, P. (1970) Shuffling, hitching, scooting or sliding: some observations in 30 otherwise normal children. *Dev. Med. Child Neurol.*, **12**, 608.

Rogers, C. (1983) *Freedom to Learn for the 80s.* Merrill, Columbus, Ohio.

Rood, M.S. (1962) Use of sensory receptors to activate, facilitate and inhibit motor response, automatic and somatic, in developmental sequence. In *Approaches to the Treatment of Patients with Neuromuscular Dysfunction* (ed. C. Sattely). *Third International Congress of World Federation of Occupational Therapists.*

Rosblad, B. & von Hofsten, C. (1992) Perceptual control of manual pointing in children with motor impairments. *Physiotherapy Theory & Practice*, **8**, 223.

Rosenbaum, P.L., King, S.M. & Cadman, D.T. (1992) Measuring processes of caregiving to physically disabled children and their families I: Identifying relevant components of care. *Dev. Med. Child Neurol.*, **34**, 103.

Rosenbloom, L. (1995) Diagnosis and management of cerebral palsy. *Arch. Dis. Child.*, **72**, 350–354.

Ross, K. & Thomson, D. (1993) An evaluation of parents' involvement in the management of their cerebral palsy children. *Physiotherapy*, **79**, 561.

Rothwell, J.C., Traub, M.M., Day, B.L., *et al.* (1982) Manual performance in a deafferented man. *Brain*, **105**, 515.

Rushworth (1961) Posture and righting reflexes. *Cerebral Palsy Bulletin*, **3**, 535.

Russell, D.J., Avery, L.M., Rosenbaum, P.L., Raina, P.S., Walter, S.D. & Palisano, R.J. (2000) Improved scaling of the Gross Motor Function Measure for children with cerebral palsy: evidence of reliability and validity. *Phys. Ther.*, **80**, 873–885.

Russell, D.J., Rosenbaum, P.L., Cadman, D.T., *et al.* (1989) The gross motor function measure: a means to evaluate the effects of physical therapy. *Dev. Med. Child Neurol.*, **31**, 341.

Russell, D., Rosenbaum, P., Gowland, C. *et al.* (1993) *Gross Motor Function Measure Manual*, 2nd edn. McMaster University, Hamilton.

Sahrmann, S.A. & Norton, B.J. (1977) The relationship of voluntary movement to spasticity in the upper motor neurone syndrome. *Ann. Neurol.*, **2**, 460–5.

Samilson, R.L. (ed.) (1975) *Orthopaedic Aspects of Cerebral Palsy.* Heinemann – Spastics International Medical Publications, London.

Scrutton, D. (ed.) (1984) *Management of the Motor Disorders of Children with Cerebral Palsy.* SIMP, Blackwell Scientific Publications, Oxford.

Scrutton, D. & Baird, G. (1997) Surveillance measures of the hips of children with bilateral cerebral palsy. *Arch. Dis. Child.*, **76**, 381–384.

Scrutton, D., Baird, G. & Smeeton, N. (2001) Hip dysplasia in bilateral cerebral palsy: incidence and natural history in children aged 18 months to 5 years. *Dev. Med. Child Neurol.*, **43**, 586–600.

Seglow, D. (1984) A pattern of early intervention. In *Paediatric Developmental Therapy.* (ed. S. Levitt), pp. 76–87. Blackwell Scientific Publications, Oxford.

Seligman, M.E.P. (1992) *Helplessness: On Development, Depression and Death.* Freeman, San Francisco.

Sharrard, W.J.W. (1971) *Paediatric Orthopaedics and Fractures.* Blackwell Scientific Publications, Oxford.

Shepherd, R.B. (1995) *Physiotherapy in Paediatrics*, 3rd edn. Butterworth-Heinemann, Oxford.

Sheridan, M.D. (1973) *Children's Developmental Progress. Birth – 5 years.* NFER Publishing Company, Windsor.

Sheridan, M.D. (1974) *Manual for the Stycar Hearing Tests*, revised edition. NFER Publishing Company, Windsor.

Sheridan, M.D. (1975) *The Developmental Progress of Infants and Young Children*, 3rd edn. HMSO, London.

Shumway-Cook, A. & Woollacott, M.H. (2001) *Motor Control: Theory and Practical Applications*, 2nd edn. Lippincott Williams & Wilkins, Baltimore.

Siebes, R.C., Wijnroks, L. & Vermeer, A. (2002) Qualitative analysis of therapeutic motor intervention programmes for children with cerebral palsy: an update. *Dev. Med. Child Neurol.*, **44**, 593–603.

Simeonsson, R.J. & McHale, S.M. (1981) Review: research on handicapped children: sibling relationships. *Child: Care, Health Develop.*, **7**, 153.

Slominski, A.H. (1984) Winthrop Phelps and the Children's Rehabilitation Institute. In *Management of the Motor Disorders of Children with Cerebral Palsy* (ed. D. Scrutton), p. 59. SIMP, Blackwell Scientific Publications, Oxford.

Sluys, E.M., van der Zee, J. & Kok, G.J. (1993) Differences between physical therapists in attention paid to patient education. *Physiotherapy Theory and Practice*, **9**, No. 2.

Soames, R. (2003) *Joint Motion: Clinical measurement and evaluation.* Churchill Livingstone, Edinburgh.

Solomons, G. & Solomons, H.C. (1975) Motor development in Yucatan infants. *Dev. Med. Child Neurol.*, **17**, 41.

Sonksen, P. (1979) Sound and the visually handicapped baby. *Child: Care, Health Develop.*, **5**, 413.

Sonksen, P., Levitt, S. & Kitzinger, M. (1984) Identification of constraints acting on motor development in young visually disabled children and principles of remediation. *Child: Care, Health Develop.*, **10**, 273.

Sowell, E.R., Trauner, D.A., Gamst, A. & Jernigan, T.L. (2002) Development of cortical and subcortical brain structures in childhood and adolescence: a structural MRI study. *Dev. Med. Child Neurol.*, **44**, 14–16.

Sparrow, S. & Zigler, E. (1978) Evaluation of a patterning treatment for retarded children. *Pediatrics*, **62**, 137.

Stanley, F. & Alberman, E. (eds) (1984) *The Epidemiology of the Cerebral Palsies.* SIMP, Blackwell Scientific Publications, Oxford.

Steel, S. (1993) Individual learning programmes. In *Elements of Paediatric Physiotherapy* (ed. P.M. Eckersley), p. 369. Churchill Livingstone, Edinburgh.

Steinbok, P., Reiner, A.M., Beauchamp, R., Armstrong, R.W. & Cochrane, D.D. (1997) A randomized clinical trial to compare selective posterior rhizotomy plus physiotherapy with physiotherapy alone in children with spastic diplegic cerebral palsy. *Dev. Med. Child Neurol.*, **39**, 178–184.

Stern, D.N. (1985) *The Interpersonal World of the Infant.* Basic Books, New York.

Stewart, P.C. & McQuilton, G. (1987) Straddle seating for the cerebral palsied child. *Br. J. Occup. Ther.*, **50**, 136.

Stockmeyer, S.A. (1967) The Rood approach. *Am. J. Phys. Med.*, **46**, No. 1, 900.

Stockmeyer, S.A. (1972) A sensorimotor approach to treatment. In *Physical Therapy Services in the Developmental Disabilities* (eds P.H. Pearson & C.E. Williams), Chapter 4. Thomas, Springfield, Illinois.

Stone, S. (1991) Qualitative research methods for physiotherapists. *Physiotherapy*, 77, 449–452.

Stroh, K. & Robinson, T. (1991) Developmental delay in young children: redressing the balance for child and parents. *Child Language Teaching and Therapy*, 7, 1.

Stroh, K., Robinson, T. & Stroh, G. (1986) A therapeutic feeding programme. *Dev. Med. Child Neurol.*, 28, 3.

Stuberg, W.A. (1992) Considerations related to weight-bearing programs in children with developmental disabilities. *Phys. Ther.*, 72, 35–40.

Stuberg, W.A., Fuchs, R.H. & Miedaner, J.A. (1988) Reliability of goniometric measurements of children with cerebral palsy. *Dev. Med. Child Neurol.*, 30, 657.

Sugden, D.A. (1992) Postural control: developmental effects of visual and mechanical perturbations. *Physiotherapy Theory & Practice*, 8, 165.

Sussman, M.D. (ed.) (1992) *The Diplegic Child*. American Academy of Orthopedic Surgeons, Rosemont.

Sykanda, A.M. & Levitt, S. (1982) The physiotherapist in the developmental management of the visually impaired child. *Child: Care, Health Develop.*, 8, 261.

Tabary, J.C., Tardieu, C., Tardieu, G. & Goldspink, G. (1972) Physiological and structural changes in the cat's soleus muscles due to immobilisation at different lengths by plaster casts. *J. Physiol. (Lond.)*, 224, 231.

Tabary, J.-C., Tardieu, C., Tardieu, G. & Tabary, C. (1981) Experimental rapid sarcomere loss with concomitant hypo-extensibility. *Muscle Nerve*, 4, 198–203.

Tardieu, C., Huet de la Tour, E., Bret, M.D., *et al.* (1982) Muscle hypoextensibility in children with cerebral palsy. *Arch. Phys. Med. Rehab.*, 63, 97.

Tardieu, C., Lespargot, A., Tabary, C. & Bret, M.D. (1988) For how long must the soleus muscle be stretched each day to prevent contracture? *Dev. Med. Child Neurol.*, 30, 3–10.

Tarran, E.C. (1981) Parents' views of medical and social work services for families with young cerebral-palsied children. *Dev. Med. Child Neurol.*, 23, 173.

Taub, E. (1980) Somatosensory deafferentation research with monkeys: implications for rehabilitation medicine. In *Behavioral Psychology in Rehabilitation Medicine: Clinical implications* (ed. L.P. Ince), p. 371. Williams & Wilkins, Baltimore.

Tecklin, J.S. (1999) *Pediatric Physical Therapy*, 3rd edn. Lippincott, Williams and Wilkins, Philadelphia.

Thelen, E., Kelso, J.A.S. & Fogel, A. (1987) Self-organising systems and infant motor development. *Dev. Rev.*, 11, 39–65.

Thelen, E., Ulrich, B.D. & Jensen, J.L. (1989) The developmental origins of locomotion. In *Development of Posture and Gait Across the Life Span* (eds M.H. Woollacott & A. Shumway-Cook), p. 25. University of South Carolina Press, Columbia.

Thomas, A.P., Bax, M.C.O. & Smyth, D.P.L. (1989) *The Health and Social Needs of Young Adults with Physical Disabilities*. Mac Keith Press, Blackwell Scientific Publications, Oxford.

Tirosh, E. & Rabino, S. (1989) Physiotherapy in children with cerebral palsy: Evidence for its efficacy. *Am. J. Dis. Child*, 143, 552.

Titchener, J. (1983) A preliminary evaluation of Conductive Education. *Physiotherapy*, 69, 313–315.

Tizard, J.P.M., Paine, R.S. & Crothers, B. (1954) Disturbances of sensation in children with hemiplegia. *J. Amer. Med. Assoc.*, 155, 628–632.

Touwen, B.C.L. (1976) *Neurological Development in Infancy*. Heinemann, London.

Touwen, B.C.L. (1978) Variability and stereotypy in normal and deviant development. In *Care of the Handicapped Child* (ed. J. Apley), p. 99. SIMP, Heinemann, London.

Touwen, B.C.L. (1987) The significance of neonatal neurological diagnosis. In *Early Detection and Management of Cerebral Palsy* (eds H. Galjaard, H.F.R. Prechtl & M. Velickovic), p. 69. Martinus Nijhoff, Dordrecht.

Trefler, E., Hanks, S., Huggins, P., *et al.* (1978) A modular seating system for cerebral-palsied children. *Dev. Med. Child Neurol.*, 20, 199.

Turker, R.J. & Lee, R. (2000) Adductor tenotomies in children with quadriplegic cerebral palsy: Longer term follow-up. *J. Pediatr. Orthoped.*, 20, 370–374.

Twitchell, T.E. (1961) The nature of the motor deficit in double athetosis. *Arch. Phys. Med.*, 42, 63.

Twitchell, T.E. (1965) Variation and abnormalities of motor development. *Phys. Ther. Rev.*, 45(5), 424.

Umphred, D. (1984) An integrated approach to treatment of the pediatric neurologic patient. In *Pediatric Neurologic Physical Therapy* (ed. S.K. Campbell), Chapter 3. Churchill Livingstone, New York.

Umphred, D.A. (2000) *Neurological Rehabilitation*, 4th edn. Mosby, St Louis.

Van Blankenstein, M., Welbergen, U.R. & de Haas, J.H. (1975) *Development of the Infant*. Heinemann, London.

Van Vliet, P. (ed.) (1992) Special issue: issues in the training of postural control. *Physiotherapy Theory & Practice*, **8**, (3).

Vojta, V. (1984) The basic elements of treatment according to Vojta. In *Management of the Motor Disorders of Children with Cerebral Palsy* (ed. D. Scrutton), p. 75. SIMP, Blackwell Scientific Publications, Oxford.

Vojta, V. (1989) *Die Cerebralen Bewegungsstorungen im Sauglingsalter*, 5th edn. Ferdinand Enke Verlag, Stuttgart.

Von Aufschnaiter, D. (1992) Vojta: A neurophysiological treatment. In *Movement Disorders in Children* (eds H. Forssberg & H. Hirschfeld), p. 7. Karger, Basel.

Voss, D.E. (1972) Proprioceptive neuromuscular facilitation. In *Physical Therapy Services in the Developmental Disabilities* (eds P.H. Pearson & C.E. Williams), Chapter 5. Thomas, Springfield, Illinois.

Voss, D.E., Ionta, M. & Meyers, B. (1985) *Proprioceptive Neuromuscular Facilitation Patterns and Techniques*. Harper & Row, New York.

van der Weel, F.R., van der Meer, A.L. & Lee, D.N. (1991) Effect of task on movement control in cerebral palsy: implications for assessment and therapy. *Dev. Med. Child Neurol.*, **33**, 419–426.

von Wendt, L., Ekenberg, L., Dagis, D. & Janlert, U. (1984) A parent-centred approach to physiotherapy for their handicapped children. *Dev. Med. Child Neurol.*, **26**, 445.

Whalley Hammell, K., Carpenter, C. & Dyck, I. (eds) (2000) *Using Qualitative Research*. Churchill Livingstone, Edinburgh.

Wiley, M.E. & Damiano, D.L. (1998) Lower-extremity strength profiles in spastic cerebral palsy. *Dev. Med. Child Neurol.*, **40**, 100–107.

Wilner, L. (ed.) (1996) *Getting On with Cerebral Palsy: From Adolescence to Old Age*. Scope, London.

Wilson, B. (1987) Single-case experimental designs in neuropsychological rehabilitation. *J. Clin. Exp. Neuropsych.*, **9**, 527.

Winnicott, D.W. (1964) *The Child, the Family and the Outside World*. Penguin Books, London.

Winstein, C.J. & Schmidt, R.A. (1990) Reduced frequency of knowledge of results enhances motor skill learning. *J. Exp. Psychol. Learn. Memory*, **16**, 677.

Winstein, C.J., Gardner, E.R., McNeal D.R., *et al.* (1989) Standing balance training: effect on balance and locomotion in hemiparetic adults. *Arch. Phys. Med. Rehabil.*, **70**, 755–762.

Winstein, C.J. & Schmidt, R.A. (1989) Sensorimotor feedback. In *Human Skills* (ed. D.H. Holding), 2nd edn, p. 17. Wiley, Chichester.

Winstock, A. (2003) *Eating and Drinking Difficulties in Children: A guide for practitioners*. Speechmark, Bicester.

Wishart, M.C., Bidder, R.T. & Gray, O.P. (1981) Parents' report of family life with a developmentally delayed child. *Child: Care, Health Develop.*, **7**, 267.

Wright, F.V., Sheil, E., Drake, J., Wedge, J.H. & Naumann, S. (1998) Evaluation of selective dorsal rhizotomy for the reduction of spasticity in cerebral palsy: a randomized controlled trial. *Dev. Med. Child Neurol.*, **40**, 239–247.

Wright, T. & Nicholson, J. (1973) Physiotherapy for the spastic child: An evaluation. *Dev. Med. Child Neurol.*, **15**, 146–163.

Yekutiel, M., Jariwala, M. & Stretch, P. (1994) Sensory deficit in the hands of children with cerebral palsy: a new look at assessment and prevalence. *Dev. Med. Child Neurol.*, **36**, 619–624.

Young, N.L., Wright, J.G., *et al.* (1998) Windswept deformity in spastic quadriplegic cerebral palsy. *Pediatr. Phys. Ther.*, **10**, 94–100.

Young, R.R. & Wiegner, A.W. (1987) Spasticity. *Clin. Orthopaed. Rel. Res.*, **219**, 50.

Zacharkow, D. (1988) *Posture, Sitting, Standing, Chair Design and Exercise*. Thomas, Springfield, Illinois.

Zinkin, P. (1979) The effect of visual handicap on early development. In *Visual Handicap in Children* (eds V. Smith & J. Keen), p. 132. Spastics Int. Med. Publ., London.

Index